Psychopharmacology

A Biochemical and Behavioral Approach

Lewis S. Seiden

The University of Chicago
Departments of Pharmacology and Physiological
Sciences and Psychiatry

Linda A. Dykstra

The University of North Carolina
Departments of Psychology and Pharmacology

 VAN NOSTRAND REINHOLD COMPANY
NEW YORK   CINCINNATI   ATLANTA   DALLAS   SAN FRANCISCO
LONDON   TORONTO   MELBOURNE

Van Nostrand Reinhold Company Regional Offices:
New York Cincinnati Atlanta Dallas San Francisco

Van Nostrand Reinhold Company International Offices:
London Toronto Melbourne

Library of Congress Catalog Card Number: 76–53019
ISBN: 0–442–27481–5

Manufactured in the United States of America

Published by Van Nostrand Reinhold Company
450 West 33rd Street, New York. N.Y. 10001

Published simultaneously in Canada by Van Nostrand Reinhold Ltd.

15 14 13 12 11 10 9 8 7 6 5 4 3 2 1

Library of Congress Cataloging in Publication Data

Seiden, Lewis S
    Psychopharmacology.

    Includes bibliographies and index.
    1. Psychopharmacology. I. Dykstra, Linda A.,
joint author. II. Title. [DNLM: 1. Psychopharmacology. 2. Psychotropic drugs—Pharmacodynamics.
3. Behavior—Drug effects. QV77 S458p]
RC483.S4   615'.78   76–53019
ISBN 0–442–27481–5

Preface

The number and use of behaviorally active drugs has increased tremendously during the past twenty-five years. As a result, interest in the scientific investigation of these drugs has also increased. The investigation of behaviorally active drugs draws on a number of disciplines, including pharmacology, psychology, psychiatry, biochemistry, anatomy and physiology. Research in this area has included the investigation of drug-neurochemical interactions (neuropharmacology) and drug-behavior interactions (behavioral pharmacology), and investigations of the effectiveness and toxicity of drugs in humans (clinical psychopharmacology). We will use the term psychopharmacology to refer to a combination of disciplines concerned with describing and examining the ways in which behaviorally active drugs exert their effects. Most of the basic biochemical, behavioral and neuropharmacological data have been obtained using nonhuman organisms; therefore, data from these nonhuman studies will be emphasized.

This book is intended as an introduction to the research literature in experimental psychopharmacology for students and professionals in psychology, pharmacology, psychiatry and the general biological and medical sciences. Since research in experimental psychopharmacology draws upon procedures and knowledge from several disciplines, a book in this area cannot be self-contained; however, some of the most fundamental principles in experimental psychopharmacology are presented as an introduction into this young and exciting field. Basic texts in each relevant discipline are suggested for those who want further background.

Facts and ideas from neurochemical, neuropharmacological and behavioral approaches to the investigation of drug action will be presented. Since only a fraction of the vast literature in experimental psychopharmacology can be examined, attention will focus on salient data and methodological issues. Background material and exemplary data from original research will be presented, as well as inferences and interpretations drawn from these data. The data and their interpretations will be critically analyzed in order to illustrate the complex methodological issues involved in this interdisciplinary field.

In preparing this book, we have relied mainly on primary literature sources and have chosen to discuss those areas where some convergence of data and interpretations exists or where disagreements and problems are clear-cut. Not all important areas of research in this field have been explored, and those that have been explored are not always treated with equal intensity. Answers to the questions posed will not always be readily found; and when conclusions are advanced, difficulties and limitations will be noted.

The subject matter as well as the organization of this book partially evolved from a formal course in psychopharmacology at The University of Chicago. The material has been taught to both undergraduate and graduate students with differing backgrounds and interests. While students have come mainly from the fields of neurobiology, pharmacology and medicine, students from the social sciences and humanities have also taken the course. A basic background in biology as well as chemistry has been routinely required, but extra reading has been suggested for students who have a difficult time with any phase of the course.

Section I of the book is concerned with the behavioral, biochemical and pharmacological methods used in psychopharmacology. In Section II biochemical and pharmacological interrelationships of drug action and behavior are discussed. This section focuses on the way in which endogenous neurochemicals in the central nervous system (neurotransmitters and macromolecules) function in the regulation of behavior and on the way in which these chemicals interact with drugs. The literature dealing with drug-behavioral-neurochemical interactions is vast; therefore only some of the many behaviors that have been examined are discussed. Motor behavior, ingestive behavior and behavior under schedule-control are emphasized. In addition, consideration is made of some aspects of aggressive behavior, sexual behavior, sensory function and sleep. Similarly, only the role of serotonin, catecholamines and acetylcholine in the mediation of these behaviors is discussed. It should be emphasized that this selection of behaviors and neurochemicals is not inclusive. Section III deals with the behavioral analysis of drug action and examines the environmental, sensory and behavioral variables that are important determinants of drug action.

LEWIS S. SEIDEN
LINDA DYKSTRA

Acknowledgments

Many colleagues and students assisted us in the preparation of this book. In particular, we gratefully acknowledge the thoughtful comments of Robert C. MacPhail, J. David Leander, Philip C. Hoffmann, Robert Balster, A. B. Campbell, Michael Emmett-Oglesby, and Ronald G. Pearl as well as those of Arvid Carlsson, Jorgen Engel and the Göteborg group. We also acknowledge numerous informal and formal discussions with colleagues and students in our respective departments as sources of constructive criticism, advice and ideas. Special thanks are due to Barbara Knight for her infinite patience in helping us to prepare this manuscript through its many revisions. Her good humor helped keep a measure of sanity and her efficiency helped us get the job finished. In addition, we wish to thank John Andressen, Fred Miller, Jeff Witkin, Richard Carter and Margaret Healey for help with references and proof reading, and Ann L. Osborn and Juan Sanchez-Ramos for help with the artwork. To our spouses, families and V. S. Dimas we are indebted for encouragement and forebearance.

Lewis Seiden is supported on a Research Career Development Award (5-KO2 MH 10562) from the National Institute of Mental Health, ADAMHA.

Contents

I METHODS

II THE PHARMACOLOGICAL AND BIOCHEMICAL
BASIS OF PSYCHOPHARMACOLOGY

III DRUG-BEHAVIOR INTERACTIONS

I
METHODS

1
Behavioral Methods for Assessing Drug Action

This chapter will present methodology used to describe the effects of drugs on behavior. In measuring drug-induced changes in behavior, it is important to have a sensitive and reliable baseline behavior. Therefore, the first task of the experimenter is to establish experimental control over an appropriate behavior. When all variables which affect that behavior are controlled (i.e., held constant), drug effects are measured as changes from control levels of performance. Since most drug effects are reversible, performance usually returns to its pre-drug level after a certain time. The concept of *control* and measurement of change from control is common to many scientific investigations. Drug effects are usually examined on behaviors which recur frequently and consistently and which can be maintained or observed over a long period of time; however, drug effects can also be examined on transitional behavior. For example, there has been considerable interest in the effects of a variety of drugs on the acquisition of behavior (see Chapters 7 and 8).

Precise behavioral control and quantification is important for the understanding of drug effects on behavior. Behavioral variables play just as important a role in the determination of a drug effect as pharmacological variables. Indeed, it is impossible to describe a drug effect on behavior without specifying how the behavior was measured and what relationship that behavior had to events in the environment which preceded, accompanied or followed it.

A thorough review of the methods used to examine drug effects on behavior goes beyond the scope of this book; therefore, only the methods which are discussed in subsequent chapters will be summarized here. In some cases, precise methods have been developed for controlling and quantifying behavior. In other cases, measurements are obtained from experimenter observation. This chapter will describe methodology for investigating motor behavior, sensory function, food and water intake, aggressive behavior, sexual behavior and sleep. The techniques of operant conditioning will also be discussed.

MOTOR BEHAVIOR

The importance of motor function in the expression and assessment of behavior is often overlooked relative to other processes; however, it is obvious that impairment of motor function can be responsible for alterations in both simple and complex behavioral patterns. Inability of an animal to perform a motor task may be quite as disruptive to behavior as loss of discriminative function, alteration in food and water consumption or factors interfering with conditioning. Motor behavior may become repetitive, grossly exaggerated or diminished and thereby interfere with the performance of another behavior through the expression of competing motor responses.

Motor activity has been assessed with a number of different techniques, each of which varies in terms of what it measures. For example, some methods record slight body or limb tremors, while others record the number of times an animal moves from one end of a cage to the other end. Therefore it is important to specify the method of assessment and to be familiar with its relative advantages and limitations. In addition, there are a number of variables whose parametric alteration influences levels of motor activity, including food and water deprivation, sex, lighting conditions, noises, species or strain, novelty of the experimental situation, duration of testing and pre-test housing conditions. These factors should always be considered in the measurement of motor behavior. The techniques used most commonly to assess motor behavior are discussed here. They are the running wheel, the rotorod, the stabilimeter and the photocell apparatus (see Finger, 1972 for a more thorough discussion of these techniques).

The running wheel is a cylinder adapted to rotate around its axle when an animal (usually a rodent) walks or runs in it. A record is made of the number of times the wheel is rotated. Since the wheel will not turn unless the animal walks or runs, coordinated locomotor activity can also be measured with the running wheel. Typically, animals only engage in a small amount of activity at first exposure to the wheel, but activity increases dramatically after a few sessions. Further exposure over prolonged periods of time may decrease activity.

The rotorod, like the running wheel, has been used to measure coordinated motor activity. Usually a mouse is placed on a rotating rod. In order to stay on the rod, the mouse must walk in a direction opposite to the direction of rotation. Coordinated motor behavior is measured by determining the amount of time the behavior is maintained (see Moore and Rech, 1967).

The stabilimeter is a cage supported by a central transverse axis that shifts position when an animal moves inside it. The types of movements recorded depend on the shape of the cage and the axis of tilt. For example, if a rectangular cage is used, movement from one side of the cage to the other causes the cage to tilt, and displacement is recorded. The stabilimeter generally does not record movements which only occur in one part of the cage.

The photocell apparatus is similar to the stabilimeter. A rectangular cage is often used, and the axis of the cage is bisected by a beam of light that shines onto a photosensitive cell. Interrupting the light beam produces a count. In some photocell chambers, a series of photocells are used so that intense motor activity occuring in a limited portion of the box can be detected. The number of counts in a photocell device is usually proportional to the number of times that the beams are interrupted by locomotion; however, a beam could be broken frequently if an animal were stationary and engaging in small movements of the head or limbs.

Movement may also be monitored by placing the animal in a field of ultrasonic waves. Movement in the field distorts the standing wave pattern, and the resulting energy changes are electronically recorded. This apparatus can record a wide range of movements in several species ranging from fine muscle tremors to gross locomotor activity. The ultrasonic devices are difficult to calibrate however, and one apparatus may not record the same level of activity as another. Moreover, a distinction is not made between locomotion, small head and limb movements, tremors and coordinated motor behavior. While direct experimenter observation can readily classify and quantify these different types of motor activity, it is subject to experimenter bias and can be very time-consuming. There problems are partially solved by having the experimenter blind to the treatment and sampling behavior for short time periods.

Stereotypic behavior can only be recorded by direct experimenter observation. Stereotypic behavior consists of the spontaneous occurrence of a repeated sequence of motor responses. For example, in the rat, stereotypy consists of head bobbing, continual biting or licking of the cage and rearing, although there may be considerable variability between individual rats. It should be emphasized that so-called stereotypic behaviors are not outside the animals normal repertoire. They are only considered as stereotyped when they occur at a frequency that is several times the normal frequency. (See Ayhan and Randrup, 1972; Dandiya et al., 1969; and Scheel-Krüger, 1971, for examples of rating scales used to quantify stereotyped behavior.)

SENSORY FUNCTION

The integration and execution of every behavior an organism engages in requires sensory function in one or more of the primary sensory modalities, which include audition, vision, taste, smell, proprioception and tactile sensation. Obviously a drug can affect sensory function and thereby alter behavior; therefore, the effects of drugs on sensation are of considerable interest. By and large this area of psychopharmacology is not as advanced as are some of the other areas, and presently the issues are mainly methodological. The difficulties encountered in measuring drug effects on sensory function are discussed in Chapter 10. There is one area of sensory function—sensitivity to painful stimuli—which has received considerable attention in pharmacology. Three procedures commonly used to examine sensitivity to painful stimuli are the hot plate test, the flinch-jump test and the titration schedule. (See Fraser and Harris, 1967, for a review of these and other techniques.)

The hot plate test was originally devised by Woolfe and Macdonald (1944). They measured the ability of drugs to inhibit reflex responses of mice placed in contact with a hot surface maintained at constant temperatures between 55° and 70°C. A temperature of 55°C is now customarily used for performing the test; however, recently it has been suggested that the analgesic effectiveness of a variety of non-narcotic analgesics and of some narcotic antagonists might be more easily identified at other temperatures (Ankier, 1974). In the flinch-jump test (Evans, 1961; Harvey and Lints, 1965; Tenen, 1967), a rat is placed on an electrified grid. The shock intensity at which the rat *flinches* and the intensity at which the rat *jumps* are determined by increasing and decreasing the shock intensity. A flinch is defined as a noticeable convulsion-like movement (crouch or startle) in response to the shock. A jump is defined as a movement in which the rear paws leave the grid in response to the shock. Since both the hot plate and flinch-jump procedures require experimenter observation, careful specification of response topography is required.

Another procedure for measuring sensitivity to painful stimuli is the titration procedure (Weiss and Laties, 1958). In this procedure, shock is delivered continuously to rats or monkeys. Increments in the shock intensity are scheduled to occur at specified intervals. Shock intensity is decreased when the animal responds on a lever. The effect of drugs on this procedure has been shown to depend on variables such as the length of the interval between shock increments and the number of responses required to produce a decrease in shock intensity.

FOOD AND WATER INTAKE

The measurement of food and water intake involves monitoring the amount of food or water an organism consumes in a specified time. The analysis of ingestion can be a simple matter of measuring food and fluid intakes once a day, or during some limited ingestion period. A more fine-grained analysis is provided by measuring meal patterns and the relationship between bouts of eating and drinking. Measurement techniques often vary from laboratory to laboratory. In some laboratories, food intake is measured by placing several pieces of pelleted diet of known total weight on the cage floor of an individual animal. The remaining food is simply weighed after some fixed time period. This procedure has certain undesirable features. As an animal chews off pieces of food pellet, variable amounts fall through the mesh floor. These crumbs and residue are sometimes difficult to collect, and their weight may be difficult to estimate if the crumbs become soaked with urine. Methods for presenting food as a powder in a feeding cup or as pellets have also been developed. While these methods facilitate intake measurements, differences do occur when food texture is altered.

Water intake is usually measured with calibrated drinking tubes which are clipped to the front of the animal's cage. A record of when drinking occurs can be obtained with a device called a drinkometer which counts the number of times the animal licks the drinking tube. While this can be used to record number of licks, it does not necessarily indicate amount of fluid ingested per lick, as different solutions may yield different ingestion volumes per lick.

Other considerations of importance in measuring food and water intake are light-dark cycles, ambient temperature, amount of time the animal has access to food or water, positioning of water bottles and positioning of the animals cage on the rack. (See Falk, 1971, for a discussion of these factors.)

AGGRESSIVE BEHAVIOR

Aggressive behavior is usually measured by direct experimenter observation. For example, aggressive behavior can be measured by observing the incidence of spontaneous fighting or by counting the number of times an animal assumes an attack posture or a submissive posture or engages in physical contact or biting. These behaviors can be further broken down into several subclasses, depending on the species observed. While various aspects of fighting behavior in wild and laboratory rats have been described in detail by ethologists, few pharmacological studies use these descriptions. (For a thorough specification of the various postures and acts that are characteristic of aggressive encounters, see Miczek, 1974.)

In some cases, experimental manipulations are made to elicit aggressive behavior within species. For example, isolation is known to induce aggressive behavior in mice. Another way to elicit aggressive behavior is by placing two animals together in a cage and shocking them by applying electric shock to the cage floor. The fighting which occurs following this procedure is called shock-induced fighting. Shock-induced fighting is measured by counting (1) the number of typical pre-fight postures that the rats exhibit toward one another, (2) the number of physical contacts made by the rat in this pre-fight posture and (3) the number of bites that occur between the two rats (see Moyer, 1968).

In other instances, two animals of different species such as a mouse and a rat are placed together in a small enclosure. Under normal circumstances the rat will not kill the mouse, but mouse killing (muricide) sometimes occurs following the administration of certain drugs.

Since aggressive behavior is defined and measured in different ways, and since the situation that generates the behavior is often not specified, care should be taken in interpreting work in this area.

SEXUAL BEHAVIOR

Sexual behavior is difficult to analyze quantitatively because it involves a variety of behavioral responses. The most prevalent approach to sexual behavior relies on direct observation and recording of behavioral responses of a sexual nature. For example, one feature of female copulatory behavior (especially in rodents and cats) is the adoption of a lordosis posture characterized by a stretching of the body in which the back is curved forward and the tail is lifted to facilitate intromission. This behavior is not observed following ovariectomy but can be restored by injection of estrogen and progesterone (Beach, 1967).

In the male rat or cat, the frequency of behaviors such as mounting, intromission and ejaculation are usually observed. These behaviors decline following castration, but they can be restored to the pre-castration level by the administration of testosterone (Beach, 1967). Attempts have also been made to assess sexual behavior on the basis of frequency of sexual responses to other stimuli. For instance, one might observe the frequency of sexual responses of a male cat to other male cats and compare it to frequency of sexual response to a female cat.

In general, there is considerable dissatisfaction with observational methods such as these. Therefore it is important to remember the difficulties involved in measuring sexual behavior when interpreting experimental data in which observational techniques have been used.

SLEEP

While all mammals spend a large portion of their time engaged in sleep, the function of sleep is not well understood. With the advent of the electroencephalogram (EEG) (Bremer, 1936) the investigation of various mechanisms related to sleep advanced. In early work with the electroencephalogram, Bremer (1936) discovered that there were rhythms that could be recorded from the cerebral cortex in man which were associated with different behavioral states. The alpha-rhythm which consists of predominantly 10-cycle-per-second EEG, was associated with a resting or relaxed state. The beta-rhythm, which is composed of activity of 14 cycles per second and upward, was associated with activation, tension or behavioral alertness. The delta-rhythm, which is 1–3.5 cycles per second, was associated with sleep in normal adults. These three rhythms were correlated with specific behavioral activity in man and in lower animals.

Early work on sleep and dreaming also demonstrated that slow waves characteristic of sleep were correlated with relaxation of the musculature, particularly in the neck. Furthermore, it was demonstrated that a phenomenon known as paradoxical sleep occurred. Paradoxical sleep is characterized by continued relaxation of the musculature accompanied by low voltage fast activity similar to beta activity (that is, wakefulness); the subject appears to be sleeping—hence, the name paradoxical sleep. If the subject awakens or is awakened during this phase of sleep, dreaming is almost invariably reported. Further work showed that this paradoxical or dream state of sleep is accompanied by frequent movements of the eyes known as rapid eye movements (REM).

Today, four EEG stages are considered in the investigation of sleep: (1) waking, which consists of a low voltage, fast cortical EEG accompanied by an active electromyogram (EMG); (2) slow wave sleep, which consists of high voltage cortical and subcortical spindles with slow waves accompanied by a relaxed EMG; (3) pre- and postparadoxical sleep, which consists of slow wave sleep as in (2), accompanied by ponto-geniculo-occipital (PGO) spikes with a more active EMG; and (4) paradoxical sleep, which consists of a tonic component characterized by fast, low voltage activity and a phasic component consisting of rapid eye movements (50–60 per minute) and bursts of PGO spikes. In most species, PGO activity almost invariably precedes paradoxical sleep for a period of 30–60 seconds.

CLASSICAL AND OPERANT CONDITIONING

Classical or respondent conditioning was formalized by the work of Pavlov (1927) in his studies of the physiology of gastric secretions. Pavlov used the following procedure: First, dogs were prepared with gastrointestinal fistulae in order that the rate and amount of gastric secretions could be measured following different types of food. Then an animal caretaker appeared with the food to be used in the experiment. After several days of the repeated appearance of the caretaker with the food, Pavlov noticed that the dogs secreted gastric juices when the caretaker appeared in the room. Pavlov called the food an *unconditioned stimulus* (*UCS*), in that it naturally elicited the gastric response. The caretaker, on the other hand, had become a *conditioned stimulus* (*CS*), in that the caretaker elicited salivation only after having been paired with the food. When a CS, such as the caretaker, and a USC, such as food, are repeatedly presented in the temporal relationship described above, the CS comes to elicit the response that in the beginning was elicited by the UCS alone. This response is called a CR (*conditioned response*). Therefore, in classical conditioning, the controlling events precede the response, and the response is said to be elicited by them. The development and maintenance of a conditioned response are determined by such factors as stimulus intensity, stimulus duration and the temporal presentation of the stimulus (see Corson and Corson, 1967).

While some psychologists have attempted to explain all behavior in terms of the classical conditioning model, B. F. Skinner (1938) observed that the relationship between behavior and its consequences was also very important for understanding behavior. For example, to say that Mr. Smith goes to work every morning for the paycheck that he receives at the end of the week is more reasonable than analyzing this complex behavior as a series of respondents with money as the final UCS. Through a series of experiments, Skinner showed that behavior could be maintained by the consequences it produced. He called this type of behavior *operant behavior*. In operant conditioning, a response is emitted by an organism, and some event (consequence) follows the response. These consequences are said to be *contingent* upon the response, since their occurrence depends on the response having occurred. In turn, the rate and form of the response are modified by these consequences.

The techniques of operant conditioning constitute a highly sophisticated and complex body of principles and ideas and methods which have proved useful in the investigation of drug effects on behavior (see Skinner, 1938; Ferster and Skinner, 1957; Keller and Schoenfeld, 1950; Holland and Skinner, 1961; Reese, 1964; Catania, 1968; Honig, 1966; Ferster *et al.*, 1975). This section will focus on the methods and concepts of operant conditioning that are commonly used in psychopharmacology.

Terminology

Consequences. Operant behavior has been defined as behavior that is maintained (or reduced) by its consequences. Therefore, the nature of these consequences becomes critical in a discussion of operant behavior. If the consequences which follow a response increase the probability that a response will recur, then those consequences (or stimuli) are called reinforcers. Any event which *increases* the probability of the response it follows is called a positive reinforcer. Food, water, intracranial stimulation and heat have all been shown to function as positive reinforcers.

The conditions under which certain stimuli may acquire positive reinforcing properties are sometimes achieved by certain antecedent manipulations such as deprivation. Stimulus events can also derive reinforcing properties by being associated with reinforcing stimuli such as food. These are called conditioned reinforcers. We will see in Chapter 11 that drugs can also serve as reinforcers. There are also instances in which electric shock can function as a positive reinforcer and will maintain responding that is characteristic of other positive reinforcers (Morse *et al.*, 1967; Kelleher and Morse, 1968; McKearney, 1968, 1969, 1970; Byrd, 1969).

Positive reinforcement refers to the situation in which the presentation of some stimulus follows a response and produces an increase in the probability that the response will recur. *Negative reinforcement* refers to the situation in which the termination or avoidance of some stimulus such as shock follows a response and produces an increase in the probability that the response will recur.

The consequences which follow a response can also *decrease* the probability that the response will recur. For example, the presentation of a stimulus such as shock contingent upon a response will decrease the frequency of occurrence of that response. This is called *punishment*. Furthermore, response probability is reduced if responding eliminates a reinforcer. Time out is an example of this procedure. A time out produces conditions during which reinforcement is not available. These consequences are presented in Table 1-1.

Extinction is the situation in which a response no longer produces the consequences that had previously followed it. For example, if an organism has been reinforced with food for lever pressing and food no longer follows this response, the response will *extinguish*; i.e., after a period of time, response rate will decrease. The immediate effect of discontinuing the food, however, is often an *increase* in response rate, called an *extinction burst*. The extinction burst is commonly seen in food vending machines. An individual deposits a coin, and presses the button which produces a sweet roll. If the roll fails to appear, the individual's rate of pressing the button usually increases dramatically, but repeated experience leads to a decrease in response rate.

TABLE 1-1.   Consequences Which Follow a Response

Probability of a Response	Stimulus Presented	Stimulus Terminated Or Removed
increases	positive reinforcement	negative reinforcement
decreases	punishment	time out

The Response. Operant conditioning has been closely identified with so-called free operant procedures in which rate of performing a simple response like lever pressing or key pecking is the principal dependent variable. To illustrate, a typical operant experiment might be designed along the following lines: A pigeon is deprived of food for 23 hours and placed in an apparatus so designed that a small quantity of grain is made available to the pigeon if it pecks a key. The apparatus is the familiar operant chamber designed by B. F. Skinner (1938), i.e., the Skinner Box. An operant pigeon chamber is illustrated in Fig. 1-1. The pigeon chamber is designed so that grain is made available whenever the subject closes a circuit by means of a key or lever activated microswitch. The particular muscle movements or response topography that lead to closure of the switch are usually not specified; the pigeon may peck the key in any manner, just so it is of sufficient force to close the circuit. The key peck is defined as the operant response. The grain is the stimulus that is presented contingent on the key peck response. If presentation of the grain increases the probability of occurrence of key pecking, the grain is considered to be a positive reinforcer.

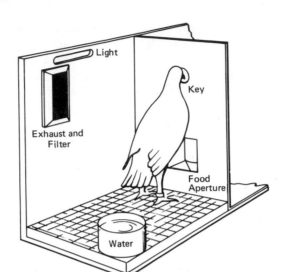

Fig. 1-1. Diagram of a typical pigeon chamber. (From Ferster *et al.*, 1975.)

Although most studies of operant conditioning employ a repeatable response such as a key peck or a lever press, any response that is maintained by the consequences which follow it is an operant response. For example, the response of running in a maze is an operant response in that reinforcement is made contingent on a particular response. In a t-maze an animal is required to run to one of two goal boxes which are arranged to the right and left of a central alley. T-maze performance is sometimes referred to as a spatial discrimination. The reinforcement is usually food or escape from shock. If food is the reinforcer, it is available in only one of the goal boxes. If shock is the reinforcer, it is terminated when the animal chooses the correct goal box. In this case, the probability or correctness of a particular response rather than the rate of responding is the dependent variable. There are many instances in which it is desirable to measure the probability or correctness of a particular response. For example, in examining drug effects on the acquisition of a response, the number of incorrect responses made in reaching a goal or the number of trials required to meet a criterion of correctness (e.g., 90% correct) might be measured. Traditionally, t-mazes with right or left turns and Y-mazes with two more choice points have been used to measure the probability of a response's occurring or the probability that a given response is correct. Operant chambers with two or more manipulanda can also be used to measure discrete responses. These are often called discrete trial procedures.

Stimulus Control.   A stimulus in operant terminology is any aspect of an organism's environment which is related to a response. Reinforcing stimuli are one kind of stimuli which relate to behavior in that they determine the probability that a response will recur. Whether or not a particular behavior is followed by reinforcement is often dependent on antecedent stimulus conditions. These are called discriminative stimuli. If reinforcement only follows a behavior when certain discriminative stimuli are present, responding will usually occur predominately in the presence of these stimuli. If this occurs, the organism is said to have made a discrimination, or, alternatively, responding is said to be under stimulus control. Stimulus control simply refers to the extent to which a stimulus determines the probability of occurrence of some response (Terrace, 1966). Stimulus generalization procedures are often used to measure the extent to which responding is controlled by a particular stimulus. (See Chapter 10 for a description of this procedure.)

The notation for a discriminative stimulus is S^D. A stimulus that is not correlated with reinforcement is called S^Δ (S-delta). Discriminative stimuli are usually visual or auditory stimuli, but they may represent any stimulus, including drug-induced stimuli (see Chapter 12). Furthermore, they can take on different dimensions—e.g., they may be lights of different intensities or colors, or they may be tones of different frequencies, intensities or durations.

Schedule-Controlled Behavior

In the procedures of operant conditioning, behavior is maintained by the consequences that follow a response. When every response is followed by reinforcement, the organism is said to be on a continuous reinforcement schedule (CRF). The amount of reinforcement delivered on a CRF schedule is high and, therefore, responding often decreases with time because of satiation. It is by no means necessary to reinforce every occurrence of a response in order to increase or maintain responding. Reinforcement can be scheduled to occur intermittently. There are a variety of intermittent schedules of reinforcement which in turn produce a variety of rates and patterns of responding. Both rate and pattern of responding are important determinants of a drug effect (Dews, 1955).

Data Collection and Analysis. In general, rate and pattern of responding generated by intermittent schedules of reinforcement are measured with digital counters and cumulative recorders. The digital counter is incremented each time a specified response (lever press, key press) occurs, and overall rate of responding is calculated from the information on the counter and an elapsed time meter. Cumulative records are made by driving paper horizontally past a marking pen; each time a response occurs, the pen moves vertically a constant distance. Reinforcement is usually indicated by a diagonal movement of the pen. Other events can be marked by a second pen, called an event pen (see Fig. 1-2). Since the paper is driven past the marking pen at a constant speed, the slope of the line at any point on the cumulative record provides a measure of rate of responding.

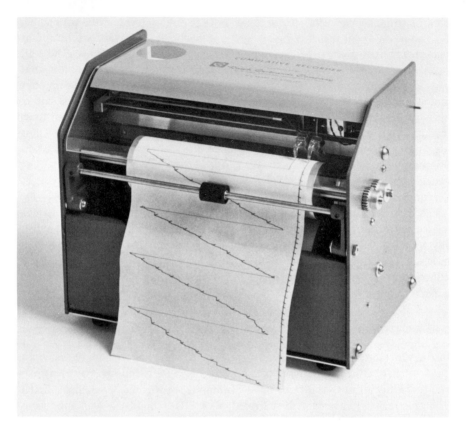

Fig. 1-2. Cumulative recorder. (Courtesy of Ralph Gerbrands Company, Arlington, Mass.)

Patterns of responding are revealed by examining large segments of the cumulative record. Inter-response times are contained on the cumulative record as the distance between two responses. The experimenter can convert these distances to units of time by hand measurements, but generally this is extremely time-consuming.

While it is possible to measure the time between individual responses (inter-response times or IRTs) on a cumulative record, the use of a digital computer facilitates the collection and analysis of inter-response time data. Some on-line digital computer systems not only record the animal's performance, but also provide instant data analysis and subsequent feedback into the behavioral system (Weiss and Laties, 1964). In this type of system, the contingencies of reinforcement can be determined by the animal's ongoing behavior. On-line systems do require, however, that there be a one-to-one correspondence between running time and computer availability. This factor can be a handicap to investigators using time-sharing computer systems.

Various off-line recording systems have also been described; these systems allow events to be recorded as they occur and also provide subsequent computer analysis (Barry *et al.*, 1966; Herrick and Denelsbeck, 1963). Seiden *et al.* (1969) have described an off-line system in which session data are recorded on an AM magnetic tape and transcribed at a later time. More recently, special computer programs have been developed in which the computer is used both to program the contingencies in the chamber as well as to acquire the data generated from the chamber; the same computer can then be used for data analysis. These systems have great flexibility and are becoming more common in operant laboratories (Snapper and Kadden, 1973; Weiss, 1973).

Positive Reinforcement Schedules.   If responding increases when the presentation of some event follows a response, positive reinforcement is said to take place.   There are numerous schedules of positive reinforcement.   The schedules which are used most often in measuring drug effects are discussed in detail below. In Fig. 1-3 characteristic rates and patterns of responding are illustrated for fixed ratio (FR), variable ratio (VR), fixed interval (FI) and variable interval (VI) schedules of reinforcement.

1. *Fixed Ratio (FR).*   Under this schedule, the organism is reinforced only after making a certain fixed number of responses.   FR 10 indicates that the animal must make 10 responses in order to be reinforced.   On the FR schedule, re-

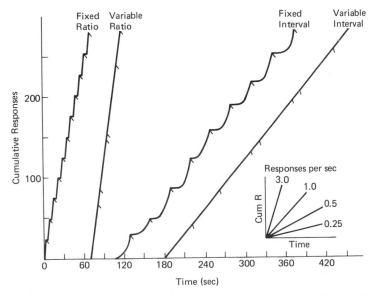

Fig. 1-3. Stylized cumulative records of responses under a fixed ratio (FR), variable ratio (VR), fixed interval (FI), and variable interval (VI), schedule of reinforcement.   Slash marks in the response record indicate reinforcement presentation.

sponses usually occur rapidly until reinforcement. After reinforcement, the animal usually pauses (post-reinforcement pause). The response rate engendered by an FR schedule is usually proportional to the FR requirement; the response rate under an FR 10 schedule will be higher than under an FR 2. Very high FR requirements, however, often engender slower overall response rates because the animal usually pauses for a long time before initiating the FR requirement. Responding on FR schedules with high response requirements is often characterized by bursts of responses at the normal FR rate intermixed with long pauses that are unrelated to reinforcement. This is called FR straining. The size of the fixed ratio at which stable performance can be maintained depends on several factors: the species of animal, the nature of the operant (weight and position of lever), deprivation conditions and the animal's conditioning history. Performance on an FR schedule may be developed from a CRF schedule provided that the progression of the ratio is not too sudden. When shaping an FR schedule with a high response requirement, it is best to raise the response requirement slowly to avoid extinction or straining.

2. *Variable Ratio (VR)*. Under this schedule, reinforcement occurs after a variable number of responses have occurred. For example, on a VR 10 schedule, the average number of responses required for reinforcement is 10, but reinforcement could occur after 2, 4, 6, 8, 10, 12, 14, . . . 18 responses. The particular number of responses required for reinforcement varies in a nonorderly manner.

3. *Variable Interval (VI)*. Under the VI schedule, responses are intermittently reinforced over time. For example, on a VI 1-min schedule (variable interval one minute) responding is reinforced on the average of once per minute; at some times reinforcement may follow the first response after 10 seconds, while at other times it may follow the first response after 120 seconds. The VI schedule produces a relatively steady response rate (see Fig. 1-3) which is resistant to extinction. Response rate on the VI schedule is dependent on both the mean reinforcement interval and the minimum reinforcement interval. As the mean and minimum interval become shorter, the response rate increases (Catania and Reynolds, 1968).

4. *Fixed Interval (FI)*. Under the fixed interval schedule, the first response that occurs after a fixed length of time has elapsed is reinforced. The schedule engenders low rates of responding at the beginning of the interval. Response rates increase as the time for reinforcement approaches. The pattern of responding which appears on the cumulative record is referred to as the FI "scallop" (Fig. 1-3). It can be quantified by the quarter-life statistic. The quarter-life is a measure of the proportion of time taken in the FI for the first quarter of the FI responses to occur (Herrnstein and Morse, 1957a; Gollub, 1964). For example, if responding occurred at an equal rate throughout an FI interval, the quarter-life would be 0.25, i.e., one quarter of the response would occur in the first 25% of the interval. A quarter-life greater than 0.25 describes an initial low rate of responding followed by accelerated responding which is characteristic of FI per-

formance.   Quarter-life values of 0.60 and 0.75 are frequently obtained and represent good control by the FI over the temporal pattern of responding.

Under most FI schedules, no stimuli are present to signal reinforcement. In some experiments, stimuli (e.g., a sequential pattern of lights) have been presented that signal the availability of reinforcement. Such stimuli are sometimes considered to serve as clocks, in that they indicate when reinforcement is due. Laties and Weiss (1966) have shown that the presence of time-correlated discriminative stimuli facilitate the development of sharply discriminated FI responding.

5. *Differential Reinforcement of Low Rate (DRL)*. The DRL schedule is very similar to an FI schedule in that only the first response after a specific interval is reinforced. There is an added requirement, however, that no response may occur during the interval. If responses do occur during the interval, the timing of the interval is started over. Responding on the DRL is usually measured in terms of inter-response times (IRT, the time between two responses). IRTs are usually grouped into several time categories or "bins." For example, all responses having an inter-response time of 1–2 sec are placed in the 1–2 sec IRT bin.

When a DRL schedule is in effect, reinforcement occurs only if responses are separated by a certain minimal time. For example, on a DRL 20-sec schedule, only IRTs of 20 sec or longer are reinforced. In terms of IRTs, one usually sees a distribution of IRTs clustered around a value that is close to the minimum time for reinforcement. Figure 1-4 illustrates this effect on a DRL 20-sec schedule. A large percentage of responses occur in the 20 sec IRT bin. Fewer responses occur in IRT bins farther removed from the reinforced IRT, except that a large percentage of responses usually also occur in the 0–2 sec IRT bin.

It is possible to influence the rate of responding on all the schedules above by placing other constraints on the schedule. For example, a limited hold can be employed. A limited hold makes reinforcement available for only a specified time; for example, in an FI 5-min limited hold (LH) 10-sec, the first response after 5 min will produce reinforcement. If however, the animal does not respond within 10 sec after the 5 min has elapsed, reinforcement will no longer be available.

6. *Schedules Employing More Than One Schedule of Reinforcement.* It is common to combine two or more schedules of reinforcement. Some of the more common combinations are described here. In a *multiple schedule*, two or more schedule components are presented, with each component signaled by a different discriminative stimulus. Reinforcement follows the completion of each component. For example, responding during the presence of a red light may be reinforced on an FI 1-min schedule. In the presence of a blue light, responding is reinforced on an FR 10 schedule. With repeated exposure, the characteristic patterns of FI and FR responding will occur in the presence of each stimulus.

A *mixed schedule* also has two or more component schedules, but there are no discriminative stimuli associated with the components. Reinforcement follows completion of each component. With a *chain schedule*, two or more sched-

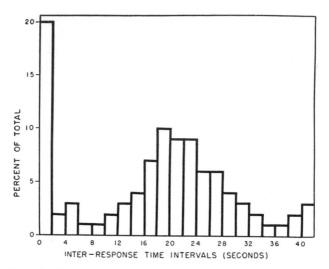

Fig. 1-4. Distribution of IRTs on a DRL 20-sec schedule. (Sidman, 1956.)

ules are also used, and a discriminative stimulus is correlated with each schedule. Reinforcement, however, only occurs after both schedule components have been completed. For example, on a chained FI 1-min FR 10 schedule, completion of the initial FI 1-min requirement would be followed by presentation of a stimulus that would signal the FR component. When the FR requirement was completed, reinforcement would be delivered. A *tandem schedule* is identical to the chained schedule, except that there are no discriminative stimuli associated with each component. Another way to characterize a sequence of schedules is as *second-order schedules*. In second-order schedules, the behavior specified by a schedule contingency is treated as a unitary response that is itself reinforced according to some schedule of reinforcement. For example, reinforcement might be contingent upon the completion of three successive FI 2-min schedules. Discriminative stimuli may or may not follow completion of each component.

One additional schedule that is used in psychopharmacology is the *concurrent schedule*. In a concurrent schedule, responding is reinforced by separate schedules *simultaneously*. For example, responses may be reinforced on an FR 10 schedule on one lever and at the same time on an FI 5-min schedule on another lever. A more detailed description of response characteristics under each schedule as well as methods of shaping the different performances will be found in Ferster and Skinner (1957), Reese (1964) and Ferster *et al.* (1975).

Negative Reinforcement Schedules. If responding increases when the removal of some event follows a response, negative reinforcement is said to take place. Negative reinforcement schedules can maintain behavior for long periods of time without the problems of deprivation and satiation which are often encountered with positive reinforcement. Electric shock is the stimulus most commonly used as a negative reinforcer, but heat, cold and loud noises are other examples of stimuli that will increase the probability of occurrence of a response which terminates or avoids their presentation. Moreover, a reduction in overall frequency of electric shock can also serve as a negative reinforcer (Sidman, 1962; Herrnstein and Hineline, 1966).

Shock is typically administered through the feet of smaller animals (such as rats, mice and cats) or through implanted or attached electrodes in larger animals, such as monkeys and pigeons. Shock intensity may range from 0.1 to 5.0 milliamperes (mA). The species involved, the duration of shock and the conditions of temperature and relative humidity are relevant determinants of the conductivity of electrical current from the shock source to the surface area of the animal. (See Campbell and Masterson, 1969, for a discussion of these variables.)

There are a number of important parameters to be considered when negative reinforcement is used to maintain responding. If the intensity of the shock is too high, it can elicit freezing behavior which is incompatible with the development of avoidance behavior (Meyer and Korn, 1964). On the other hand, shock intensities that are too low will not serve as effective negative reinforcers. Pulsating shock has been found to be more effective than continuous shock for the development of avoidance behavior (D'Amato and Schiff, 1964; D'Amato et al., 1964, 1965). Other crucial variables include the duration of the preshock stimulus (Myers, 1962; Meyer et al., 1960), the spacing of trials, the handling of the animals (Herz, 1960), the time between shocks and the time each response postpones a shock (Sidman, 1953b).

1. *Escape.* Electric shock is administered at certain intervals for a given duration of time. The animal terminates the shock by emitting an appropriate response (pressing a lever, running down one arm of a t-maze). For example, the experimental animal may receive a two-second shock once every 20 seconds; the shock can be terminated by a lever press. Sometimes it is difficult to shape escape responding. Rats, for example, may respond to shock in one of two mutually exclusive ways. They may either run when the shock is presented, or they may freeze. The freezing response consists of crouched posture along with sympathetic discharge, including piloerection, urination and defecation (see Chapter 3, p. 74). The running response makes it far more likely that the rat will accidentally hit the lever. When the rat accidentally hits the lever, this response is reinforced since it terminates shock. Therefore, the lever press is more likely to occur the next time the shock is presented. When freezing occurs, the rat is less likely to make the appropriate response. The shock will eventually terminate after a specified interval. Therefore, the freezing response will also be reinforced, even though this is not the "correct" escape response. Unless this pattern can be changed, these animals are usually excluded from the experiment.

Escape responding can also be maintained under schedules similar to those used for food presentation. Cook and Catania (1964) used an FI escape schedule in which the first response after 10 minutes terminated a shock which continuously pulsed throughout the FI interval. This schedule engendered response rates and patterns similar to a conventional FI schedule maintained by food. The termination of a stimulus paired with shock can also maintain responding. Kelleher and Morse (1964) trained monkeys on a multiple FR FI schedule. Responding terminated a stimulus correlated with occasional electric shocks.

2. *Avoidance.* Escape responding *terminates* a negative reinforcer once it has been presented. Avoidance responding, on the other hand, decreases the frequency of occurrence of the negative reinforcer by *postponing* its occurrence. In the *discrete trial avoidance procedure* (or signalled avoidance) a preshock stimulus is presented at some time prior to the occurrence of a shock. The preshock stimulus usually is a buzzer, tone or light. Initially the preshock stimulus has little effect on the animal's behavior, while the shock elicits a freezing response or running.

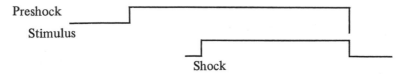

The time interval between the onset of the stimulus and the onset of the shock is set at a specified value (usually about 10 seconds); the stimulus usually remains on during the shock and the two terminate at the same time. A response which occurs during this interval terminates the stimulus and also prevents the occurrence of the shock. Experiments using this paradigm are often designed so that a response that occurs during the time when both the preshock stimulus and shock are present will also terminate the shock; this is an escape response.

The stimulus which precedes the shock is often called a warning stimulus or a conditioned stimulus (because it has been paired with the shock), and the procedure itself is often called the CAR (conditioned avoidance response). Escape responses have also been called unconditioned responses, and avoidance responses conditioned responses. As Dews and Morse (1961) have pointed out, this terminology can be misleading. Therefore, we will simply use the following terms: avoidance response, escape response and preshock stimulus.

Early investigators of discrete trial avoidance usually employed either a pole jump or a shuttle box response to measure avoidance. The pole jump apparatus consists of a metal grid floor with an insulated pole. The animal escapes the shock by jumping from the floor to the pole; or he avoids the shock by jumping from the floor to the pole in the presence of the preshock stimulus. The shuttle box procedure usually makes use of a two-compartment box with a grid floor. A stimulus is presented prior to the shock. The animal avoids shock by jumping from one compartment to the other across a low hurdle. Both one-way and two-way avoidance procedures are used. In the two-way avoidance procedure, the animal shuttles from the left to the right compartment or from the right to the left compartment, depending on where he is when a trial is initiated. In the one-way avoidance prodecure, the animal only shuttles in one direction. For example, if the animal is required to shuttle from the right to the left compartment to avoid shock, the experimenter returns the animal to the right compartment after each trial. These procedures are often called active avoidance. Some investigators use the term passive avoidance to refer to the situation in which an animal avoids shock by *not* responding. This can be classified as a punishment procedure in that the animal is shocked contingent on making some response, i.e., exploring the second chamber (see the next section for a discussion of punishment procedures). Many avoidance procedures now use a bar-press response or a wheel-turning response.

In the *continuous avoidance procedure* (Sidman, 1953a) shocks are scheduled to occur at regular intervals in the absence of a response. The interval between two shocks is referred to as the SS interval (shock-shock interval) and is often about 20 seconds long. A response that occurs within the SS interval delays the next shock for a fixed amount of time (this is the response-shock or RS interval). By pressing the lever at suitable intervals, shock can be postponed indefinitely. Sometimes a signal is added prior to the shock. This paradigm has been referred to by several different names: Sidman, free-operant, continuous, or non-discriminated or discriminated avoidance. We will use the term continuous avoidance. The continuous avoidance schedule may or may not have an escape component. In some procedures the shock can be avoided by responding on one lever and escaped by responding on another lever (Heise and Boff, 1962).

Procedures Which Produce a Decrease in Response Rate. Generally, two procedures are used to decrease response rate. In one procedure an event such as electric shock is presented contingent on a response. This is called a punishment procedure. In the other procedure (conditioned suppression) an event such as electric shock is presented noncontingently. While shock is the stimulus used most often in these procedures, a variety of stimuli can be used to suppress responding, including blasts of air (Masserman, 1946) and noise (Holz and Azrin, 1962). Many of the same variables that were discussed above regarding the use of shock in negative reinforcement procedures apply to its use in punishment and conditioned suppression procedures.

1. *Punishment.* In order to produce a decrease in responding by presenting shock contingent on a response, there must be some pre-existing level of responding. Schedules of positive reinforcement are therefore usually used to maintain responding, and punishment is superimposed on this baseline behavior. In some instances periods of punished responding alternate with periods of unpunished responding (Geller and Seifter, 1960).

The reduction in responding following punishment has been shown to be a function of a number of variables including the schedule of reinforcement on which punishment is superimposed, the deprivation level of the experimental subject and the intensity and the frequency of delivery of the punishing stimulus. For example, when response-contingent shocks are superimposed on a fixed ratio schedule of responding for food presentation, punishment lengthens the pause preceding the usual run of responses (Azrin, 1959), while punishment produces a general lowering of response frequency when it is superimposed on variable-interval (Azrin, 1960), fixed-interval (Azrin and Holz, 1961) and differential reinforcement of low rate (Holz et al., 1963) schedules of food presentation. (For a thorough review of the variables affecting punished responding see Azrin and Holz, 1966.)

2. *Conditioned Suppression.* The conditioned suppression procedure first described by Estes and Skinner (1941) has been called by various names, including the Estes-Skinner Procedure, conditioned suppression and the conditioned fear or conditioned emotional response. Conditioned suppression is typically established in the following way: Behavior is maintained by positive reinforcement. After lever pressing has stabilized, a stimulus is presented; when the stimulus terminates, an unavoidable shock occurs. If the preshock stimulus and the shock are paired repeatedly, response suppression will occur during the preshock stimulus. Suppression usually begins with the onset of the stimulus and ends upon termination of the shock. Conditioned suppression can also be produced by a stimulus (prefood stimulus) which signals food presentation (Azrin and Hake, 1969; Miczek and Grossman, 1971), although others have observed facilitation during a prefood stimulus (Brady, 1961; Henton and Brady, 1970; Herrnstein and Morse, 1957b; LoLordo, 1971).

Numerous variables have been shown to affect responding in the conditioned suppression paradigm. The duration of the preshock stimulus has been shown to determine the degree of suppression. In general, brief stimuli produce greater degrees of suppression (Miczek and Grossman, 1971; Stein et al., 1958) than longer stimuli. Moreover, Stein et al. (1958) have shown that suppression also depends on the extent to which opportunities for reinforcement are reduced. Blackman (1968) has presented data which indicate that conditioned suppression may depend on the rate of responding maintained by the baseline schedule of positive reinforcement.

Adjunctive Behavior. While a variety of behaviors can be maintained by schedules of reinforcement or punishment, it has been observed that other behaviors sometimes accompany schedule-maintained behavior although these behaviors are not part of the response-reinforcement relationship. For example, Falk (1961) observed that rats drank large quantities of water immediately after consuming a food pellet on an FI schedule of reinforcement. Under certain conditions rats increased liquid consumption 10-fold. This pattern of excessive drinking that occurs after pellet presentation has been called scheduled-induced polydipsia or, more generally, adjunctive behavior. A variety of behaviors have been cited as examples of adjunctive behavior, including attack or biting behavior and wheel-running. (See Falk, 1972, and Wayner, 1974, for a review of adjunctive behavior.)

SUMMARY

In most cases a drug's effect on behavior is examined by establishing experimental control over a behavior, administering a drug and measuring changes from control performance. In this chapter, a variety of behavioral techniques were discussed, and the importance of defining the details of each technique was noted. It was also noted that parametric variation in the variables of an experimental situation is a primary determinant of a drug effect. In order to describe and understand the actions of drugs on behavior, these parameters must be investigated. Therefore, the examination of drug-behavior interactions requires strict behavioral as well as pharmacological controls.

REFERENCES

Ankier, S. I. 1974. New hot plate tests to quantify antinociceptive and narcotic antagonist activities. *Eur. J. Pharmacol.* 27: 1–4.
Ayhan, I. H. and A. Randrup. 1972. Role of brain noradrenaline in morphine-induced stereotyped behaviour. *Psychopharmacologia* 27: 203–212.
Azrin, N. H. 1959. Punishment and recovery during fixed-ratio performance. *J. Exp. Anal. Behav.* 2: 301–305.
Azrin, N. H. 1960. Effects of punishment intensity during variable-interval reinforcement. *J. Exp. Anal. Behav.* 3: 123–142.
Azrin, N. H. and D. F. Hake. 1969. Positive conditioned suppression: conditioned suppression using positive reinforcers as the unconditioned stimuli. *J. Exp. Anal. Behav.* 12: 167–173.
Azrin, N. H. and W. C. Holz. 1966. Punishment. *In* W. K. Honig (ed.), *Operant Behavior: Areas of Research and Application.* Appleton-Century-Crofts, New York, pp. 380–447.
Azrin, N. H. and W. C. Holz. 1961. Punishment during fixed-interval reinforcement. *J. Exp. Anal. Behav.* 4: 343–347.
Barry, H., III, W. J. Kinnard, Jr., N. Watzman and J. P. Buckely. 1966. A computer-oriented system for high-speed recording of operant behavior. *J. Exp. Anal. Behav.* 9: 163–171.
Beach, F. A. 1967. Cerebral and hormonal control of reflexive mechanisms involved in copulatory behavior. *Physiol. Rev.* 47: 289–316.
Blackman, D. 1968. Effects of drugs on conditioned "anxiety." *Nature* 217: 769–770.
Brady, J. V. 1961. Motivational-emotional factors and intracranial self-stimulation. *In* D. E. Sheer (ed.), *Electrical Stimulation of the Brain.* University of Texas Press, Austin, Texas. pp. 413–430.
Bremer, F. 1936. Nouvelles recherches sur le mechanisme du sommeil. *C. R. Soc. Biol. (Paris)* 122: 460–483.

Byrd, L. D. 1969. Responding in the cat maintained under response-independent electric shock and response-produced electric shock. *J. Exp. Anal. Behav.* **12**: 1–10.

Campbell, B. A. and F. A. Masterson. 1969. Psychophysics of punishment. *In* B. A. Campbell and R. M. Church (eds.), *Punishment and Aversive Behavior.* Appleton-Century-Crofts, New York. pp. 3–42.

Catania, A. C. (ed.). 1968. *Contemporary Research in Operant Behavior.* Scott, Foresman & Co., Glenview, Illinois.

Catania, A. C. and G. S. Reynolds. 1968. A quantitative analysis of the responding maintained by interval schedules of reinforcement. *J. Exp. Anal. Behav.* **11**: 327–383.

Cook, L. and A. C. Catania. 1964. Effects of drugs on avoidance and escape behavior. *Fed. Proc.* **23**: 818–835.

Corson, S. A. and E. Corson. 1967. Pavlovian conditioning as a method for studying the mechanisms of action of minor tranquilizers. *Neuropsychopharmacology*, Proceedings of the International Congress of College Instruction and Neuropsychopharmacology, 5th, Washington, D.C., pp. 857–878.

D'Amato, M. R., D. Keller and G. Beiderman. 1965. Discriminated avoidance learning as a function of parameters of discontinuous shock. *J. Exp. Psychol.* **70**: 543–548.

D'Amato, M. R., D. Keller and L. DiCara. 1964. Facilitation of discriminated avoidance learning by discontinuous shock. *J. Comp. Physiol. Psychol.* **58**: 344–349.

D'Amato, M. R. and D. Schiff. 1964. Long-term discriminated avoidance performance in the rat. *J. Comp. Physiol. Psychol.* **57**: 123–126.

Dandiya, P. C., B. D. Gupta, M. L. Gupta and S. K. Patni. 1969. Effects of LSD on open field performance in rats. *Psychopharmacologia* **15**: 333–340.

Dews, P. B. 1955. Studies on behavior I. Differential sensitivity to pentobarbital of pecking performance in pigeons depending on the schedule of reward. *J. Pharmacol. Exp. Ther.* **113**: 393–401.

Dews, P. B. and W. H. Morse. 1961. Behavioral pharmacology. *Ann. Rev. Pharmacol.* **1**: 145–174.

Estes, W. K. and B. F. Skinner. 1941. Some quantitative properties of anxiety. *J. Exp. Psychol.* **29**: 390–400.

Evans, W. O. 1961. A new technique for the investigation of some analgesic drugs on a reflexive behavior in the rat. *Psychopharmacologia* **2**: 318–325.

Falk, J. L. 1971. Determining changes in vital functions: Ingestion. *In* R. D. Myers (ed.), *Methods in Psychobiology*, Vol. 1. Academic Press, New York, pp. 301–329.

Falk, J. L. 1961. Production of polydipsia in normal rats by an intermittent food schedule. *Science* **133**: 195–196.

Falk, J. L. 1972. The nature and determinants of adjunctive behavior. *In* R. M. Gilbert and J. D. Keehn (eds.), *Schedule Effects: Drugs, Drinking and Aggression.* University of Toronto Press, Toronto, pp. 148–173.

Ferster, C. B. and B. F. Skinner. 1957. *Schedules of Reinforcement.* Appleton-Century-Crofts, New York.

Ferster, C. B., S. Culbertson and M. C. P. Boren. 1975. *Behavior Principles.* Prentice-Hall, Englewood Cliffs, New Jersey.

Finger, F. W. 1972. Measuring behavioral activity. *In* R. D. Myers (ed.), *Methods in Psychobiology*, Vol. 2, Academic Press, New York, pp. 1–18.

Fraser, H. F. and L. S. Harris. 1967. Narcotic and narcotic antagonist analgesics. *Ann. Rev. Pharmacol.* **7**: 277–300.

Geller, I. and J. Seifter. 1960. The effects of meprobamate, barbiturates, *d*-amphetamine and promazine on experimentally-induced conflict in the rat. *Psychopharmacologia* **1**: 482–492.

Gollub, L. R. 1964. The relations among measures of performance of fixed-interval schedules. *J. Exp. Anal. Behav.* 7: 337–343.

Harvey, J. A. and C. E. Lints. 1965. Lesions in the medial forebrain bundle: Delayed effects on sensitivity to electric shock. *Science* 148: 250–252.

Heise, G. A. and E. Boff. 1962. Continuous avoidance as a baseline for measuring behavioral effects of drugs. *Psychopharmacologia* 3: 264–282.

Henton, W. W. and J. V. Brady. 1970. Operant acceleration during a pre-reward stimulus. *J. Exp. Anal. Behav.* 13: 205–209.

Herrick, R. M. and J. S. Denelsbeck. 1963. A system for programming experiments and for recording and analyzing data automatically. *J. Exp. Anal. Behav.* 6: 631–635.

Herrnstein, R. J. and P. N. Hineline. 1966. Negative reinforcement as shock-frequency reduction. *J. Exp. Anal. Behav.* 9: 421–430.

Herrnstein, R. J. and W. H. Morse. 1957a. Effects of pentobarbital on intermittently reinforced behavior. *Science* 125: 929–931.

Herrnstein, R. J. and W. H. Morse. 1957b. Some effects of response-independent positive reinforcement on maintained operant behavior. *J. Comp. Physiol. Psychol.* 50: 461–467.

Herz, A. 1960. Drugs and the conditioned avoidance response. *Int. Rev. Neurobiol.* 2: 229–277.

Holland, J. G. and B. F. Skinner. 1961. *The Analysis of Behavior: A Program for Self-Instruction.* McGraw-Hill, New York.

Holz, W. C. and N. H. Azrin. 1962. Recovery during punishment by intense noise. *Psychol. Rep.* 11: 655–657.

Holz, W. C., N. H. Azrin and R. E. Ulrich. 1963. Punishment of temporally spaced responding. *J. Exp. Anal. Behav.* 6: 115–122.

Honig, W. K. (ed.). 1966. *Operant Behavior: Areas of Research and Application.* Appleton-Century-Crofts, New York.

Kelleher, R. T. and W. H. Morse. 1964. Escape behavior and punished behavior. *Fed. Proc.* 23: 808–817.

Kelleher, R. T. and W. H. Morse. 1968. Schedules using noxious stimuli. III. Responding maintained with response-produced electric shocks. *J. Exp. Anal. Behav.* 11: 819–838.

Keller, F. S. and W. N. Schoenfeld. 1950. *Principles of Psychology*, Appleton-Century-Crofts, New York.

Laties, V. G. and B. Weiss. 1966. Influence of drugs on behavior controlled by internal and external stimuli. *J. Pharmacol. Exp. Ther.* 152: 388–396.

LoLordo, V. M. 1971. Facilitation of food-reinforced responding by a signal for response-independent food. *J. Exp. Anal. Behav.* 15: 49–55.

Masserman, J. H. 1946. *Principles of Dynamic Psychiatry.* Saunders, Philadelphia.

McKearney, J. W. 1968. Maintenance of responding under a fixed-interval schedule of electric shock presentation. *Science* 160: 1249–1251.

McKearney, J. W. 1969. Fixed-interval schedules of electric shock presentation: extinction and recovery of performance under different shock intensities and fixed-interval schedules. *J. Exp. Anal. Behav.* 12: 301–313.

McKearney, J. W. 1970. Responding under fixed ratio and multiple fixed-interval fixed-ratio schedules of electric shock presentation. *J. Exp. Anal. Behav.* 14: 1–6.

Meyer, K. E. and J. H. Korn. 1964. Effect of UCS intensity on the acquisition and extinction of an avoidance response. *J. Exp. Psychol.* 67: 352–359.

Meyer, D. R., C. Chungsoo and A. F. Wesemann. 1960. On problems of conditioning discriminated lever-press avoidance responses. *Psychol. Rev.* 67: 224–228.

Miczek, K. A. 1974. Intraspecies aggression in rats: effects of *d*-amphetamine and chlordiazepoxide. *Psychopharmacologia* 39: 275–301.

Miczek, K. A. and S. P. Grossman. 1971. Positive conditioned suppression: effects of CS duration. *J. Exp. Anal. Behav.* **15**: 243–247.

Moore, K. E. and R. H. Rech. 1967. Antagonism by monoamine oxidase inhibitors of α-methyltyrosine-induced catecholamine depletion and behavioral depression. *J. Pharmacol. Exp. Ther.* **156**: 70–75.

Morse, W. H., R. N. Mead and R. T. Kelleher. 1967. Modulation of elicited behavior by a fixed-interval schedule of electric shock presentation. *Science* **157**: 215–217.

Moyer, K. E. 1968. Kinds of aggression and their physiological basis. *Commun. Behav. Biol., Part A* **2**: 65–87.

Myers, A. K. 1962. Effects of CS intensity and quality in avoidance conditioning. *J. Comp. Physiol. Psychol.* **55**: 57–61.

Pavlov, I. P. 1927. *Conditioned Reflexes: An Investigation of the Physiological Activity of the Cerebral Cortex.* Oxford University Press, London.

Reese, E. P. 1964. *Experiments in Operant Behavior.* Appleton-Century-Crofts, New York.

Scheel-Krüger, J. 1971. Comparative studies of various amphetamine analogues demonstrating different interactions with the metabolism of the catecholamines in the brain. *Eur. J. Pharmacol.* **14**: 47–59.

Seiden, L. S., R. Schoenfeld and D. Domizi. 1969. A system for the recording and analysis of interresponse time data using an AM tape recorder and digital computers. *J. Exp. Anal. Behav.* **12**: 289–292.

Sidman, M. 1953a. Avoidance conditioning with brief shock and no exteroceptive warning signal. *Science* **118**: 157–158.

Sidman, M. 1953b. Two temporal parameters of the maintenance of avoidance behavior by the white rat. *J. Comp. Physiol. Psychol.* **46**: 253–261.

Sidman, M. 1962. Reduction of shock frequency as reinforcement for avoidance behavior. *J. Exp. Anal. Behav.* **5**: 247–257.

Sidman, M. 1956. Time discrimination and behavioral interaction in a free operant situation. *J. Comp. Physiol. Psychol.* **49**: 469–473.

Skinner, B. F. 1938. *The Behavior of Organisms.* Appleton-Century-Crofts, New York.

Snapper, A. G. and R. M. Kadden. 1973. Time-sharing in a small computer based on a behavioral notation system. *In* B. Weiss (ed.), *Digital Computers in the Behavioral Laboratory*. Appleton-Century-Crofts, New York, pp. 41–97.

Stein, L., M. Sidman and J. V. Brady. 1958. Some effects of two temporal variables on conditioned suppression. *J. Exp. Anal. Behav.* **1**: 153–162.

Tenen, S. S. 1967. The effects of *p*-chlorophenylalanine, a serotonin depletor, on avoidance acquisition, pain sensitivity and related behavior in the rat. *Psychopharmacologia* **10**: 204–219.

Terrace, H. S. 1966. Stimulus control. *In* W. K. Honig (ed.), *Operant Behavior: Areas of Research and Application*. Appleton-Century-Crofts, New York.

Wayner, M. J. 1974. Specificity of behavioral regulation. *Physiol. Behav.* **12**: 851–869.

Weiss, B. and V. G. Laties. 1964. Drug effects on the temporal patterning of behavior. *Fed. Proc.* **23**: 801–807.

Weiss, B. and V. G. Laties. 1958. Fractional escape and avoidance on a titration schedule. *Science* **128**: 1575–1576.

Weiss, B. (ed.). 1973. *Digital Computers in the Behavioral Laboratory*. Appleton-Century-Crofts, New York.

Woolfe, G. and A. D. Macdonald. 1944. The evaluation of the analgesic action of pethidine hydrochloride (Demerol). *J. Pharmacol. Exp. Ther.* **80**: 300–307.

2
Pharmacological and Biochemical Methods in Psychopharmacology

PHARMACOLOGICAL TECHNIQUES

In this chapter, we will review pharmacological and biochemical procedures which are used to examine mechanisms of action of behaviorally active drugs. The methods discussed are drawn primarily from the disciplines of pharmacology and biochemistry. Detailed information concerning these methods and procedures may be found in various textbooks (Goodman and Gilman, 1970; Goldstein *et al.*, 1974; also see below, Tables 2-2 and 2-3). The methods outlined below will help the reader understand the fundamental techniques and evaluate research discussed in the following chapters.

Drug Dosage

The effect of a drug on behavior is a function of several variables including the amount (i.e., the dose) of the drug administered. In determining the dose range of the drug, it must be realized that all drugs are toxic in sufficient doses, and high doses are often lethal. The psychopharmacologist has little interest in the lethal dose of a drug, but it must be taken into consideration in behavioral studies. Toxicity of a drug is usually expressed as the LD50; LD standing for lethal dose and the 50 indicating that the dose will kill 50% of a population of animals (Goldstein *et al.*, 1974). Generally, the LD50 of a drug is available prior to behavioral experiments. The ED50 is a statistic similar to the LD50, which is used to express the effectiveness of a drug (i.e., the effective dose 50). The ED50 is the dose which is effective in achieving a certain end point in 50% of the animals.

The effect of a drug in relationship to its dose can also be expressed in a dose-response function. In order to obtain a dose-response function, a wide range of drug doses is examined in order to span a dose range that reflects both minimum and maximum effects. In general, a dose-response curve is generated by plotting the dose of a drug on the abscissa and the response (i.e., drug effect) on the ordinate. When the dose-response function is plotted on an arithmetic basis, the shape of the function is sigmoidal and often has a low slope. Plotting the function with the drug doses on a logarithmic scale (base varies depending on the experimental procedures) often produces a linear dose-response function. The linear function obtained is amenable to statistical analysis, and, therefore, drug dosage is often varied logarithmically. An example of a behavioral dose response function is illustrated by the effect of various doses of amphetamine on the rate of responding maintained by an FI schedule of reinforcement. Low doses of amphetamine usually increase response rate, some intermediate doses may not affect rate, and high doses usually decrease the rate (i.e., the dose-response curve is an inverted U). Complex dose-response functions of this type are by no means atypical in psychopharmacology. The complex nature of the dose-response function emphasizes the importance of obtaining dose-response information over a broad range of doses, since generalities based on a single dose can be misleading.

In specifying the drug dose, it is important to know whether the quantity administered is expressed as a function of the *base* or of the *salt*. The *base* refers to the pharmacologically active component of the compound, whereas the salt usually refers to the base plus some inorganic salt (or ion) to which the base is ionically bound. In most cases the inorganic salt is pharmacologically inert. Drugs are most often administered as *salts* (i.e., base plus inorganic salt), since the salt form of the drug is usually much more soluble in aqueous media than the base. For example, amphetamine is always administered as an amphetamine salt (e.g., amphetamine sulfate). The salt is readily soluble in aqueous solutions, whereas amphetamine base is much less soluble. However, amphetamine rather than sulfate is the active compound. In order to determine the dose of amphetamine when it is given as a salt, the molecular weight (M.W.) of amphetamine alone and of the sulfate anion alone must be obtained. For example, the molecular weight of amphetamine alone is approximately 135 and the molecular weight of the sulfate anion is about 96. Since there are 2 (N) molecules of amphetamine to one molecule of sulfate, over 25% of the weight of amphetamine sulfate consists of the sulfate anion.

In order to determine the concentration of free base in a solution containing 1.0 mg/ml of amphetamine sulfate, the following calculations are carried out:

$$\frac{N \text{ (M. W. of Free Base)}}{N \text{ (M. W. of Free Base)} + \text{(M. W. of Inactive Ion)}} \text{(concentration of salt)}$$

$$= \frac{2\,(135)}{2\,(135) + 96} \times 1.0 \text{ mg amphetamine sulfate/ml} = 0.74 \text{ mg amphetamine/ml}$$

The type of salt must also be expressed (for example, sulfate, hydrochloride, bitartrate), because each salt has a different molecular weight.

Drug Administration

There are several routes by which a drug may be administered. We will confine our discussion to administration routes used experimentally in psychopharmacology with nonhumans; some of these routes are also applicable to human studies (for a thorough discussion of routes of administration in humans, see Goodman and Gilman, 1970; Goldstein *et al.*, 1974). The routes of administration most frequently used for animal studies include intraperitoneal (ip), intravenous (iv), subcutaneous (sc), intramuscular (im), oral (po, meaning per oral), intraventricular (ivt), intracerebral (ic) and intracisternal (ict). The relative advantages, disadvantages and special problems concerning each route of administration are discussed below. Several considerations are involved in choosing the administration route of a behaviorally active drug, including solubility in various liquids (commonly referred to as vehicles), ability to be absorbed by physiological systems (capillaries, gastrointestinal tract and mucous membranes), the extent and rate of metabolism, the extent and rate of uptake by organs (such as brain, liver, and muscle and fat) and duration of time over which the drug is tested.

Generally, drugs used in psychopharmacological research are nonpolar organic compounds which are relatively insoluble in aqueous vehicles. When a drug in the form of salt is soluble in an aqueous medium at a pH of 7 or close to neutrality (pH between 5.5 and 8.5), the vehicle most commonly used is physiological saline (0.9% sodium chloride in water), since its osmolarity is close to the osmolarity of blood plasma. Compounds in vehicles with an osmolarity or pH differing greatly from that of blood must be administered cautiously. Strongly acidic or basic injections may cause irritation, as evidenced by writhing and squealing of the animals, and this reaction may affect behavior under examination. In addition, injections of low or high pH solutions may change blood pH and lead to behavioral effects by changing the concentration of blood components such as oxygen or carbon dioxide. For both of these reasons, the pH of an administered solution must be taken into account (Goodman and Gilman, 1970).

Many nonpolar drugs are soluble in organic solvents such as ethanol (ethyl alcohol), glycerin or polyethylene glycol. Many organic solvents are toxic and therefore cannot be considered as vehicles for drug injection. Ethanol has the drawback of being a psychopharmacological agent itself, and therefore cannot be used as a vehicle. Frequently, nonpolar, water-insoluble compounds are administered as suspensions rather than solutions. Water and physiologic saline are not good suspension vehicles since insoluble drugs sediment rapidly in them. A viscous inert organic liquid may be combined with water as the suspension vehicle (polyethylene glycol, methyl cellulose and Tween-80). Special care must be exercised when a viscous liquid such as polyethylene glycol is used for the vehicle. These liquids generally have a high viscosity and must be injected with a large-bore needle which may produce puncture wounds, especially with repeated dosing. In addition, the rate of absorption of a drug in a viscous vehicle may be slower than that of a drug in an aqueous vehicle. As with aqueous solutions, consideration of pH and irritation caused by the suspension must be taken into account.

Routes of Administration

The route of administration depends in part upon the vehicle used to prepare the drug, and the solubility of the drug in that vehicle. Absorption, metabolism and excretion of the drug are other important considerations. Some drugs are completely inactivated by enzymes or acidity in the stomach and therefore cannot be administered orally. Others are metabolized by the liver; therefore, an administration route in which the drug passes through the liver before going to the heart and arterial blood supply would decrease its pharmacologic effect.

The existence of the "blood-brain barrier" is a special problem in psychopharmacology. A large number of compounds diffuse easily from the blood to the extra- and intracellular spaces of various organs but not to brain. In general, primary, secondary and tertiary amines penetrate the blood-brain barrier, whereas quaternary amines do not. For example, atropine sulfate, a teritary amine, diffuses readily from the blood to the brain. On the other hand, methylatropine, a quaternary amine, does not readily permeate the brain. There are several compounds which enter the brain readily, others moderately and some not at all, with a spectrum of relative permeabilities in between. The blood-brain barrier is not an absolute barrier. Its permeability to different compounds is determined to a great extent by the physical and chemical properties of a given drug (e.g., fat solubility, electric charge, etc.). Anatomically, this barrier is not uniform. Some compounds which generally do not enter the brain may penetrate regions of the brain with a particularly rich blood supply like certain parts of the hypothalamus (Zimmerman and George, 1974). In spite of the above qualifications, there is little doubt that many drugs and endogenous chemical compounds of interest to the experimental psychopharmacologist do not penetrate the brain to a significant degree. Thus, in order to introduce a drug into the brain, it may be necessary to administer the drug directly (intraventricular, intracerebral injections—see below) or to use a chemical precursor which does enter the brain (Lajtha and Ford, 1968; Myers, 1974).

Oral (po). Not all drugs can be administered orally. Some are converted to inactive compounds by enzymes or acids in the gastrointestinal tract. Drugs absorbed across the GI tract enter the hepatic circulation and pass through the liver before going to the heart and eventually the brain. Some drugs may be metabolically inactivated by liver enzymes. In humans, oral administration is a common route, but in animals it presents difficulties. A drug frequently tastes bitter, and animals generally will not ingest it unless it is combined with food to mask the taste. Spilling or partial ingestion make it difficult to deliver a specified dose. In addition, depending on the pH of the stomach and its contents, the degree and the time course of drug absorption by blood may vary. Inaccurate delivery can be alleviated by gastric intubation, in which a tube is inserted into the mouth, down the esophagus and into the stomach. This process can cause enough trauma to disrupt behavior, however. Oral administration of drugs mixed with food is a convenient method for sustaining drug levels over time if precise dosage is not crucial.

Intraperitoneal (ip). This is a frequently used route of drug administration in animal studies. The peritoneal cavity is bounded above by the diaphragm, and below by the bladder, and contains all the abdominal organs except the kidney. The peritoneal cavity is highly vascularized, and drugs are rapidly absorbed from it. Both suspensions and solutions can be injected, provided that their pH and the compounds they contain do not cause undue irritability in the peritoneal cavity. Since intraperitoneal injections entering the bloodstream pass through the liver before reaching the heart, metabolism in the liver may present problems. In addition, the needle tip may penetrate one of the structures contained in the peritoneal cavity. This hazard can be avoided by using a needle of the proper length, and withdrawing the plunger of the syringe before injection. If the needle is located correctly, the plunger will return to its original position. If the needle is in a vein or artery, blood will appear in the syringe; if it is in the bladder, urine will appear. If the needle is in the GI tract, one frequently notes bubbles of air. One of the advantages of ip injections, particularly in rodents, is that they can be done quickly and repeatedly without damaging effects.

Intravenous (iv). Unlike other routes of drug administration, there is little delay in absorption from tissues to bloodstream with the iv route. Moreover, drugs injected iv do not pass through the hepatic circulation first. Solutions reasonably similar in pH and osmolarity to blood (i.e., physiologic saline) are suitable for iv injections. However, suspensions or nonaqueous solutions present problems if injected into a vein. In small animals such as rodents, and to a lesser extent in larger animals such as monkeys, dogs and cats, it is difficult to inject intravenously while the animal is conscious. In rodents, superficial veins are small and collapse when punctured with a needle. In addition, small clots in the vein may form, making repeated injections difficult.

A catheter can be surgically implanted into a vein, provided patency of the catheter is maintained, and compounds can be injected iv on a routine basis. A surgically implanted catheter often requires elaborate restraints to prevent the animal from removing it. The tissue around the catheter eventually becomes infected and necrotic, and the catheter does not remain in place. In monkeys, catheters can remain in place for several months at a time, while in rats they usually remain in place for a matter of weeks (see Weeks, 1972, for further details). The chronically implanted catheter has been used for studying self-administration of drugs such as morphine and amphetamine (see Chapter 11).

Intramuscular (im). One of the main advantages of the im route is a relatively even absorption of the drug. Drugs injected by the im route are absorbed by capillaries in the muscle and go through the venous system to the heart. Unlike oral and ip administration, the drug does not go through the liver before reaching the heart. Most im injections are with aqueous or inert oil base solutions. Absorption tends to be slower than it is in other routes of administration, particularly with oil or other viscous solutions. Injections must be done with care, as it is possible to cause muscle injury. To minimize the extent of muscle trauma, im injection volumes should be small. Repeated injection by the im route is difficult, since even carefully performed injections cause some trauma, and daily injections produce cumulative muscle injury.

Subcutaneous (sc). The rate of absorption after subcutaneous administration varies with the site of injection, but is usually slow. The rate of absorption is similar to that after im administration. Aqueous solutions and oil vehicles are most frequently used. Oil vehicles may be quite viscous, even in the form of pellets, and provide long and sustained drug release into the bloodstream.

Intracerebral (ic). Intracerebral injections have been used to apply drugs to specific brain areas. Two techniques are used for introducing a drug directly into cerebral tissue. The first involves implanting a cannula into a specific brain region with the aid of a stereotaxic apparatus which gives the exact coordinates in the brain (Booth, 1968; Grossman, 1960). The cannula is fixed to the top of the skull and injections can be made into it periodically. This technique is used to study the effects of drugs at central nervous system (CNS) sites. Some investigators inject small quantities of crystalline chemicals through the cannula, while others inject aqueous solutions. Unfortunately, it is not possible to estimate dose when the compound is introduced in crystalline form. The concentrations are very high at the tip of the cannula and decrease as one moves away from the cannula tip. Moreover, effective concentrations of the drug may diffuse some distance from the cannula.

Furthermore, injection of crystals tends to produce lesions near the cannula tip. Injection of aqueous solutions reduces the extent of lesions, but it is difficult to assess the extent of diffusion. At first glance, the intracerebral injection technique would seem to be the method of choice for localizing the site of drug action, but in view of the above problems, this method must be approached with caution. Myers (1974) has given a detailed account of the methods and principles of, and the conclusions that can be drawn from, direct injections of chemicals into the brain.

The other intracerebral injection technique involves injecting drugs directly through the skull. Mice, rats and goldfish are usually used (Agranoff *et al.*, 1966; Glassman and Wilson, 1973; Flexner *et al.*, 1964). One must be particularly careful when making these injections, since a hand-held syringe is likely to produce brain damage. The problem of neural tissue destruction is not completely obviated by control injections, since it is uncertain whether the location and extent of the damage is the same for vehicle- and drug-treated animals.

Intraventricular (ivt). There are several methods for implanting cannulae into the lateral ventricles of rats, cats and monkeys (Hayden *et al.*, 1966). This technique cannot readily be used in animals smaller than the rat. Since the ventricular system in the rat is quite small (approximately 200 μl), exact location must be used to implant the cannula.

Intraventricular injections are done with aqueous solutions (generally an artificial cerebral spinal fluid or saline) (Lewy and Seiden, 1972). A cannula is placed in the ventricle and anchored to the skull so that it remains in place for months. The main problem with this procedure is in interpreting drug effects. Drugs injected into the ventricular system are mainly taken up by neuroanatomical structures surrounding the ventricles. Some drugs have different effects when given by the intraventricular route rather than systemically. On the other hand, drugs that ordinarily do not reach the CNS when administered systemically can be examined with this technique.

Intracisternal (ict). Intracisternal injections are used to introduce substances into the cerebrospinal fluid. The advantage of this technique is that no surgery is required. Animals are usually lightly anesthetized prior to the procedure, but it is not necessary to anesthetize them. A needle is inserted into the cisterna magna through the foramen magnum. The needle is inserted at the posterior margin of the foramen magnum and directed toward a point on the dorsal surface of the head (Schanberg *et al.*, 1967).

PHARMACOLOGICAL AND BIOCHEMICAL PRINCIPLES

Section II of this text (Chapters 3–8) deals with the biochemical basis of psychopharmacology. The primary objective of this section is to investigate interactions between drugs, behavior and biochemistry in brain. Drugs are chemicals and logically would be expected to exert their effects on CNS function by interacting with other chemicals in the central nervous system. The problem lies in determining which CNS chemicals a drug acts upon, and which of these chemicals is responsible for the drug effect.

Chemical Transmission

The notion of chemical transmission of a nerve impulse across a synapse is of
central importance to research in neurophysiology, neuropharmacology and
psychopharmacology. The basic phenomena are conceptually simple, but difficult to demonstrate experimentally. The following example illustrates the concept of synaptic transmission. Consider two neurons with the axon of one (A)
synapsing with the dendrite of another (B). When neuron A is stimulated, the
action potential propagates itself down the axon until it reaches the synapse
(Fig. 2-1). Neurophysiological and neurochemical research (see Eccles, 1964)
provides evidence that an action potential, on reaching the synapse, causes release of a chemical by neuron A. The area from which secretion occurs is called
the *presynaptic terminal*. The released chemical diffuses across the *synaptic
cleft* and causes permeability changes in B (the *postsynaptic membrane*), which
in turn may cause neuron B to fire. In summary, transmission across synapses requires the following sequence: nerve impulse—secretion of the transmitter—
altered permeability—nerve impulse.

We will be concerned with four different compounds believed to be chemical
transmitters in the central nervous system. These compounds are serotonin, norepinephrine, dopamine and acetylcholine. (See Table 2-1 for chemical structures.)
In Chapters 3-7, we will discuss the evidence that these compounds are transmitters in the peripheral and central nervous system, as well as the criteria a
compound must fulfill in order to be designated a transmitter. The evidence for
chemical transmission of the nerve impulse has been worked out in some detail,
and it is widely accepted that norephinephrine and acetycholine are transmitters
in the peripheral nervous system. Inferences concerning the nature of transmitter compounds in the central nervous system are extrapolated, at least in part,
from this function in the peripheral nervous system.

In spite of the fact that there is substantial evidence that these chemicals are
transmitters, all of the data required to prove their function in this role has not
been gathered; therefore, it has become traditional to refer to a central nervous
system transmitter as a *putative* transmitter. Although we will refer to them as
transmitters, the reader should be aware that serotonin, norepinephrine, dopamine and acetylcholine are considered to be putative transmitters. It should be
noted that other compounds are also considered to be putative transmitters;
these include glycine, histamine, phenylethylamine and various polypeptides.
Research into the neurochemistry, neuropharmacology and biochemistry of
acetylcholine, norepinephrine, dopamine and serotonin in relationship to behavioral function has been far more extensive than with any of the other putative transmitters; we will, therefore, confine our attention to these transmitters
in the following chapters (see Chapters 4, 5, 6 and 7).

Chapter 8 outlines the possible role of ribonucleic acid (RNA) and protein in

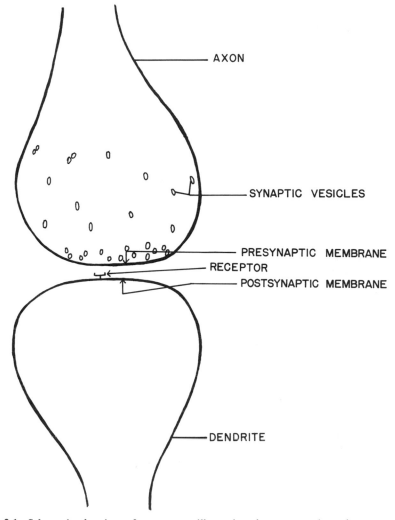

Fig. 2-1. Schematic drawing of a synapse illustrating the presynaptic and postsynaptic terminals. This is an axodendritic synapse. Axosomatic and axoaxonic synapses also exist in the central nervous system. The synaptic cleft is the area between the presynaptic and postsynaptic membranes. Transmitters are believed to be stored in synaptic vesicles, and following release into the synaptic cleft, they are thought to act on receptors.

CNS function related to behavior. These compounds exist in all cells but their special importance in brain function may lie in their ability to alter permanently the discharge patterns or permeability of nerve cells. It has been suggested that long-term changes in RNA and/or proteins in the CNS may be caused by experiences involved in learning and memory.

TABLE 2-1.   Chemical structures of some biogenic amines

DOPAMINE	
NOREPINEPHRINE	
EPINEPHRINE	
SEROTONIN	
ACETYLCHOLINE	

Terminology

Throughout the next five chapters, certain terms will be used repeatedly, and it will be of use to define the terms here.

Agonist   A drug or naturally occurring endogenous chemical (e.g., neurotransmitter) capable of combining with a receptor to initiate a response. The response may be initiation of a nerve impulse at the postsynaptic membrane.

Antagonist   A drug that tends to block or reverse the action of an agonist.

Biogenic amine	A naturally occurring amine (e.g., dopamine, norepinephrine, serotonin) which may serve as a synaptic transmitter in the CNS.
Cholinergic	A system of neurons which contain the compound acetylcholine and in which acetylcholine functions as a transmitter substance.
Dopaminergic	A system of neurons which contain dopamine and in which dopamine functions as a transmitter substance.
Noradrenergic	A system of neurons which contain the compound norepinephrine and in which norepinephrine functions as a transmitter. In some instances, the word *adrenergic* is used synonymously with noradrenergic.
Catecholaminergic	A general term referring to either dopaminergic and/or noradrenergic neurons.
Serotonergic	A system of neurons which contain the compound serotonin and in which serotonin functions as a transmitter substance.
Receptor	Reactive components in effector tissues such as muscle or nerves. These receptors when activated, result in physiological responses such as increased muscle contraction or increases or decreases in the rates of nerve discharge. The receptor may be activated chemically and is presumed to undergo conformational (i.e., structural) changes which initiate the subsequent physiological response. Example: norepinephrine can cause increased contraction of smooth muscle in blood vessels.

Drug-Chemical Interactions

One criterion for attributing the behavioral action of a drug to a brain biochemical system is measurement of chemical changes produced by the drug. Ideally, both behavioral measures and CNS biochemical measures are made in the same laboratory using the same strain of animal, a similar range of doses, the same pretreatment times and both cerebral and extracerebral tissue for chemical assay purposes. While this represents the ideal case, the chemical mechanism of action of a drug is often inferred from neurochemical studies which may involve different species of animals, doses and pretreatment times from those used in behavioral studies. Inferences concerning the biochemical mechanism of drug action are strengthened if a good correlation exists between the chemical and behavioral changes. However, while correlations between biochemical and behavioral data may exist, they do not prove the existence of a causal relationship between the observed behavioral and biochemical changes. It is a basic tenet of scientific reasoning that a correlation *does not* prove cause and effect. The tenuousness of correlative data is emphasized by the fact that a drug affects more than one and perhaps several different chemical systems. Since several systems can be affected by a particular drug, a prodigious amount of experimental work is required to determine which of these systems is best correlated with the drug's behavioral actions. While there is no foolproof experimental method to prove that an endogenous chemical system mediates a drug action, there are procedures that take into account the problems cited above and add weight to inferences concerning causal mechanisms.

Replacement Studies.   If the behavioral action of a drug is thought to be due to drug-induced depletion of one or more transmitters within the CNS, then the chemical(s) presumed to be depleted can be replaced. This approach is similar to the experimental approach used by endocrinologists over the past 20 years. If an endocrine gland is removed and the effects of its removal on a target organ can be reversed by either an extract or purified hormone obtained from the gland, evidence that the hormone secreted by the gland was essential for maintenance of normal function of the target organ is obtained.

Replacement of a transmitter is complicated, however, by the fact that most transmitters do not readily penetrate the blood-brain barrier. Therefore, the natural precursor of a transmitter, which is capable of entering the brain, is used for replacement. If replacing the drug-depleted chemical by administration of its precursor antagonizes the drug's behavioral effects, the chemical initially depleted may be responsible for the maintenance of the behavior. Moreover, it may be the chemical that mediates the drug effect. Specific examples of this approach will be given in Chapters 4, 5 and 7.

Replacement of a drug-depleted chemical requires certain considerations. Replacement should take place with doses close to the physiological range, i.e., final concentration should be in the order of 1–10 μg/g of tissue. If function can only be restored when the depleted transmitter is raised to a level much greater than its natural or physiological level, it is questionable whether it is acting as a physiological agent. The question of determining what constitutes the physiological range for a transmitter compound in the brain must be tempered by the fact that although it is possible to determine the normal level or content of a transmitter in the whole brain, or even in an anatomical section of brain, the level of transmitter at a synapse is difficult to measure. Since transmitters are concentrated in certain neurons and further concentrated at specific loci within synaptic endings, their levels are much higher at the synapse than in whole brain. In spite of the difficulties posed by these technical problems, the question is legitimate and should be considered, especially in light of new techniques as they are made available. Furthermore, it is important to distinguish between central and peripheral effects of the replaced transmitter, as well as to determine whether the administered chemical precursors themselves, independent of their products, have effects on the behavior in question.

Drug-Drug Interactions. Not all behaviorally active drugs are thought to act by depleting transmitter compounds. Some drugs are thought to interfere with receptors or enzymes or with other processes responsible for inactiviation of endogenous chemicals. Replacement of the neurochemical compound is not applicable to this situation, but there are other means to determine whether a drug affects behavior by receptor blockade or enzyme inhibition. One approach is to test a number of drugs having a similar mechanism at the biochemical level; if this biochemical mechanism is important to the behavior, these drugs should have similar behavioral effects. Another method is to examine compounds with chemical mechanisms of action opposite to the first drug. Such a drug would be expected to antagonize the behavioral effects of the first drug.

There is no single approach toward the problem of fully delineating a drug's biochemical mechanism of action. Many experiments, both behavioral, biochemical and pharmacological, are needed to provide evidence for biochemical mechanisms of drug action, as well as evidence for the role of endogenous CNS transmitters in the maintenance of behavior. The remainder of this chapter discusses biochemical assays used in the neurochemical side of this work. Detailed explanations of the methods are not reviewed here, but references are supplied (Tables 2-2 and 2-3).

TABLE 2-2. Methods of biochemical analysis commonly used in analytical neurochemistry

Thin-layer chromatography	Touchstone (1973); Niederwieser and Pataki (1970); Heftmann (1967); Stahl (1969); Fleming and Clark (1970)
Paper chromatography	Morris and Morris (1963); Heftmann (1967)
Column chromatography	Weinstein and Laurencott (1964); Morris and Morris (1963); Heftmann (1967); Kirchner (1967)
Gas chromatography	Schupp (1968); Kroman and Bender (1968)
Electrophoresis	Morris and Morris (1963); Whitaker (1967)
Centrifugation/ultracentrifugation	Wattiaux (1971); Trautman (1964); Appel *et al.* (1972)
Spectrophotometry	Newman (1964)
Spectrofluorometry	Udenfriend (1969); Guilbault (1973); White and Argauer (1970)
Radiochemistry	Manara (1971); Aronoff (1967)
Mass spectrometry	Hammar (1971); Hill (1966); Milne (1971); Waller (1972)
Theory, basic biochemistry, kinetics	Goldstein *et al.* (1974); Karlson (1965); Lehninger (1975)

TABLE 2-3.   Specific assay procedures

Catecholamine concentrations	Anton and Sayre (1964); Axelrod and Kopin (1961); Bertler *et al.* (1958, 1959); Carlsson and Waldeck (1958); Häggendal (1963, 1966); Shore and Olin (1958); Snyder *et al.* (1966); Nagatsu (1973); Neff *et al.* (1971)
Catecholamine turnover/changes in metabolism	Sedvall *et al.* (1968); Neff *et al.* (1969, 1971); Gordon *et al.* (1966); Spector *et al.* (1963, 1965); Costa and Neff (1966); Brodie *et al.* (1966)
Enzymes involved in catecholamine metabolism Tyrosine hydroxylase Dopamine decarboxylase Monoamine oxidase (MAO) Dopamine-beta-hydroxylase (DBH) O-methyl-transferase	D'Iorio (1961); Axelrod *et al.* (1959); Nagatsu (1973)
Serotonin and metabolites	Twarog (1961); DoAmaral (1973); Udenfriend and Weissbach (1963); Bogdanski *et al.* (1956); Udenfriend *et al.* (1958); Garattini and Valzelli (1965); Hanson (1966); Erspamer (1966); Hagen and Cohen (1966); Blaschko and Levine (1966)
Serotonin turnover	Tozer *et al.* (1966); Grahame-Smith (1973); Cheney *et al.* (1971); Shen *et al.* (1970); Lin *et al.* (1969); Neff *et al.* (1971)
Enzymes related to serotonin metabolism	Renson (1973); Lovenberg *et al.* (1962); Garattini and Valzelli (1965); Hagen and Cohen (1966); Blaschko and Levine (1966)
Acetylcholine and metabolites	Crossland (1961); Jenden *et al.* (1973); Hanin (1969, 1974); Reid *et al.* (1971)
Acetylcholine turnover	Jenden *et al.* (1974); Hanin (1974)
Enzymes involved in the metabolism of acetylcholine	Smallman (1961); Suszkiw (1973)
RNA concentrations and metabolism	Von Hungen *et al.* (1968); Rappoport *et al.* (1969); Hydén (1966); Koenig (1969)
Protein and protein metabolism	Schneider *et al.* (1973); Colewick and Kaplan (1962); Lowry *et al.* (1951); Lajtha (1970); Koenig (1969)
Enzyme kinetics	Liébecq (1971).

BIOCHEMICAL TECHNIQUES

In order to examine relationships between neurochemistry and behavior one must be able to measure the tissue contents of biogenic amines and macromolecules as well as alterations in activity of enzymes that regulate synthesis and degradation of biogenic amines.

General Considerations

The tissue content of a compound is defined as the quantity of that compound per unit weight of tissue. In the case of the biogenic amines, brain contents are low and are therefore expressed as micrograms per gram of tissue (i.e., $\mu g/g$) (one microgram is equal to 10^{-6} g), or nanograms per gram of tissue (ng/g) (one nanogram is equal to 10^{-9} g). The terms concentration or levels are used interchangeably to refer to the quantity of the transmitter per unit weight of brain. As we shall see in subsequent chapters, alterations in the content of a transmitter in the brain can lead to changes in brain function and behavior.

Alterations in function are also possible without changes in the transmitter content. In the latter case, the metabolism of the synthetic and degradative processes may be so altered as to cause an increase or decrease in transmitter availability, while the overall contents are unchanged. For example, consider the following set of reactions where B is the transmitter:

$$A \; \rightleftharpoons \; B \; \rightleftharpoons \; C$$

The rate of turnover of transmitter (B) with a level that is constant over time can be considered a combination of the rate of synthesis of the transmitter from a precursor (A) and rate of degradation to a metabolite (C). The turnover rate of B is often expressed as the time required to metabolize or synthesize one-half the amount of B ($T\frac{1}{2}$), assuming that content does not change with time. When synthesis and degradation proceed at equal rates, equilibrium (i.e., steady-state) is reached and the content of B does not change with time. Any change in the utilization of B will be reflected, not as an increase or decrease in the total content of B, but as a change in $T\frac{1}{2}$ (i.e., a change in the turnover of B). Changes in metabolism include changes in turnover. In the above example, there are only two pathways, synthesis and degradation. The compounds discussed in the following chapters present a more complex situation because there are multiple pathways, each of which must be taken into account when measuring turnover. For example:

$$
\begin{array}{c}
\overset{\displaystyle B \;(\text{storage})}{\Big\updownarrow} \\[4pt]
A \; \rightleftharpoons \; B \; \rightleftharpoons \; C \\[4pt]
\Big\updownarrow \\[2pt]
D
\end{array}
$$

In this situation, B exists in two forms, each of which can turn over at a different rate. A is the precursor of the transmitter B. C and D are both metabolites. B (storage) is a transmitter that is in a different subcellular fraction (or pool) than B. The turnover rates of B (storage) and B may be different. This complex situation holds for many compounds of interest to the neuro- and psycho-pharmacologists, but this complexity is difficult to deal with on both theoretical and experimental bases.

Variations have been reported in brain amine contents of animals due to species or strain differences, age, sex and environmental lighting and temperature. Certain compounds however, have been studied in a number of different laboratories and there is reasonably good agreement as to "normal" brain content. In addition, there are often enough data in the research literature to estimate the variability of an assay among laboratories. Different assay procedures often yield different estimates of endogenous chemicals. In evaluating neurochemical data, it is important to know the absolute content (μg/g) obtained in control animals in order to compare these with other values reported in the literature. For example, the absolute content of norepinephrine in rat brain is reported to be around 0.4 μg/g of brain in normal adult rats. An experiment reporting a value of 0.2 μg/g would not be consistent with the literature, and the author(s) should recognize this discrepancy and attempt to explain it. Research reports that describe data as a percent of control values without reporting the absolute value or the control are unsatisfactory because there is no way to determine whether the assay values are consistent with values reported by other investigators.

The Assay Technique

The purpose of an assay is to determine content of a neurochemical or amount of an enzyme in brain. Even for the relatively low number of compounds and enzymes of primary interest, there are a large variety of assay techniques and a detailed account of precise methods would go far beyond the scope of this chapter (see Table 2-3). Many of the technical methods used are complicated in execution as well as theoretical foundation. Research reports describing basic techniques are generally not complete enough to allow an inexperienced chemist to carry them out successfully. It may be necessary for investigators to work in a laboratory where a technique is in use in order to learn the detailed manipulations necessary for proper assay of these chemicals.

The technical methods for determining contents and/or turnover rates of chemicals in the brain involve many steps using analytical chemistry. Animals are first killed, and the brain is removed. Once the experimental animal has been killed and the brain removed, there are three phases of the assay: (1) isolation; (2) identification; (3) quantification of the compound.

Depending upon the compound analyzed (dopamine, norepinephrine, etc.), analytical procedures differ in detail; but the general procedures are the same. Specific analytical techniques for a particular substance will not be included, but references are listed in Tables 2-2 and 2-3. The references in Table 2-2 are examples of common methods.

Isolation. The first step in an assay is to extract the compound(s) and to isolate them in a purified or partially purified form so as to remove compounds that interfere with either identification or quantification. The first step of the isolation procedure requires homogenization of the brain in a solvent. Further isolation can be achieved by a number of methods:

A. Solvent extraction: Certain chemicals are more soluble in one solvent than in another. The compound of interest can be separated by use of different solvents.

B. Column chromatography: In this procedure, materials having an affinity for binding certain chemicals are used. Different compounds attach to complexes in the column with greater or lesser affinity and can be removed with different solvents. In many cases, the solvent determines which compound is removed from the column. This procedure has high resolution and is used to separate different chemical compounds which may have similar chemical structures.

C. Ultracentrifugation: In viscous media, insoluble compounds sediment at a rate proportional to their density. This procedure is used for separating proteins, RNA and subcellular organelles.

D. Gas chromatography: In gas chromatography, a liquid is volatilized to a gas, and the various constituents of the gas can be separated on a column. The gas chromatographic procedure has been used to estimate the quantity of compounds in extremely low concentrations (10^{-15} M).

E. Electrophoresis: Charged compounds placed in an electric field will migrate toward opposite poles. The speed and the direction of their migration are functions of their net charge. Electrophoresis is particularly useful for isolating various species of ribonucleic acid or protein.

Identification. The procedure most frequently used for identification of compounds of low molecular weight involves comparing the behavior of the unknown compound with the behavior of a compound of known structure (i.e., a standard). If the compound shows properties identical to those of the standard in several test systems, then the compound being assayed is assumed to be the same as the standard. The most frequently used techniques are:

A. Thin-layer chromatography
B. Paper chromatography
C. Spectrophotometry
D. Spectrofluorometry

Quantification. Once a compound has been separated from other constituents of the extract that might interfere with its identification, the amount present may be determined in several ways. Some of the techniques are listed on the following page.

    A. Spectrophotometry
    B. Spectrofluorometry
    C. Mass spectrometry
    D. Bioassay

The first three techniques are useful for both quantification and identification. Each depends on measuring some physical-chemical aspect of the compound such as absorption of light at certain wavelengths (spectrophotometry). Bioassay techniques, on the other hand, apply compounds to an *in vitro* tissue preparation and measure a physiological reaction (i.e., contraction of muscle suspended in nutrient media). Bioassay is more sensitive (i.e., it will detect lower concentrations of a compound) than either of the photometric methods, but is very slow and laborious because the preparation used in the assay is not stable in terms of its responses. Mass spectrographic techniques used in more recent neurochemical investigations are very sensitive, but instrumentation is expensive.

The Turnover Technique

Estimates of the rate at which a compound is synthesized and degraded or otherwise utilized in a system are a measure of its turnover rate. Estimation of turnover makes certain assumptions about the number of forms in which a compound may exist and the number of synthetic and degradative pathways operative in maintaining its level at a steady state. Estimation of turnover rate is frequently used as an indicator of the physiological activity of a compound. The level of the compound may remain constant, but its turnover rate may change. The change in turnover rate may indicate a change in the activity of the compound. There are two approaches to turnover measurement: (1) the isotopic technique and (2) the enzyme inhibition technique.

Isotopic Techniques. Radioactive isotopes, such as tritium (^{3}H) and carbon (^{14}C), are useful for measuring biochemical functions, both *in vivo* and *in vitro*.* These isotopes are biologically indistinguishable from naturally occurring, nonradioactive hydrogen and carbon; however, their presence in a tissue extract is detectable. It is possible to incorporate one of these labeled atoms into the structure of an endogenous compound and follow its metabolism over time. The labeled compound is introduced into the brain via the intraventricular or the intracisternal route of administration, or, if the compound readily passes the blood-brain barrier, it can be administered systemically. Turnover measures are obtained by killing the animal and assaying the brain tissue.

    Liquid scintillation counting is most frequently used to detect radioactively tagged (or labeled) substances. Counting techniques are extremely sensitive, and

---

In vivo refers to processes occurring within the living organism as distinguished from those biological events that can occur outside the living organism (i.e., *in vitro*).

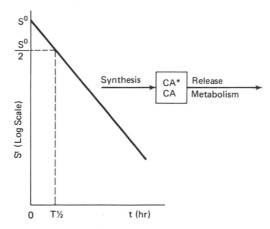

Fig. 2-2. Estimation of the turnover rate of a catecholamine (CA) by the isotopic method. (From Nagatsu, 1973.)

If [CA] = the amount of CA in the CA pool (pool size)
[CA*] = the amount of labeled CA

$$S^t = \text{the specific activity of CA at time } t = \frac{CA^*}{CA}$$

S^0 = the specific activity of CA at zero time
$T_{1/2}$ = half-life (the time in which specific activity of CA is halved)
k = rate constant (the percentage of the CA pool that is renewed per unit of time)

then $S^t = S^0 e^{-kt}$

log $S^t = \log S^0 - 0.4343\, kt$

$$k = \frac{\log S^0 - \log S^t}{0.4343\, t} = \frac{1}{1.44\, T_{1/2}}$$

Turnover rate = $k \cdot [CA]$

only small amounts of labeled compound need be introduced into a biological system for detection. Usually, the amount of labeled compound is less than one percent of the total quantity of endogenous compound. This small amount is called a *tracer dose*.

Figure 2-2 describes turnover calculations: a precursor substrate is converted to a catecholamine (CA), which is then metabolized to an inactive metabolite. Under ideal circumstances, labeled CA (CA*) is introduced into the system. The time of injection is considered zero time, and we assume that CA* mixes rapidly with the endogenous CA pool. The specific activity of a compound is the fraction of total compound (radioactive plus nonradioactive) that is radioactive. Thus, at zero time, the specific activity of CA is

$$\frac{CA^*}{CA + CA^*}$$

Since the labeled catecholamine is less than one percent of the endogenous amine, the denominator essentially represents endogenous amine. Radioactivity in the numerator is most commonly expressed as disintegrations per minute (DPM), and the endogenous catecholamine level is expressed as either micrograms or micromoles.

The radioisotope labeling process is as follows. Labeled CA is introduced, and at zero time equilibrates with the endogenous pool. Synthesis and destruction of CA continue as usual, and labeled CA is destroyed at the same rate as endogenous CA. Since destroyed CA is replaced with "cold" (nonlabeled) CA, the denominator of the specific activity expression $(CA^* + CA)$ remains constant under steady-state conditions. However, the numerator (CA^*) becomes smaller because additional labeled CA is not synthesized or added; therefore, specific activity (S) declines. The decline in specific activity is thus a measure of the percentage of CA that is used and replaced per unit time. By following the decline in specific activity after pulse labeling (i.e., quickly administering the labeled compound to obtain rapid mixing), one can obtain a biological half-life $(T_{1/2})$ as well as rate constant (k) for catecholamine synthesis under steady-state conditions. The steady-state condition may be altered by injecting a quantity of labeled CA large enough to increase significantly the quantity of brain CA. In such a case, k_1 may temporarily decrease. (For more information, see Goldstein et al., 1974; Westley, 1969; Nagatsu, 1973.)

As previously stated, this method involves many assumptions, some of which may not hold. It has however, been used to estimate turnover and changes in catecholamine biochemistry induced by drugs or other variables. Other isotopic techniques using labeled precursor have also been used; their advantages and disadvantages have been described by Nagatsu (1973).

Enzyme Inhibition Techniques. Several drugs inhibit enzymes involved in synthesis or degradation of some endogenous chemicals. Many investigators have studied the effects of these enzyme inhibitors on behavior, and have attempted to correlate drug-induced enzyme inhibition with behavioral changes. An enzyme inhibitor can block either synthesis or destruction of a compound. Consider:

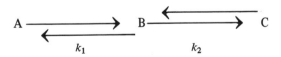

where k_1 and k_2 are rate constants indicating the rate at which A is converted to B and B to C, respectively. If enzymatic conversion of A to B is blocked, k_2 may be estimated by measuring the decline of B over time, assuming that k_2 does not change as a result of inhibiting conversion of A to B. Information concerning the use of various enzyme inhibitors for estimating turnover may be found by consulting Table 2-3. Enzyme activity is generally determined *in vitro* and expressed as amount of substrate converted/weight of tissue/unit time. This measures the velocity of reaction.

A basic consideration in determining enzyme activity is the law of mass action, which for enzymes assayed *in vitro* is best handled with Michaelis-Menton kinetics (see Westley, 1969). Michaelis-Menton kinetics is a set of mathematical formulae relating the rate of enzymatic catalysis to the amount of substrate present, assuming that the amount of enzyme remains constant. The velocity of the reaction increases asymptotically with the increase in substrate concentration (see Fig. 2-3).

The essential hypothesis underlying the kinetics of enzyme action is that the enzyme binds the substrate:

Enzyme (E) + Substrate (S) $\longrightarrow$ Enzyme-Substrate $\longrightarrow$ E + Product (P)

or:

$$E + S \longrightarrow (ES) \longrightarrow E + P$$

Applying the mass action law,

$$K = \frac{(S)\,(E)}{(ES)},$$

where (E), (S) and (ES) denote the content of enzyme, substrate and the enzyme-substrate complex, respectively $^\circ$K is the rate of the reaction. At the maximum velocity (V_{max}), the concentration of enzyme is rate-limiting (i.e., the

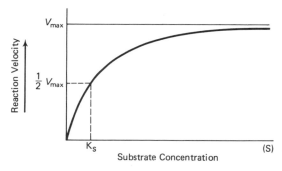

Fig. 2-3. Dependency of reaction rate on substrate concentration (at constant enzyme concentration). (S) is the substrate concentration. V is the reaction velocity at any given (S). V is expressed in moles of substrate reacted per unit weight of enzyme or tissue per unit of time. K_s (the Michaelis-Menton constant) is the substrate concentration at half the maximum velocity ($\frac{1}{2} V_{max}$). (From Nagatsu, 1973.)

enzyme limits the velocity at which the reaction can occur), and substrate is in excess. The quantity K_m is the substrate concentration at one-half maximum velocity. It can be seen from Fig. 2-3 that varying the substrate concentration around K_s (K_s approximately equals K_m) causes a change in the reaction velocity. Therefore, substrate concentration is rate-limiting. The major point of practical importance in Michaelis-Menton kinetics is that a range of concentrations of substrate is crucial in determining enzyme activity. A single substrate concentration will not adequately characterize the activity of an enzyme. Rather, enzyme activity is best determined by using several substrate concentrations from which a K_m may be derived.

In various chapters of Section II, we will consider enzyme activity in the presence of enzyme-inhibiting drugs. Enzymatic activity *in vitro* is often expressed as a percentage of control enzyme activity. Under most circumstances these assays are carried out with substrate concentrations that yield the maximum velocity; however, it is important in analyzing the literature to be aware of whether or not this has been done.

There are two types of enzyme inhibitors, competitive and noncompetitive. The competitive inhibitor competes with substrate for the active site of the enzyme, so that the relative amounts of substrate and inhibitor determine enzyme activity. With a noncompetitive inhibitor, however, the degree of inhibition is determined by the amount of inhibitor, regardless of the amount of substrate. Theory and practical techniques of distinguishing competitive from noncompetitive inhibition can be found in Westley (1969) and Lehninger (1975).

Methods for isolating and partially purifying enzymes and assaying their activity can be found in literature cited in Table 2-3. Extraction of active enzymes differs considerably from substrate extraction. It is desirable to extract the enzyme in a medium that will not destroy enzyme activity; however, substrate extraction is improved by inactivation of enzymes which normally degrade the substrate.

Incorporation Techniques

In Chapter 8, we will discuss the incorporation of radioactive amino acids into protein and the incorporation of labeled bases into RNA. The basic methodology, as in turnover studies and concentration measurements, involves separation, identification and quantification as described above.

Other Disciplines of Importance

Neuroanatomy. Even the most cursory examination of the anatomical structure of the CNS goes beyond the scope of this book. However, knowledge of brain structure is important in dealing with brain function. The student is urged to consult a text on neuroanatomy for an overview of brain structure (see Truex and Carpenter, 1969; Matzke and Foltz, 1972).

Histochemistry. This technique is at the interface of several disciplines: anatomy, biochemistry, histology and pharmacology. Histochemistry is important for localization of drugs and endogenous biochemicals in the CNS. The techniques of freeze-dried autoradiography (Roth, 1971) and fluorescence histochemistry (Falck *et al*., 1962) have been invaluable tools for the cellular localization and gross anatomical distribution of compounds.

SUMMARY

In this chapter we have tried briefly to outline some biological and physiological techniques useful in determining behavioral and biochemical mechanisms of drug action. As we have seen, these techniques draw on many disciplines including chemistry, biochemistry, enzymology, physical chemistry, physics and mathematics. Although expertise in all these fields is not necessary for understanding this book, background in the material is useful. This chapter should supply the knowledge necessary for understanding what follows, but the student is encouraged to explore these matters further. It does provide source material to which the student may refer when more information is desired.

REFERENCES

Agranoff, B. W., R. E. Davis and J. J. Brink. 1966. Chemical studies on memory fixation in goldfish. *Brain Res.* **1**: 303–309.

Anton, A. H. and D. F. Sayre. 1964. The distribution of dopamine and dopa in various animals and a method for their determination in diverse biological material. *J. Pharmacol. Exp. Ther.* **145**: 326–336.

Appel, S. H., E. D. Day and D. D. Mickey. 1972. Cellular and subcellular fractionation. *In* R. W. Albers, G. J. Siegel, R. Katzman and B. W. Agranoff (eds.), *Basic Neurochemistry*. Little, Brown and Co., Boston, pp. 425–448.

Aronoff, S. 1967. *Techniques of Radiobiochemistry*. Hafner Publishing Co., New York.

Axelrod, J., W. Albers and C. D. Clemente. 1959. Distribution of catechol-O-methyl transferase in the nervous system and other tissues. *J. Neurochem.* **5**: 68–72.

Axelrod, J. and I. J. Kopin. 1961. Estimation of O-methylated metabolites of catecholamines. *In* J. H. Quastel (ed.), *Methods in Medical Research* **9**: 153–158. Year Book Medical Publishers, Inc., Chicago.

Bertler, A., A. Carlsson and E. Rosengren. 1958. A method for the fluorimetric determination of adrenaline and noradrenaline in tissues. *Acta Physiol. Scand.* **44**: 273–292.

Bertler, A., A. Carlsson and E. Rosengren. 1959. Fluorimetric method for differential estimation of the 3-O-methylated derivatives of adrenaline and noradrenaline (metanephrine and norametanephrine). *Clin. Chim. Acta* **4**: 456–457.

Blaschko, H. and W. G. Levine. 1966. Metabolism of indolealkylamines. *In* V. Erspamer (ed.), *Handbook of Experimental Pharmacology* **19**: 212–244. Springer-Verlag, New York.

Bogdanski, D. F., A. Pletscher, B. B. Brodie and S. Udenfriend. 1956. Identification and assay of serotonin in brain. *J. Pharmacol. Exp. Ther.* **117**: 82–88.

Booth, D. A. 1968. Mechanism of action of norepinephrine in eliciting an eating response on injection into the rat hypothalamus. *J. Pharmacol. Exp. Ther.* **160**: 336–348.

Brodie, B. B., E. Costa, A. Dlabac, N. H. Neff and H. H. Smookler. 1966. Application of steady state kinetics to the estimation of synthesis rate and turnover time of tissue catecholamines. *J. Pharmacol. Exp. Ther.* **154**: 493–498.

Carlsson, A. and B. Waldeck. 1958. A fluorimetric method for the determination of dopamine (3-hydroxytyramine). *Acta Physiol. Scand.* **44**: 293–298.

Cheney, D. L., A. Goldstein, S. Algeri and E. Costa. 1971. Narcotic tolerance and dependence: lack of relationship with serotonin turnover in the brain. *Science* **171**: 1169–1170.

Colewick, S. P. and N. O. Kaplan (eds.). 1962. *Methods in Enzymology* 5. Academic Press, New York.

Costa, E. and N. E. Neff. 1966. Isotopic and non-isotopic measurements of the rate of catecholamine biosynthesis. *In* E. Costa, L. Côté and M. D. Yahr (eds.), *Biochemistry and Pharmacology of the Basal Ganglia*. Raven Press, New York, pp. 141–156.

Crossland, J. 1961. Biologic estimation of acetylcholine. *In* J. H. Quastel (ed.), *Methods in Medical Research* 9: 125–129. Year Book Medical Publishers, Inc., Chicago.

DoAmaral, J. 1973. An approach to the assay of serotonin using gas-liquid chromatography and mass fragmentography–the pineal gland as a model system. *In* J. Barchas and E. Usdin (eds.), *Serotonin and Behavior*. Academic Press, New York, pp. 201–207.

D'Iorio, A. 1961. Method for measurement of O-methyl-transferase activity. *In* J. H. Quastel (ed.), *Methods in Medical Research* 9: 208–209. Year Book Medical Publishers, Inc., Chicago.

Eccles, J. C. 1964. *The Physiology of Synapses*. Springer, New York.

Erspamer, V. 1966. Bioassay of indolealkylamines. *In* V. Erspamer (ed.), *Handbook of Experimental Pharmacology* 19: 113–131. Springer-Verlag, New York.

Falck, B., N. A. Hillarp, G. Thieme and A. Torp. 1962. Fluorescence of catecholamines and related compounds condensed with formaldehyde. *J. Histochem. Cytochem.* **10**: 348–354.

Fleming, R. M. and W. G. Clark. 1970. Quantitative thin-layer chromatographic estimation of labeled dopamine and norepinephrine, their precursors and metabolites. *J. Chromatog.* **52**: 305–312.

Flexner, L. B., J. B. Flexner, R. B. Roberts and G. de la Haba. 1964. Loss of recent memory in mice as related to regional inhibition of cerebral protein synthesis. *Proc. Nat. Acad. Sci.* **52**: 1165–1169.

Garattini, S. and L. Valzelli. 1965. *Serotonin*. Elsevier Publishing Co., New York.

Glassman, E. and J. E. Wilson. 1973. RNA and brain function. *In* G. B. Ansell and P. B. Bradley (eds.), *Macromolecules and Behavior*. University Park Press, Baltimore, pp. 81–92.

Goldstein, A., L. Aronow and S. M. Kalman. 1974. *Principles of Drug Action*. John Wiley & Sons, New York.

Goodman, L. S. and A. Gilman. 1970. *The Pharmacological Basis of Therapeutics*. Macmillan, New York.

Gordon, R., J. V. O. Reid, A. Sjoerdsma and S. Udenfriend. 1966. Increased synthesis of norepinephrine in the rat heart on electrical stimulation of the stellate ganglia. *Mol. Pharmacol.* **2**: 610–613.

Grahame-Smith, D. G. 1973. Does the total turnover of brain 5-HT reflect the functional activity of 5-HT in brain? *In* J. Barchas and E. Usdin (eds.), *Serotonin and Behavior*. Academic Press, New York.

Grossman, S. P. 1960. Eating or drinking elicited by direct adrenergic or cholinergic stimulation of hypothalamus. *Science* 132: 301–302.

Guilbault, G. G. (with contributions by R. F. Chen, G. Govindjee, G. Papageorgiou, E. Rabinowitch, E. L. Wehry). 1973. *Practical Fluorescence: Theory, Methods and Techniques*. Marcel Dekker, Inc., New York.

Hagen, P. B. and L. H. Cohen. 1966. Biosynthesis of indolealkylamines. Physiological release and transport of 5-hydroxytryptamine. *In* V. Erspamer (ed.), *Handbook of Experimental Pharmacology* 19: 182–211. Springer-Verlag, New York.

Häggendal, J. 1963. An improved method for fluorimetric determination of small amounts of adrenaline and noradrenaline in plasma and tissues. *Acta Physiol. Scand.* 59: 242–254.

Häggendal, J. 1966. Newer developments in catecholamine assay. *Pharmacol. Rev.* 18: 325–329.

Hammar, C. G. 1971. Mass spectrometry. *In* Z. M. Bacq, R. Capek, R. Paoletti and J. Renson (eds.), *Fundamentals of Biochemical Pharmacology*. Pergamon Press, New York, pp. 21–28.

Hanin, I. 1969. A specific gas chromatographic method for assaying tissue acetylcholine: present status. *Advances in Biochemical Psychopharmacology* 1: 111–130.

Hanin, I. (ed.). 1974. *Choline and Acetylcholine: Handbook of Chemical Assay Methods*. Raven Press, New York.

Hanson, A. 1966. Chemical analysis of indolealkylamines and related compounds. *In* V. Erspamer (ed.), *Handbook of Experimental Pharmacology* 19: 66–112. Springer-Verlag, New York.

Hayden, J. F., L. R. Johnson and R. P. Maickel. 1966. Construction and implantation of a permanent cannula for making injections into the lateral ventricle of the rat brain. *Life Sci.* 5: 1509–1515.

Heftmann, E. 1967. *Chromatography* (2nd edition). Van Nostrand Reinhold Co., New York.

Hill, H. C. 1966. *Introduction to Mass Spectrometry*. Heyden and Son, London.

Hydén, H. 1966. Production of RNA in neurons and glia in Parkinson's disease indicating genic stimulation. *In* E. Costa, L. J. Côté and M. D. Yahr (eds.), *Biochemistry and Pharmacology of the Basal Ganglia*. Raven Press, New York, pp. 195–204.

Jenden, D. J., L. Choi, R. W. Silverman, J. A. Steinborn, M. Roch and R. A. Booth. 1974. Acetylcholine turnover estimation in brain by gas chromatography/mass spectrometry. *Life Sci.* 14: 55–63.

Jenden, D. J., M. Roch and R. A. Booth. 1973. Simultaneous measurement of endogenous and deuterium-labeled tracer variants of choline and acetylcholine in subpicomole quantities by gas chromatography/mass spectrometry. *Anal. Biochem.* 55: 438–448.

Karlson, P. 1965. *Introduction to Modern Biochemistry*. Academic Press, New York.

Kirchner, J. G. 1967. *Thin-layer Chromatography Technique of Organic Chemistry* XII, Perry, E. S. and A. Weissberger, eds. Interscience publishers, Div. of John Wiley and Sons, New York.

Koenig, E. 1969. Nucleic acid and protein metabolism of the axon. *In* A. Lajtha (ed.), *Handbook of Neurochemistry* 2: 423–434, Plenum Press, New York.

Kroman, H. S. and S. R. Bender (eds.) 1968. *Theory and Application of Gas Chromatography in Industry and Medicine*. Grune & Stratton, New York and London.

Lajtha, A. (ed.). 1970. *Protein Metabolism of the Nervous System*. Plenum Press, New York.

Lajtha, A. and D. H. Ford (eds.). 1968. *Brain Barrier Systems*. Elsevier Publishing Co., New York.

Lehninger, A. L. 1975. *Biochemistry: The Molecular Basis of Cell Structure and Function*. Worth Publishers, New York.

Lewy, A. J. and L. S. Seiden. 1972. Operant behavior changes norepinephrine metabolism in rat brain. *Science* 175: 454–456.

Liébecq, Cl. 1971. Introduction to enzyme kinetics. *In* Z. M. Bacq, R. Capek, R. Paoletti and J. Renson (eds.), *Fundamentals of Biochemical Pharmacology*. Pergamon Press, New York, pp. 59–86.

Lin, R. C., E. Costa, N. H. Neff, C. T. Wang and S. H. Ngai. 1969. *In vivo* measurements of 5-hydroxytryptamine turnover rate in the rat brain from the conversion of C^{14}-tryptophan to C^{14}-5-hydroxytryptamine. *J. Pharmacol. Exp. Ther.* 170: 232–238.

Lovenberg, W., H. Weissbach and S. Udenfriend. 1962. Aromatic L-amino acid decarboxylase. *J. Biol. Chem.* 237: 89–93.

Lowry, O. H., N. J. Rosebrough, A. L. Farr and R. J. Randall. 1951. Protein measurement with the folin phenol reagent. *J. Biol. Chem.* 193: 265–275.

Manara, L. 1971. Isotopic methods and activation analysis. *In* Z. M. Bacq, R. Capek, R. Paoletti and J. Renson (eds.), *Fundamentals of Biochemical Pharmacology*. Pergamon Press, New York, pp. 29–34.

Matzke, H. A. and F. M. Foltz. 1972. *Synopsis of Neuroanatomy.* Oxford University Press, New York.

Milne, G. W. (ed.). 1971. *Mass Spectrometry: Techniques and Applications*, John Wiley, New York.

Morris, C. J. O. R. and P. Morris. 1963. *Separation Methods in Biochemistry*. Interscience Publishers, New York.

Myers, R. D. 1974. *Handbook of Drug and Chemical Stimulation of the Brain*, Van Nostrand Reinhold Co., New York.

Nagatsu, T. 1973. *Biochemistry of Catecholamines*. University Park Press, Baltimore.

Neff, N. H., S. H. Ngai, C. T. Wang and E. Costa. 1969. Calculation of the rate of catecholamine synthesis from the rate of conversion of tyrosine-^{14}C to catecholamines. Effect of adrenal demedulation on synthesis rates. *Mol. Pharmacol.* 5: 90–99.

Neff, N. H., P. F. Spano, A. Groppetti, C. T. Wang and E. Costa. 1971. A simple procedure for calculating the synthesis rate of norepinephrine, dopamine and serotonin in rat brain. *J. Pharmacol. Exp. Ther.* 176: 701–710.

Newman, D. W. 1964. Ultraviolet and visible absorption spectroscopy. *In* D. W. Newman (ed.), *Instrumental Methods of Experimental Biology*. Macmillan, New York, pp. 324–359.

Niederwieser, A. and G. Pataki. 1970. *Progress in Thin-layer Chromatography and Related Methods*, Vol. I. Humphrey Science Publishers, Inc., Ann Arbor, Michigan.

Rappoport, D. A., R. R. Fritz and J. L. Myers. 1969. Nucleic acids. *In* A. Lajtha (ed.), *Handbook of Neurochemistry* 1: 101–119, Plenum Press, New York.

Reid, W. D., D. R. Haubrich and G. Krishna. 1971. Enzymic radioassay for acetylcholine and choline in brain. *Anal. Biochem.* 42: 390–397.

Renson, J. 1973. Assays and properties of tryptophan 5-hydroxylase. *In* J. Barchas and E. Usdin (eds.), *Serotonin and Behavior*. Academic Press, New York, pp. 19–32.

Roth, L. J. 1971. The use of autoradiography in experimental pharmacology. *In* B. B. Brodie and J. R. Gillette (eds.), *Handbook of Experimental Pharmacology* 28: 286–316. Springer-Verlag, New York.

Schanberg, S. M., J. J. Schildkraut and I. J. Kopin. 1967. The effects of pentobarbital on the fate of intracisternally administered norepinephrine-H^3. *J. Pharmacol. Exp. Ther.* 157: 311–318.

Schneider, D. J., R. H. Angeletti, R. A. Bradshaw, A. Grasso and B. W. Moore (eds.). 1973. *Proteins of the Nervous System*. Raven Press, New York.

Schupp, O. E., III. 1968. *Gas Chromatography Technique of Organic Chemistry*, **XIII**, Perry, E. S. and A. Weissberger, eds. Interscience Publishers, Div. of John Wiley and Sons, New York.

Sedvall, G. C., V. K. Weise and I. J. Kopin. 1968. The rate of norepinephrine synthesis measured *in vivo* during short intervals: influence of adrenergic nerve impulse activity. *J. Pharmacol. Exp. Ther.* **159**: 274–282.

Shen, F., H. H. Loh and E. L. Way. 1970. Brain serotonin turnover in morphine tolerant and dependent mice. *J. Pharmacol. Exp. Ther.* **175**: 427–434.

Shore, P. A. and J. S. Olin. 1958. Identification and chemical assay of norepinephrine in brain and other tissues. *J. Pharmacol. Exp. Ther.* **122**: 295–300.

Smallman, B. N. 1961. Determination of choline acetylase activity. *In* J. H. Quastel (ed.), *Methods in Medical Research* **9**: 203–207. Year Book Medical Publishers, Inc., Chicago.

Snyder, S. H., R. J. Baldessarini and J. Axelrod. 1966. A sensitive and specific enzymatic isotopic assay for tissue histamine. *J. Pharmacol. Exp. Ther.* **153**: 544–549.

Spector, S., A. Sjoerdsma and S. Udenfriend. 1965. Blockade of endogenous norepinephrine synthesis by alpha-methyl-tyrosine, an inhibitor of tyrosine hydroxylase. *J. Pharmacol. Exp. Ther.* **147**: 86–95.

Spector, S., A. Sjoerdsma, P. Zaltman-Nirenberg, M. Levitt and S. Udenfriend. 1963. Norepinephrine synthesis from tyrosine-C^{14} in isolated perfused guinea pig heart. *Science* **139**: 1299–1301.

Stahl, E. (ed.). 1969. *Thin-layer Chromatography, A Laboratory Handbook* (2nd edition). Springer-Verlag, New York.

Suszkiw, J. B. 1973. Quantitation of acetylcholinesterase and acetylcholine-binding sites in excitable membrane fragments from electric eel. *Biochim. Biophys. Acta* **318**: 69–77.

Touchstone, J. C. (ed.). 1973. *Quantitative Thin Layer Chromatography*. John Wiley and Sons, New York.

Tozer, T. N., N. H. Neff and B. B. Brodie. 1966. Application of steady state kinetics to the synthesis rate and turnover time of serotonin in the brain of normal and reserpine-treated rats. *J. Pharmacol. Exp. Ther.* **153**: 177–182.

Trautman, R. 1964. Ultracentrifugation. *In* D. W. Newman (ed.), *Instrumental Methods of Experimental Biology*. Macmillan, New York, pp. 211–297.

Truex, R. C. and M. B. Carpenter. 1969. *Human Neuroanatomy*. Williams and Wilkins, Baltimore.

Twarog, B. M. 1961. Notes on the bioassay of serotonin. *In* J. H. Quastel (ed.), *Methods in Medical Research* **9**: 183–185. Year Book Medical Publishers, Inc., Chicago.

Udenfriend, S. 1969. *Fluorescence Assay in Biology and Medicine* **2**. Academic Press, New York.

Udenfriend, S. and H. Weissbach. 1963. 5-hydroxytryptophan and derivatives. *In* S. P. Colowick and N. O. Kaplan (eds.). *Methods in Enzymology* **6**: 598–605. Academic Press, New York.

Udenfriend, S., H. Weissbach and B. B. Brodie. 1958. Assay of serotonin and related metabolites, enzymes and drugs. *In* D. Glick (ed.), *Methods of Biochemical Analysis* **6**: 95–130. Interscience Publishers, New York.

Von Hungen, K., H. R. Mahler and W. J. Moore. 1968. Turnover of protein and ribonucleic acid in synaptic subcellular fractions from rat brain. *J. Biol. Chem.* **243**: 1415–1423.

Waller, G. W. (ed.). 1972. *Biochemical Applications of Mass Spectrometry*. J. Wiley and Sons, New York.

Wattiaux, R. 1971. Centrifugation of subcellular components. *In* Z. M. Bacq, R. Capek, R. Paoletti and J. Renson (eds.), *Fundamentals of Biochemical Pharmacology*. Pergamon Press, New York, pp. 87–96.

Weeks, J. R. 1972. Long-term intravenous infusion. *In* R. D. Myers (ed.), *Methods in Psychobiology* **2**: 155–168. Academic Press, New York.

Weinstein, L. H. and H. J. Laurencott. 1964. Column chromatography. *In* D. W. Newman (ed.), *Instrumental Methods of Experimental Biology*. Macmillan, New York, pp. 113–135.

Westley, J. L. 1969. *Enzymic Catalysis*. Harper and Row, New York.

Whitaker, J. R. 1967. Electrophoresis in stabilizing media. *In* G. Zweig and J. R. Whitaker (eds.), *Paper Chromatography and Electrophoresis*. Academic Press, New York.

White, C. E. and R. J. Argauer. 1970. *Fluorescence Analysis; A Practical Approach*. Marcel Dekker, Inc., New York.

Zimmerman, E. and R. George. 1974. *Narcotics and the Hypothalamus*. KROC Foundation Symposium No. 2. Raven Press, New York.

II
THE PHARMACOLOGICAL AND BIOCHEMICAL BASIS OF PSYCHOPHARMACOLOGY

Behaviorally active drugs interact with neurochemicals in brain to produce an effect. The alterations in behavior caused by the interaction of a drug with neurochemical systems is the "drug effect." The site at which a drug or neurochemical alters neural activity is called the receptor. In considering drug receptors and drug effects, two important considerations must be borne in mind. First, very few drugs interact solely with a single receptor, even though a few drug effects may be the result of just one drug-receptor interaction. Second, the nature of most drug receptors has not been characterized. The usefulness of considering a receptor derives from its utility as a unifying and explanatory concept, but the drug receptor, *per se*, has no observable physical dimensions. For the present discussion, it will suffice to envision the receptor as an entity with which a chemical or drug interacts, the ultimate consequence of this interaction being the drug effect.

AIMS

The main focus of the following chapters will be on biochemicals normally present in the nervous system that either act as neural transmitters or play a role in the regulation of the electrical activity of the nervous system. Norepinephrine (NE), dopamine (DA), serotonin (5-hydroxytryptamine, 5-HT) and acetylcholine (ACh) will be considered in detail because the biochemistry, physiology and pharmacology of these compounds as well as their role in the maintenance of nervous system function and behavior have been examined extensively. In particular their role in motor behavior, behavior under schedule control and ingestive behavior will be examined. In addition, some aspects of their role in sexual behavior, aggressive behavior, sleep and sensory function will be considered.

A clear understanding of the functional role of naturally occurring substances located in brain and other nervous tissue will not only facilitate the understanding of the way in which certain classes of drugs affect behavior, but may also enable one to understand the important biochemical and physiological processes that play a role in behavior.

Because of the complexity of the central nervous system, the autonomic nervous system (ANS) will be reviewed in Chapter 3 as a model of biochemical and physiological events that may occur in the central nervous system (CNS). Chapters 4, 5 and 6 will be concerned with the role of the biogenic amines (5-HT, NE and DA) in the regulation of behavior, as well as the role of behavior in the regulation of the metabolism and distribution of the biogenic amines. Chapter 7 will be devoted to the role of ACh in the regulation of behavior and Chapter 8 to the role of various long-chain macromolecules in memory and learning.

HISTORICAL BACKGROUND

The function of the brain in the mediation of behavior dates back to the eighteenth century—an era in which basic experiments in physics, chemistry and anatomy led to the emergence of concepts and data in both neurophysiology and neuroanatomy. Further developments in these fields in the eighteenth and nineteenth centuries supported the notion that sensory perception, motor activity and integration of perception and motor activity (i.e., behavior) occurred in the brain. M. A. Brazier (1959, p. 58) has provided a comprehensive historical outline of the major developments in this area beginning with Aristotle. She concludes:

> ... With the recognition that sensation and motion were mediated by the nerves their position becomes unassailable, for movement was regarded as the sign of life. Slowly the concept of neural organization began to be pieced together and levels of integration were postulated, in the spinal cord, in the cortex and in the deeper structures of the brain. The period of analysis of the function of each structural unit, of each sector of the nervous system, was followed by a shift of emphasis towards a synthetic consideration of neural activity. The search began for the physiological mechanisms of mental processes, of consciousness of memory—all terms and concepts that had belonged to another domain of thought. In the neurophysiology of today we find both angles of approach, ranging from analysis of the intimate physicochemical basis of nervous structure and dynamics to the synthesis of actions that we call behavior of the organism.

Interest in naturally occurring chemicals in brain, and their relationship to brain function and behavior, began at the turn of the century. Anthropologists working in Mexico and the southwestern part of the United States found that certain tribes used peyote as a sacrament in religious ceremonies. The peyote button when chewed, or dissolved in hot water and consumed in tea, was found to be capable of producing visual and auditory hallucinations thought to be similar to those occurring during acute psychotic episodes associated with schizophrenia. In 1896 the active substance (mescaline) was isolated from the button of the peyote cactus (*Lophophora williamsii*), and its chemical structure was determined in 1918 (Fig. 1). Mescaline was the first purified chemical substance that, when consumed in small amounts, was able to produce hallucinations and change in affect; and therefore it generated interest in a possible biochemical basis for the etiology of schizophrenia.

There have been many accounts of the use of mescaline in anthropological, social, behavioral and pharmacological literature. Klüver (1966) has written an elegant account of the sensory experience that occurs after mescaline ingestion, and has discussed the importance of chemical agents as tools in the elucidation of brain function and behavioral processes.

In 1943 Hofmann discovered that lysergic acid diethylamide (LSD) (Fig. 1) produced psychological effects very similar to those occurring after mescaline ingestion. Hofmann accidently ingested a small quantity of LSD while working with a series of indole derivatives. Shortly thereafter, he began to experience unusual sensations of vertigo and restlessness; his perception of the size and shape

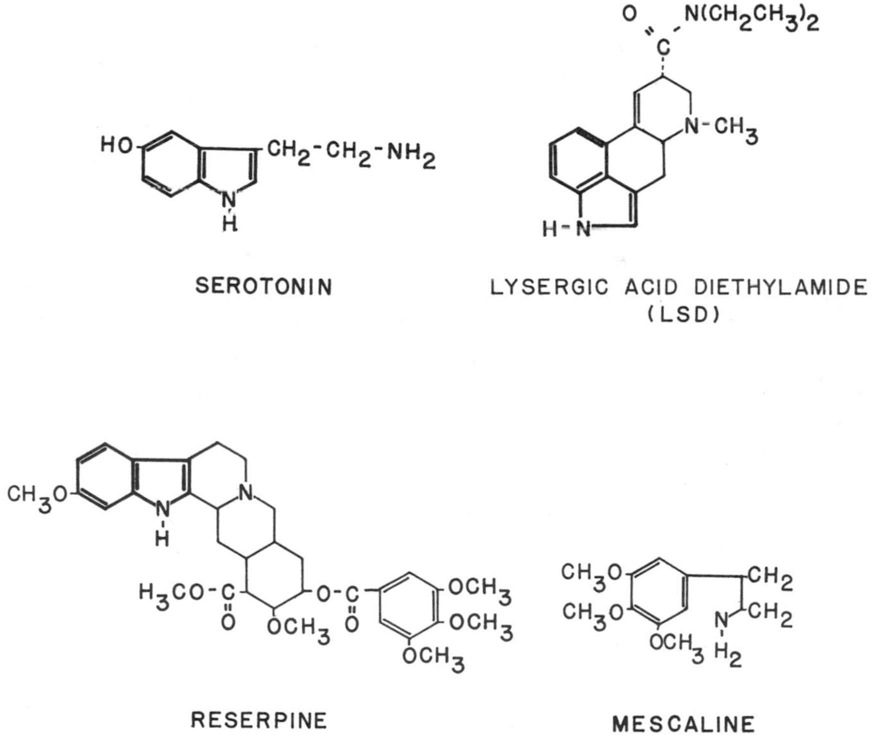

SEROTONIN

LYSERGIC ACID DIETHYLAMIDE
(LSD)

RESERPINE

MESCALINE

Fig. 1. Structures of serotonin, reserpine, LSD and mescaline. Serotonin, reserpine and LSD contain the basic indole nucleus.

of objects was distorted, and he was unable to concentrate on his work. He decided to return to his home, where he went to bed and experienced a dreamlike state partially characterized by vivid imagery. Later, after Hofmann recognized the similarities between LSD and mescaline, he attempted to repeat the "trip" by intentionally ingesting LSD. Unfortunately, he used the dose for mescaline as his guide for the dose of LSD and took 0.25 mg of LSD, which is recognized today as a rather large dose. These experiments were repeated later with smaller doses of LSD, replicating Hofmann's original findings. Hofmann's experience further reinforced interest and speculation as to a possible chemical basis for the symptomatology and etiology of schizophrenia, and throughout the years a variety of theories were advanced. At the time of Hofmann's discovery, however, it was not known what naturally occurring endogenous substrate LSD or mescaline acted upon, nor was it known whether a psychotic episode might be caused by the presence of an abnormal metabolite of an endogenous substance or an abnormal rate of metabolism of the endogenous substrate (Stoll and Hofmann, 1943; Stoll, 1947).

In the late 1940s, clinical investigators hypothesized that there is a substance in blood responsible for hypertension. It was thought that if the substance responsible for hypertension could be isolated and identified, the search for an antagonist to its action on the smooth muscle of the circulatory system would be facilitated. Possessing the compound in a relatively purified form would enable investigators to perform experiments on isolated smooth muscle organ systems *in vitro*. A compound was isolated from the gut which caused contraction of smooth muscle and elevation of blood pressure. Rapport (1949) identified the compound as 5-hydroxytryptamine (serotonin, 5-HT); it was later found that 5-HT is an amine distributed widely in tissues. Since 5-HT was an indolealkylamine, it was thought that other compounds differing in structure but containing the same indole nucleus might conceivably interfere with the action of 5-HT on blood pressure (see Fig. 1). Since 5-HT in small amounts elicits contraction in the uterus of an estrous rat, this system was used as an *in vitro* test for various antagonists. When some of these antagonists were tested in man, they proved to be psychotomimetic; one of these compounds was LSD.

In 1957 Brodie and his colleagues found that reserpine, a hypotensive drug as well as a tranquilizer, depleted 5-HT from brain and other tissues in which it occurs. Based on this finding and several others to be discussed, the hypothesis was formulated that the effects of reserpine were mediated by the release of 5-HT from the storage sites in the brain. Other workers (Gaddum, 1953; Wooley and Shaw, 1952), noting the resemblance between 5-HT and many hallucinogenic indole derivatives, advanced hypotheses relating the abnormal metabolism of 5-HT to abnormal behavioral states in man and animals.

It was found that reserpine also depleted both dopamine and norepinephrine from brain and other tissues in which they occur (Holzbauer and Vogt, 1956;

Carlsson *et al.*, 1957). This finding created an interesting, stimulating and highly productive controversy in the scientific literature as to which monoamine was responsible for the actions of reserpine. As research progressed in this area, it was found that many drugs (Chapter 3) which modified the distribution and metabolism of the biogenic amines also had profound effects on various types of behavior. Therefore, the role of the amines in behavior became important both for understanding the underlying neurochemical substances of behavior and the neurochemical basis of drug action.

REFERENCES

Brazier, M. A. 1959. The historical development of neurophysiology. *In* J. Field, H. W. Magoun, V. E. Hall (eds.), *Handbook of Physiology*, Section 1: Neurophysiology, Vol. 1. Waverly Press, Baltimore, pp. 1–58.

Carlsson, A., E. Rosengren, A. Bertler and J. Nilsson. 1957. Effect of reserpine on the metabolism of the catecholamines. *In* S. Garattini and V. Ghetti (eds.), *Psychotropic Drugs*. Elsevier Press, Amsterdam, pp. 363–372.

Gaddum, J. H. 1953. Antagonism between lysergic acid diethylamide and 5-hydroxytryptamine. *J. Physiol.* 121: 15p.

Holzbauer, M. and M. Vogt. 1956. Depression by reserpine of the noradrenaline concentration in the hypothalamus of the cat. *J. Neurochem.* 1: 8–11.

Klüver, H. 1966. *Mescal and Mechanisms of Hallucinations*. University of Chicago Press, Chicago.

Rapport, M. M. 1949. Serum vasoconstrictor (serotonin) V. The presence of creatinine in the complex. Proposed structure of the vasoconstrictor principle. *J. Biol. Chem.* 180: 961.

Stoll, W. A. 1947. Lysergäure-diathylamid ein phantastikum aus der mutterkontrgruppe. *Schweiz. Arch. Neurol. Psychiat.* 60: 279.

Stoll, W. A. and A. Hofmann. 1943. Partialsynthese von alkaloiden vom typus des ergobasins 6: Mitteilung über Mutterkornalkaloide. *Helv. Chim. Acta.* 26: 944.

Wooley, D. W. and E. Shaw. 1952. Some antimetabolites of serotonin and their possible application to the treatment of hypertension. *J. Am. Chem. Soc.* 74: 2948–2949.

3
The Autonomic Nervous System

The concept of chemical transmission of the nerve impulse in the autonomic nervous system (ANS) has been extremely important to understanding the mechanisms by which drugs act on the ANS. Most drugs that have effects on the ANS do so by affecting one, or perhaps more, of the chemicals involved in transmission. Therefore, one might think in simple terms of the following situation:

Drug $----\rightarrow$ Changes in chemical transmission
$\downarrow$
Changes in ANS function
$\downarrow$
Change in ANS activity

That is, the drug affects some transmitter(s), and the effect of the drug on the transmitter leads to a change in autonomic function. A drug's effect on transmitter function can occur at several places, including transmitter synthesis, degradation, storage or its activity at the receptor site.

Chemical transmission of nerve impulses in the central nervous system (CNS) is also a very important phenomenon, and a number of compounds are thought to be CNS transmitters. The number of transmitters in the CNS is probably larger than in the ANS; however, it is much more difficult to identify transmitters in the CNS, because of the complexity of this system. In spite of this complexity, the role of chemical transmission in the expression of the effects of centrally active drugs has been an active and viable field of study by both neuropharmacologists and biochemically oriented psychopharmacologists over the past two decades. It has been found that many centrally active drugs affect some aspect of chemical transmission across the synapse. Simply stated as an analogy to ANS drug effects, we have the following situation:

Drug -----→ Change in chemical transmission

↓

Change in CNS function

↓

Change in behavior

As we shall see, some drugs affect transmission in both the ANS and the CNS. Moreover, some transmitters occur in both systems.

The elucidation of the pharmcology of the autonomic nervous system is a classic example of research in the biological sciences. Research in this area includes an investigation of mechanisms of drug action, as well as an investigation of basic biochemical and physiological processes involved in nervous transmission, nerve-muscle conduction and maintenance of homeostasis in the organism. In addition, the model of the nerve cell as derived from ANS research, especially with regard to the way in which it synthesizes, stores, utilizes and inactivates transmitter compounds, has been used as a point of departure for understanding chemical events occurring in the central nervous system. Furthermore, drugs that affect CNS function invariably affect the ANS.

As the name *autonomic* implies, the autonomic (or visceral) nervous system is historically considered to be a network of nerves that mediates bodily functions not under voluntary control. The ANS plays an important role in regulating the function of literally every organ in the body. For instance, it regulates the size of the pupil by innervating muscles in the iris; heart rate and force of contraction are also regulated by this system, thus effecting changes in both blood pressure and the supply of blood and essential nutrients to various parts of the body. In addition, blood pressure and blood flow are regulated by the ANS innervation of blood vessels of the skin, skeletal muscle, brain, respiratory system and digestive system. Here ANS regulation is relatively specific; through a series of complicated reflexes, patterns of blood flow to different systems in the organism can be modulated as a function of the second-to-second requirements of those systems (Gellhorn, 1968). The ANS also regulates the constriction of the bronchial tubes, thus affecting air flow to the lungs. Various functions in the gastrointestinal system, including motility of the GI tract, secretions of the gall bladder and stomach and tone of various sphincters, are also under ANS control. Similarly, the ANS regulates the urinary system and the sex organs. In the skin, the ANS controls piloerector muscles and sweat glands. In the liver, glycogenolysis appears to be influenced by autonomic activity. In addition, the ANS appears to be the chief regulator of most exocrine gland secretions.

The ANS has also played an important role in the development of research and theory in psychology (see Cannon, 1927; James, 1950; Harris and Brady, 1973, 1974; Miller, 1969). Many theoretically and experimentally oriented psychologists have been concerned with the neurophysiological, the neuroanatomical and, more recently, the neurochemical basis for behavior. In particular they have investigated afferent input to CNS structures thought to control thirst, hunger, sexual arousal and fear.

BASIC PROPERTIES OF THE ANS

Anatomical and Physiological Properties

One major difference between the autonomic nerves and the somatic nerves is the muscles they innervate. The motor nerves of the ANS supply efferents to all structures with the exception of the skeletal muscles (Fig. 3-1), which are usually supplied by the somatic nervous system. These two systems also differ in several other ways. The most distal synaptic junctions in the ANS are located outside the central nervous system, while the most distal synaptic junctions in the somatic nervous system are located inside the CNS. The axons of nerves that innervate skeletal muscle travel all the way from the CNS to the skeletal muscle. On the other hand, in the ANS the axons synapse outside the CNS in specific structures called ganglia. Autonomic effector neurons with cell bodies in the spinal cord and axons emanating from the spinal cord to synapses in ganglia are called preganglionic neurons. Autonomic effector neurons that have their cell bodies in ganglia and have processes (axons) which conduct impulses away from the cell body to innervate end organs are called postganglionic neurons. In the somatic nervous system a muscle is usually supplied by a single nerve; on the other hand, autonomic neurons tend to be diffusely interconnected and form plexuses; a single autonomic nerve may supply several related muscles. Somatic nerves to skeletal muscle are myelinated, whereas post-ganglionic autonomic nerves are nonmyelinated.

Sympathetic and Parasympathetic Divisions of the ANS

The autonomic nervous system regulates the muscle tone and activity of the eye (e.g. pupillary constriction and dilation), the heart (rate), blood vessels (degree of constriction), lung (relaxation of bronchial musculature), the gastrointestinal tract (degree of motility) and salivary and sweat glands (amount of secretion). The ANS is divided into two subsystems—termed sympathetic and parasympathetic (Table 3-1). Most organs are innervated by both systems, and they usually act in opposition to each other. For instance, sympathetic activity results in relaxation of the bronchial muscles of the lung, whereas parasympathetic activity causes contraction.

The sympathetic and parasympathetic divisions of the ANS can be distinguished on an anatomical and biochemical basis, although neither method of classifica-

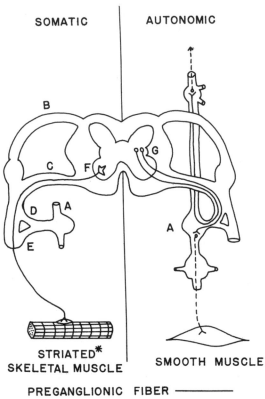

SOMATIC   AUTONOMIC

STRIATED*
SKELETAL MUSCLE   SMOOTH MUSCLE

PREGANGLIONIC FIBER ————————
POSTGANGLIONIC FIBER - - - - - - - -

*All skeletal muscle is usually striated and receives innervation from the somatic division of the nervous system. The autonomic nervous system innervates all smooth muscle; in addition, it innervates the heart, which is a striated muscle. The heart is the only striated muscle to receive its innervation from the ANS.

Fig. 3-1. An illustration of the anatomical characteristics of the autonomic and the somatic nervous system at the level of the thoracolumbar outflow. (*A*) Ganglia. (*B*) Dorsal root of the spinal cord. (*C*) Ventral root of the spinal cord. (*D*) Grey ramus communicans. (*E*) White ramus communicans.   (*F*) Motor fiber originating in the anterior column. (*G*) Autonomic preganglionic efferent fiber originating in the intermediolateral column.

tion forms a completely consistent picture. In the *sympathetic* division of the ANS, the cell bodies of the preganglionic neurons lie in the intermediolateral column of the spinal cord, and the outflow of the sympathetic system extends from the first (Fig. 3-2) thoracic to the second lumbar segment of the spinal cord. Preganglionic fibers of the sympathetic outflow are generally shorter than the postganglionic fibers (Fig. 3-2 and 3-3). Sympathetic ganglia are interconnected and form a structure known as the sympathetic chain. The synaptic

TABLE 3-1.   Responses of major effector organs to autonomic nerve impulses

Organ	Sympathetic impulses (Noradrenergic)	Parasympathetic impulses (Cholinergic)
Eye	dilate pupil	constrict pupil
Heart	increase in rate, conduction time, contractility, velocity	decrease in rate, conduction, velocity, contractility
Blood vessels	generally constrict, but dilate in skeletal muscle	
Lung	relax bronchial muscle	contract bronchial muscle stimulate bronchial glands
GI tract	decrease motility and tone, increase contraction of sphincters	increase intestinal motility decrease or relax sphincters
Gallbladder	relax	stimulate
Salivary glands	secrete thick, viscous saliva	secrete profuse, watery saliva
Sweat glands[1]	secrete	
Adrenal medulla[2]	secrete epinephrine and norepinephrine into bloodstream	
Genitalia	produce ejaculation in male	produce erection
Uterus	pregnant: increase contraction non-pregnant: increase relaxation	

[1]Sweat glands use acetylcholine as a transmitter at the neuromuscular junction except for a few areas, such as the palm of the hand, where norepinephrine is the transmitter. By chemical classification the sweat glands could be classified as parasympathetic (i.e., cholinergic), but since they are innervated by a short-preganglionic fiber emanating from the thoracolumbar section of the spinal cord, and a long postganglionic fiber, the sweat glands are classified as sympathetic.

[2]Acetylcholine is released by the preganglionic fiber onto the adrenal medulla, which causes release of epinephrine from the adrenal medulla. The adrenal medulla is a group of specialized postganglionic cells which secrete epinephrine and norepinephrine.

transmitter at ganglionic synapses is acetylcholine, and the transmitter at the nerve–smooth muscle junction (more generally defined as the neuroeffector junction) (postganglionic) is norepinephrine.

In the *parasympathetic* division of the ANS, the cell bodies of the preganglionic fibers issue from the midbrain (cranial nerve III, oculomotor), the medulla oblongata (cranial nerve VII, facial; cranial nerve IX, glossopharyngeal; cranial nerve X, vagus) and the intermediolateral column of the sacral segment of the spinal cord (Fig. 3-2). Unlike sympathetic preganglionic fibers which are short, the preganglionic fibers in the parasympathetic system are usually long, and the

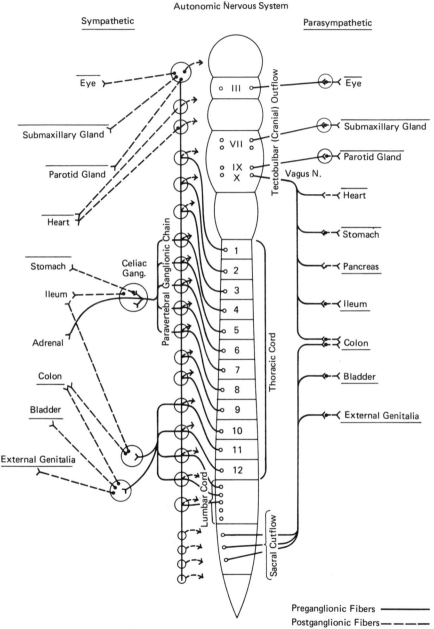

Fig. 3-2. The anatomical characteristics of the ANS showing both (1) the points of decussation from the spinal cord of the sympathetic and parasympathetic fibers and (2) the relative lengths of both pre- and postganglionic fibers in the sympathetic and parasympathetic divisions of the ANS.

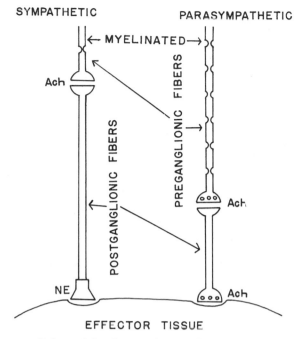

SYMPATHETIC   PARASYMPATHETIC

← MYELINATED →

Ach

PREGANGLIONIC FIBERS

POSTGANGLIONIC FIBERS

Ach

NE   Ach

EFFECTOR TISSUE

Fig. 3-3. A diagram of the peripheral sympathetic and parasympathetic nervous system. Assume an impulse in the preganglionic fiber; this leads to the release of ACh at the synapse in the ganglion. Transmitter diffuses across the synaptic cleft and acts on the postganglionic receptor, resulting in depolarization of the postganglionic neuron; the released ACh must then be inactivated. This is achieved through the action of acetylcholinesterase which is located in the postganglionic membrane.

A similar series of events takes place at the neuroeffector junction site. In this case, the predominant effect is on the end organ. Acetylcholine (ACh) is released from parasympathetic postganglionic fibers, and norepinephrine is released from sympathetic postganglionic fibers.

postganglionic parasympathetic fibers are usually short (Figs. 3-2 and 3-3). In the parasympathetic division of the ANS, acetylcholine is the transmitter at both ganglionic synapses and at the neuroeffector junction. In general, sympathetic preganglionic fibers synapse with a greater number of postganglionic cells than preganglionic parasympathetic fibers, thus producing more diffuse innervation. In the case of the parasympathetic fibers, there is a tendency toward a one-to-one correspondence between the pre- and postganglionic fibers.

CHEMICAL TRANSMISSION IN THE AUTONOMIC NERVOUS SYSTEM

The nerve impulse is a bioelectric phenomenon involving the propagation of a change in potential along a fiber which is normally polarized; this polarization of the nerve cell is maintained by active extrusion of sodium from the interior of the cell. Excitation of a nerve cell temporarily increases permeability of the cell to sodium. It was first suggested by Dubois Reymond in 1877 that the action potential is transmitted by way of chemical transmission from nerve to muscle, i.e., across the neuromuscular junction or simply the junction. The concept has been extended to include transmission from nerve to nerve as well. This is transmission across the synapse (see Chapter 2).

Although the notion of chemical transmission of a nerve impulse across a junction or synapse is appealing, it is not easy to establish. Generally speaking, four criteria must be met before a given substance can be demonstrated to be a transmitter. First, the enzymes for synthesis of the transmitter, as well as the transmitter itself, must be present in the nerve cell. Second, the substance must be shown to be released into the junction or synapse when the prejunctional or presynaptic fiber is stimulated. Third, local administration of the compound to the junction or synapse should mimic the effects of prejunctional or presynaptic stimulation. Fourth, interfering with the synthesis, degradation, storage or pharmacological action of the substance should have an effect on transmission. It is often difficult to satisfy all of these criteria. In practice, one, two or three criteria are met, and investigators proceed on the assumption that the compound is a transmitter if this concept is not contradicted by further experiments (see Cooper *et al.*, 1974).

Acetylcholine

Historical Background. Our present-day understanding of neuroeffector and synaptic transmission in the autonomic nervous system is the result of the research efforts of literally thousands of investigators over the past 60 or more years. To do justice to this topic, *vis-à-vis* the history of science, we would go beyond the scope of this chapter. However, in this section we will discuss some crucial experiments to illustrate examples of the biochemical, pharmacological and physiological techniques that, when combined, have defined the nature of synaptic transmission within the ANS.

In 1907, Dixon observed that a drug called muscarine produced physiological effects that mimicked stimulation of the vagus nerve (parasympathetic). Dixon postulated that parasympathetic (Fig. 3-3) postganglionic nerves secrete a muscarine-like substance when stimulated, perhaps even muscarine itself. Four years later, Hunt and Traveau discovered that acetylcholine, the acetic ester of choline, could cause a reduction in blood pressure, an effect similar to vagal stimulation. Dale, working during this same period, found that an extract of ergot also had very powerful parasympathomimetic effects, and he tried to isolate muscarine from the extract. The active compound that was finally isolated, however, turned out to be much more labile than muscarine. Dale demonstrated that the purified isolate was acetylcholine and speculated that it might mediate parasympathetic stimulation. In 1921, Otto Loewi demonstrated that stimulation of the vagus resulted in the secretion of a substance that mimicked vagal effects. In a modification of this classic experiment, it was found that if one connected the circulatory system of two frogs and stimulated the vagus of one frog, the heart rate of both frogs slowed, demonstrating that a chemical substance was released into the blood upon vagal stimulation (see Burn, 1968; Goodman and Gilman, 1970, for further details). The preponderance of evidence collected since that time strongly indicates that acetylcholine is a transmitter in the ANS. Neurons that secrete acetylcholine as a transmitter substance are called *cholinergic* fibers.

Muscarinic and Nicotinic Receptors. Acetylcholine has a dual action in the ANS. Under certain conditions, its administration mimics parasympathetic activity, and under others its administration mimics sympathetic activity. The parasympathetic effects of ACh are called muscarinic because they mimic the effects of muscarine administration. The sympathetic effects of ACh are called nicotinic because they mimic the initial effects of nicotine administration. If, for example, a relatively small dose of ACh (2 μg) is injected into a cat, the blood pressure and heart rate decrease (see Fig. 3-4). This decrease in blood

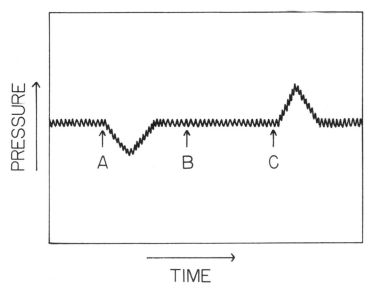

Fig. 3-4. The effects of a small and a large dose of acetylcholine on blood pressure in an anesthetized cat. (*A*) Intravenous administration of 2 μg of ACh; note the fall in blood pressure caused by slowing of the heart (a parasympathetic effect). (*B*) Administration of 2 mg of atropine followed by 2 μg of ACh; very little, if any, changes in blood pressure occur. (*C*) A large dose of ACh (1 mg) causes an increase in blood pressure that is due to stimulation of sympathetic ganglia and to stimulation of the adrenal medulla.

pressure and heart rate is classified as the vagal, parasympathetic and *muscarinic* effect of ACh. When blood pressure returns to normal, subsequent treatment of the same cat with atropine blocks the blood pressure decrease produced by 2 μg of ACh (see Fig. 3-4). However, when a relatively high dose of ACh (1 mg) is injected, blood pressure increases; this is a sympathetic and *nicotinic* effect of ACh. Atropine therefore blocks the parasympathetic (or muscarinic) effects of ACh, but does not block sympathetic stimulation of the ganglia (a nicotinic effect).

High doses of acetylcholine also stimulate receptors on the adrenal medulla, causing release of epinephrine and norepinephrine into circulating blood, which in turn can cause an increase in blood pressure. Therefore, the increase in blood pressure seen after administration of atropine and a relatively high dose of ACh (1 mg) arises from two factors: (1) acetylcholine-induced stimulation of sympathetic postganglionic neurons and (2) stimulation of the adrenal medulla which releases epinephrine and norepinephrine into the circulation. It should be noted that sympathomimetic effects besides changes in blood pressure also occur under these circumstances, but the main point to be emphasized here is the distinction between muscarinic and nicotinic receptors.

From these and other data it has been concluded that ACh is the transmitter substance at the sympathetic and parasympathetic ganglia, and at the parasympathetic neuroeffector junction (Fig. 3-3). Moreover, the effects of ACh on the ganglia are mimicked by nicotine, but not by muscarine; therefore, these actions of ACh are referred to as nicotinic. On the other hand, the action of ACh at the parasympathetic neuroeffector site is not mimicked by nicotine, but by muscarine. As we shall see, drugs which affect the ANS often act specifically at selected functional sites. For example, atropine blocks all of the muscarinic but none of the nicotinic effects of ACh.

The fact that ACh has a dual action in the ANS implies that there are two types of *receptors* that may be activated by the transmitter. One class of receptors is termed muscarinic, and the other is termed nicotinic. At the present time, as with all receptors, these two classes of receptors are defined on an operational basis; it is not now known whether two physicochemically distinct classes of ACh receptors exist. At any rate, the operational definition of muscarinic and nicotinic receptors is quite useful in explaining both drug action and normal autonomic activity.

Norepinephrine

Historical Background. In the 1920s it was established by the work of Cannon and others that stimulation of sympathetic postganglionic fibers caused the secretion of a substance that could increase blood pressure and heart rate. This substance was called "sympathin" by Cannon and was found to be secreted at many sites in the sympathetic system. It had chemical properties similar to those of epinephrine; however, it did not seem likely that epinephrine was the transmitter since it did not completely mimic the effects of sympathin. Subsequently, Von Euler (1946) identified norepinephrine as the primary transmitter at postganglionic sympathetic neuroeffector junctions. Neurons which secrete norepinephrine as a transmitter are called *noradrenergic* fibers. Norepinephrine shows a dual action similar to that produced by ACh. This dual action is thought to be due to the existence of two types of noradrenergic receptors; these receptors are termed α and β. This subject will be dealt with later in the chapter.

THE NORADRENERGIC NEURON

Experimental evidence demonstrating chemical transmission in the ANS has led to development of a model of the noradrenergic neuron which, although specifically developed from the evidence relevant to the actions of NE at the neuroeffector junction, has been applied at other areas, including sites in the CNS. In developing the model (Carlsson, 1966; Iversen, 1967) (Fig. 3-5) of the noradrenergic neuron, each process in the biochemistry and physiology of the neuroeffector junction will be explored, and the action of certain prototypic drugs on these processes will be described. There are five processes that are basic to chemical transmission: (1) synthesis, (2) storage, (3) release, (4) transmitter-receptor interaction and (5) inactivation of transmitter. Once the transmitter is synthesized and stored in the presynaptic element, it can be released in dis-

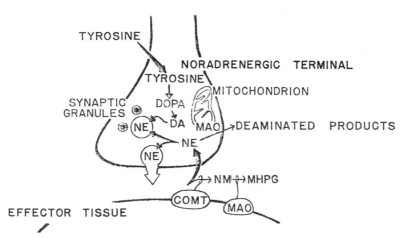

Fig. 3-5. A noradrenergic model of the nerve ending illustrating synthesis, storage in granules, release, and inactivation through reuptake and enzymatic degradation. Abbreviations—NM: normetanepherine; MHPG: methoxy-4, hydroxy-phenylglycol; DOPA: dihydroxyphenylalanine; DA: dopamine; NE: norepinephrine; COMT: catechol-O-methyltransferase ; MAO: monoamine oxidase.

crete quantities from its storage sites to cause a response in the effector cell. Termination of the effect of a transmitter can be accomplished by enzymatic degradation, diffusion away from the receptor or active uptake (called "reuptake") into the presynaptic nerve endings. Many aspects of the model have been verified through biochemical, physiological and histological techniques; much of the original data on which it is based stems from pharmacological studies.

Metabolism and Storage

Synthesis.   The most important naturally occurring catecholamines in mammals are dopamine, norepinephrine and epinephrine. The catecholamines (CAs) present in mammalian tissue are synthesized from the essential dietary amino acid, phenylalanine, or from tyrosine (Fig. 3-6). Phenylalanine may be converted to tyrosine in the liver by phenylalanine hydroxylase; tyrosine also occurs in the diet. Tyrosine is the natural precursor of catecholamines in tissue. Hydroxylation of tyrosine by tyrosine hydroxylase to form L-dihydroxyphenylalanine (L-dopa) is the first step in the biosynthesis of CAs; tyrosine hydroxylase is found in the supernatant fraction of the cell and is the rate-limiting enzyme in the formation of norepinephrine and dopamine. While dopamine is not a neural transmitter in the peripheral nervous system, it is thought to be in the CNS, and its function will be discussed in Chapters 5 and 6. L -Dopa is decarboxylated by aromatic-L-amino acid decarboxylase,* which is located in the soluble cell fraction.   The decarboxylation of L-dopa leads to the formation of dopamine, which can be hydroxylated in the *beta* position by the enzyme, dopamine-β-hydroxylase (DBH) to form norepinephrine. Current evidence indicates that this enzyme is localized in the granules that store norepinephrine (see section on storage). These reactions occur in the adrenal medulla, the sympathetic nervous system and specific neurons in the central nervous system. The amino group of norepinephrine can be methylated by phenylethanolamine-N-methyl transferase (PNMT) to form epinephrine; this reaction is largely confined to the adrenal medulla.

Inactivation.   There are two principal pathways for enzymatic degradation of the catecholamines; oxidation by the enzyme monoamine oxidase (MAO) and/ or O-methylation by the enzyme catechol-O-methyltransferase (COMT) (Fig. 3-6).   Monoamine oxidase catalyzes conversion of the amine into an aldehyde, which in turn is oxidized to the corresponding acid. Acid metabolites of biogenic amines are physiologically inert. COMT catalyzes the methylation of the

---

*This was the first enzyme (also referred to as L-Dopa decarboxylase) discovered in the synthesis of catecholamines (Holtz *et al.*, 1938); on the basis of this discovery, the pathway for catecholamine synthesis was proposed (Blaschko, 1939).

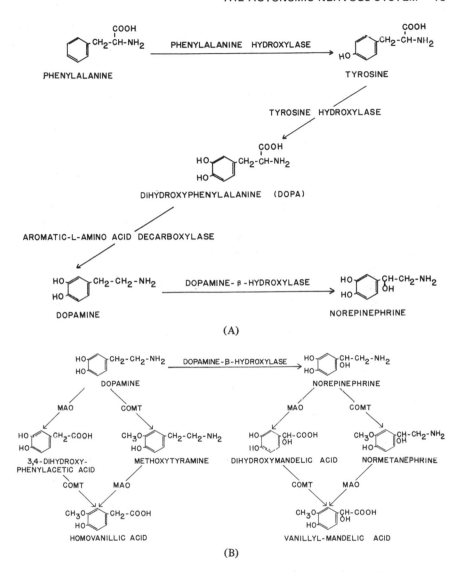

Fig. 3-6. (*A*) Catecholamine synthesis. (*B*) Catecholamine degradation.

catecholamine to form the corresponding O-methylated catecholamine derivative, which is also physiologically inert. Metabolites produced by MAO can be
methylated by COMT, and, likewise, metabolites of COMT can be oxidized by
MAO. In each case, the corresponding catechol O-methylated acid metabolite
(vanillyl-mandelic acid, homovanillic acid; see Fig. 3-6) is the product. Monoa-

mine oxidase is bound to mitochondria, and COMT is bound to muscle at the neuromuscular membrane.

There are two other mechanisms by which the catecholamines can be inactivated. The first, and probably most important, is the process of reuptake of the released compound back into the presynaptic ending. There are certain drugs that appear to block the reuptake mechanism. Secreted NE may also be inactivated by simple diffusion away from the site of action, although it does not appear that this is a major route of inactivation.

Storage. There appear to be at least two mechanisms for NE storage in nerve, and though these are not yet identifiable on a morphological basis, data obtained from radiochemical tracer studies and drug studies suggest that there are both a rapidly synthesized and released functional (or free) pool and a slowly synthesized and released reserve pool. The functional (or free) pool consists mainly of newly synthesized NE, whose storage site has not yet been determined, while the reserve pool is believed to be stored in specialized structures called granules. A granule is a subcellular organelle which is thought to take up and release neural transmitters. Norepinephrine is thought to be synthesized in the cell body and transported in granules down the axon to the synapse. Electron microscopy and flourescence histochemistry have revealed that NE is stored in visible structures. The dynamic equilibrium that exists between the two pools [i.e., the rapidly synthesized and released functional (or free) pool and the slowly synthesized and released reserve (or granular) pool], as well as factors which influence this equilibrium, are not completely understood.

Pharmacology

Physiology. Stimulation of the sympathetic nervous system which causes release of NE from neuroeffector sites also causes a certain pattern of physiological responses in the organism (see above, Table 3-1). Blood pressure, heart rate and stroke volume are increased. The blood vessels supplying skeletal muscle are dilated, while those supplying the gut and skin are constricted and there is an overall increase in peripheral resistance in the vasculature. Most of the smooth muscle of the gut is relaxed and consequently GI motility decreases. In addition, there is usually constriction of the sphincters of the GI tract. The radial muscle of the iris contracts, leading to mydriasis (enlargement of the pupil), and the ciliary muscle relaxes. Salivary and sweat glands show increased secretion. Epinephrine and norepinephrine secretion from the adrenal medulla increases, leading to increased blood levels of these amines and further effects on smooth muscle sensitive to catecholamine (see footnote in Table 3-1). Furthermore, sympathetic discharge also has metabolic effects including increased glycogenolysis (the conversion of glycogen to glucose).

Alpha and Beta Receptors. The physiological effects outlined above can be elicited by the administration of certain drugs (i.e., sympathomimetics) or natural transmitters involved in sympathetic stimulation (epinephrine or norepinephrine). While all sympathetic drugs do not show exactly the same effects, the description above closely delineates the action of NE or E. The action of sympathomimetics differs depending on the specific drug and the particular type of muscle the drug is acting on. For example, sympathetic stimulation leads to contraction of the smooth muscles in the wall of the blood vessels supplying the GI tract as well as the skin, but causes dilation of the vessels supplying striated muscle. Similarly, during sympathetic stimulation, certain parts of the gut are relaxed while some sphincters constrict. The explanation for this dual effect is that there are two types of noradrenergic receptors; α and β receptors. These were originally classified by Ahlquist (1948) on the basis of differing pharmacological responses elicited by a group of sympathomimetic amines. In brief, it was found that when various sympathomimetic amines were tested on various organ systems, they fell into two distinct groups. In one group epinephrine was the most potent and isoproterenol the least potent—this group of receptors was called α. In the β group, isoproterenol was the most potent and norepinephrine the least potent. Further evidence for the existence of α and β receptors is adduced from the fact that there are compounds which selectively block one or the other type of receptor. In general the effect of activation of α receptors is excitatory—causing contraction of the smooth muscle involved. In general, the effect of β stimulation is inhibitory—causing relaxation of the muscle involved. The important exceptions to this are discussed below.

A single sympathomimetic effector cell may contain both α and β receptors; though, generally, one or the other predominates. Blood vessels supplying striated muscle have mainly β receptors; thus, only a sympathomimetic with very strong α effects will cause contraction. The heart has only β receptors, but unlike other β receptors, activation of the β receptors in the heart causes excitation. Beta stimulation results in an increase in heart rate and an increase in stroke volume.

Drug Effects. A large number of drugs affect autonomic function at specific points in the noradrenergic neuron. We will not discuss all these drugs; rather we will confine our discussion to representative drugs which influence both autonomic and CNS function and therefore have implications in psychopharmacology. Table 3-2 presents a summary of prototypic drugs which have effects on the important processes occurring within the noradrenergic neuron. Many of these drugs have more than one effect in the noradrenergic system as well as having effects on other systems. It should also be pointed out that some of these drugs affect noradrenergic, dopaminergic and serotonergic function in the CNS. Their effects in the CNS will be reviewed in Chapters 4, 5 and 6.

TABLE 3-2. Prototypic drugs affecting processes in the noradrenergic neuron in the ANS

Process	Drug[1]
Receptor stimulation	isoproterenol
	norepinephrine
	epinephrine
Synthesis inhibition	
Tyrosine hydroxylase	α-methylparatyrosine
Aromatic-L-amino acid	Ro 4-4602-1 (N-(dl-seryl) N-
decarboxylase	(2,3,4-trihydroxybenzylhydrazine)
Dopamine-beta hydroxylase	disulfiram
Degradative inhibition	
MAO	nialamide
	pargyline
	iproniazid
COMT	pyrogallol
Reuptake blockade	cocaine
	imipramine, desipramine or
	desmethylimipramine
	amphetamine
Receptor blockade	
α	phenoxybenzamine, phentolamine, ergots
β	propranolol
Storage	reserpine
	tetrabenazine

[1] In considering the processes which these drugs affect, it must be borne in mind that these drugs affect other systems as well. For example, reserpine and tetrabenazine deplete serotonin from tissue in which they occur. In addition, not all the systems on which the drugs may possibly act have been examined.

1. *Receptor Agonists.* Sympathomimetic drugs (e.g., ephedrine, amphetamine, phenylephrine and isoproterenol) and the natural transmitters, epinephrine and norepinephrine, stimulate noradrenergic receptors and produce dilation of the pupil, relaxation of the bronchials, drying of the nasal mucosa and an increase in blood pressure. The specific drug effect is dependent on whether the compound is a more effective alpha or beta agonist. Nevertheless, even though a receptor agonist is a more effective beta or alpha agonist, its action will be mixed. For example, a weak beta agonist may affect an organ if β receptors predominate in that organ. Therefore, it is difficult to classify a drug as a pure alpha or beta agonist.

2. *Synthesis Inhibitors.* Tyrosine hydroxylase is the rate-limiting step in the synthesis of dopamine and norepinephrine. Alpha-methylparatyrosine (AMT) inhibits this enzyme, thereby causing a reduction in the tissue levels of catecholamines. Alpha-methylparatyrosine does not seem to have profound effects on the function of the ANS. Since it does seem to affect behavior, it will be considered in relation to the noradrenergic system in later chapters. The compound Ro 4-4602-1, or (N-(*dl*-seryl) N-(2,3,4-trihydroxybenzylhydrazine), an experimental compound, is a noncompetitive inhibitor of aromatic-L-amino acid decarboxylase. Disulfiram is an inhibitor of dopamine-beta-hydroxylase (DBH), the enzyme which catalyzes the conversion of dopamine to norepinephrine.

3. *Degradation Inhibitors.* There are several drugs which inhibit monoamine oxidase (MAO). Iproniazid, nialamide and pargyline are the most frequently used drugs in this category. Pyrogallol is an inhibitor of COMT. These drugs have been widely used in research concerning the role of the catecholamines in both the ANS and the CNS.

4. *Reuptake Blockers.* Axelrod *et al.* (1961) have discovered that the major mechanism of termination of the action of norepinephrine (Table 3-2) in the neuroeffector junction is by reuptake into the same cell which released the transmitter. Both cocaine and tricyclic antidepressants (e.g., imipramine) block this reuptake process. For example, sufficient concentrations of exogenously administered or endogenous secreted norepinephrine cause vasoconstriction in certain vascular beds (e.g., skin or gut). Drugs that block uptake, like cocaine, can cause vasoconstriction in these beds in response to small amounts of exogenously administered or endogenously liberated norepinephrine that normally do not produce vasoconstriction. Other drugs including pipradrol, methylphenidate, amphetamine and chlorpromazine also block reuptake. These compounds may also have other actions such as causing release or blocking receptors, and their pharmacological actions have not been solely attributed to blockade of reuptake. Even cocaine and the tricyclic compounds that are considered prototypic reuptake blocking agents have other effects which contribute to their pharmacological actions.

5. *Receptor Blockers:*

(a) *Alpha blocking drugs.* Phenoxybenzamine and certain derivatives of this drug block α receptors in the ANS. Phenoxybenzamine inhibits the excitatory response caused in smooth muscle by sympathetic stimulation, and, in so doing, allows the β effects of intrinsic NE to predominate. For example, treatment of an anesthetized cat with a small dose (2.5 μg/kg) of epinephrine will cause a transient increase in blood pressure. In the first instance, the pressor response is caused by an increase in resistance to blood flow due to constriction of the peripheral vasculature (an alpha effect). When the α receptors are blocked, however, the same dose of epinephrine causes a β effect, leading to vasodilation and a decrease in blood pressure. The effects of both α and β stimulation on the gut lead to a decrease in the motility of the gut; therefore α blockade does not have profound effects on the GI system. The main effects of α blockade are on the vascular bed; α blockers either inhibit constriction or cause dilation.

(b) *Beta blocking drugs.* Propranolol is the prototypic drug that specifically blocks β receptors. The main effects of β blockade, as with α blockade, appear to be on the cardiovascular system. Beta receptor blockade may have little effect on the heart under normal circumstances, while it can partially or completely block the effects of sympathetic stimulation which leads to increased cardiac output (as during exercise). If the organism is pretreated with a β blocker, blood pressure remains unchanged or may only increase slightly because of increased stroke volume during exercise.

6. *Drugs That Interfere with Storage.* Reserpine, which is derived from the ancient Indian drug Rauwolfia, causes depletion of amines from noradrenergic as well as serotonergic nerve cells. Reserpine-induced depletion of central and peripheral transmitters has profound physiological and behavioral consequences. Reserpine causes hypotension, constriction of the pupil, ptosis and increased gastrointestinal motility. In the ANS, these signs are typical of *decreased* sympathetic tone and, as a consequence, an increased parasympathetic force. In addition, other physiological signs occur, including hypothermia and loss of both spontaneous motor activity and feeding behavior. The latter signs are thought to be mediated by the CNS.

Reserpine is thought to deplete amines by interfering with their storage. According to the model (Fig. 3-6) of the noradrenergic neuron, intraneuronally synthesized amines, as well as those taken up into the cell, are stored in the granules (see p. 74). This implies that at any given time there exists a certain fraction of amines which are not stored in granules and therefore are "free" within the cell. Since the amount of free amine is limited through degradation by MAO, a balance exists between the free and granular fractions. Interference with granular binding can disturb this equilibrium and cause a decrease in the total amount of amine but an increase in the amount of "free" amine. In addition, reserpine administration is accompanied by an increase in MAO metabolites. While an increase in MAO metabolites implies that the transmitter is being rapidly metabolized, the pharmacological actions of reserpine are suggestive of a loss of noradrenergic transmission (i.e., depletion) rather than an increase in noradrenergic transmission (i.e., an increase in free NE). Therefore, while reserpine causes depletion of CAs by interfering with storage, in so doing it may also increase the free NE in the cell. In Chapter 4 the question of the so-called free pool will be discussed further.

Guanethidine has some pharmacological effects that are similar to those of reserpine. In addition, the mechanism of action of guanethidine is thought to be similar to that of reserpine, but it is not as well understood. Since guanethidine does not penetrate the blood-brain barrier, it is not used in psychopharmacological studies.

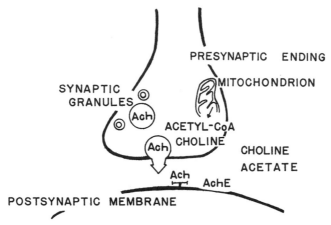

Fig. 3-7. Model of a cholinergic synapse. Abbreviations—ACh: acetylcholine; AChE: acetyl-cholinesterase.

THE CHOLINERGIC NEURON

Biochemical, pharmacological and physiological investigations into chemical transmission have established convincing evidence that acetylcholine functions as a transmitter substance at neuroeffector sites in the autonomic system as well as in skeletal musculature. Acetylcholine (ACh) also serves as a transmitter at all ganglia in the ANS. There is also evidence that it serves as a transmitter in the CNS. Acetylcholine function in terms of behavior will be discussed in Chapter 7. Current concepts of the model (Fig. 3-7) for the cholinergic neuron describe five processes that parallel processes in the noradrenergic neuron: (1) synthesis, (2) storage, (3) release, (4) transmitter-receptor interaction and (5) inactivation.

Metabolism and Storage

Synthesis. Acetylcholine (ACh) is synthesized from acetate and choline, and the reaction is catalyzed by the cytoplasmic enzyme choline acetylase (CoA),* which is localized within cholinergic neurons (see Fig. 3-8). In order for acetate to enter into the reaction with choline, it must first combine with coenzyme A to form acetyl CoA. As shown in Fig. 3-8, the formation of acetyl CoA requires adenosine triphosphate. Although the reaction is not thoroughly understood, it is presumed that acetyl CoA arises from the metabolism of glucose through glycolysis, and, therefore, acetyl CoA would be present in abundance in nerve cells. Choline can be synthesized in the liver or obtained from dietary sources. Choline is not synthesized in cholinergic nerve cells. Cholinergic neurons take up

---

*Also called choline-acetyl transferase.

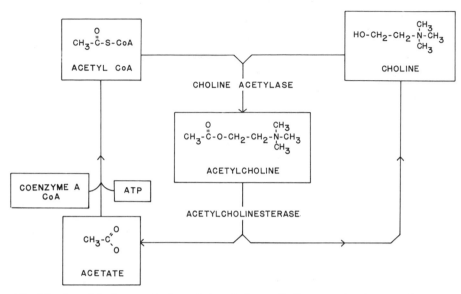

Fig. 3-8. Acetylcholine synthesis and degradation. Choline acetylase is more formally called choline-acetyl transferase. ATP: adenosine triphosphate.

choline by an active transport system which operates efficiently at low concentrations of choline.

Inactivation. Acetylcholine is rapidly degraded by the enzyme acetylcholinesterase (Fig. 3-8). This enzymatic reaction splits ACh into acetate and choline. Some of the choline is taken up in the nerve cell and used for ACh synthesis (see Cooper *et al.*, 1974; Albers *et al.*, 1972).

Generally acetylcholinesterase, the enzyme catalyzing the hydrolysis of ACh, is located in the postsynaptic membrane or in the neuroeffector junction. There are at least two types of enzymes capable of hydrolyzing other esters as well as ACh. In general, neural tissue contains acetylcholinesterase, while nonneural tissue contains pseudocholinesterase (Cooper *et al.*, 1974). A model of the cholinergic neuron is shown in Fig. 3-7.

Storage. Acetylcholine is found in cholinergic nerve endings in two forms: (1) as free ACh in the cytoplasm and (2) as stored ACh in subcellular organelles called synaptic vesicles.

Pharmacology

Acetylcholine is the transmitter at several sites in the peripheral nervous system and is a well established transmitter in the central nervous system. In the peripheral nervous system, acetylcholine is the transmitter at:

1. All parasympathetic postganglionic neural-effector junctions (the receptors at these junctions are muscarinic; see p. 70).
2. All autonomic ganglia and the splanchnic neural-adrenal medulla junction (receptors are nicotinic; see p. 70).
3. Postganglionic sympathetic neural-effector junctions with sweat glands (the receptors at these junctions are muscarinic; see p. 65).
4. All striate muscle nerve junctions (the receptors at these junctions are nicotinic).

The effects of muscarinic receptor stimulation are characterized by parasympathetic autonomic discharge (see Table 3-1). Representative pharmacological effects of muscarinic agents include bradycardia, increased secretions of the nasal mucosa, increased GI motility and constriction of the pupil.

The effects of nicotinic receptor stimulation are complicated because receptor localization is diverse. The nicotinic receptors exist in autonomic ganglia and at nerve–striate muscle junctions. Additional complexity is added by the fact that nicotine and nicotinic drugs initially stimulate at autonomic ganglia and at striate neuromuscular junctions, which effect is followed by a blockade, especially with high doses.

Drug Effects. A large number of drugs have effects on the cholinergic system. We will review some of these drugs with emphasis on agents or classes of drugs that also have effects on the central nervous system and behavior. The latter material will be more extensively reviewed in Chapter 7. A summary of the effects of prototypic drugs on cholinergic processes is presented in Table 3-3.

1. *Receptor Agonists:*

(a) *Parasympathomimetic agents.* The parasympathomimetic agents fall into two groups. The first group contains the choline esters bethanechol, carbachol and methacholine. Each of these compounds has an action very similar to the naturally occurring compound, acetylcholine. The second class of compounds is the parasympathetic alkaloids. These include pilocarpine, arecoline and muscarine. These latter agents work primarily on autonomic effector cells. Parasympathomimetic agents cause constriction of the pupil, stimulation of the GI tract (reflected by an increase in GI motility) and stimulation of various glands, such as salivary glands, pancreas and mucosal cells in the respiratory tract. In addition, the parasympathomimetic agents cause diaphoresis, with some agents being able to cause production of up to 3 liters of sweat from one injection (see Table 3-1).

(b) *Drugs acting primarily on nicotinic receptors.* The pharmacological effects of nicotine are complex because both parasympathetic and sympathetic postganglionic nerves are sensitive to the actions of nicotine. In addition, nicotine first stimulates and then depresses activity in the postsynaptic fiber. Nevertheless, since nicotine has been used to investigate central nervous system function as well as autonomic function, we will outline a few of its more prominent

TABLE 3-3. Prototypic drugs affecting processes in the cholinergic neuron in the ANS

Process	Drug
Receptor stimulation	acetylcholine[1]
	methacholine[1]
	carbachol[1]
	nicotine
	pilocarpine
	arecoline
	muscarine
Interference with release	botulinus toxin[1]
Choline uptake blockade	hemicholinium[1]
Degradative inhibition	neostigmine[1]
	physostigmine *eserine*
	diisopropylfluorophosphate
Receptor blockade	
Muscarinic	atropine
	scopolamine
Nicotinic	hexamethonium[1]
	tetraethylammonium[1]
	mecamylamine

[1] Does not cross the blood-brain barrier.

pharmacological effects. For the purposes of this brief discussion of the effects of nicotine on peripheral nerve and striated muscle, we will consider the drug to be mainly a stimulant. The stimulant action of nicotine on sympathetic ganglia leads to an increase in blood pressure and heart rate, pupil dilation, sweating and piloerection. Stimulation of the sympathetic ganglia also causes release of epinephrine and norepinephrine from the adrenal medulla. The increased circulating epinephrine and norepinephrine contribute to the sympathetic effects listed above. Nicotinic stimulation of parasympathetic ganglia also causes an increase in GI motility and bladder contractions. At very high doses, nicotine can cause paralysis of skeletal muscles. Although there are other ganglionic stimulants with properties similar to those of nicotine, these will not be considered here or elsewhere in the text (see Goodman and Gilman, 1970). Nicotine's actions on the central nervous system will be considered in Chapter 7.

2. *Synthesis, Release and Uptake Inhibitors.* There are no well known drugs that inhibit choline acetylase. Synthesis of acetylcholine, however, can be inhibited by preventing the uptake of choline by cholinergic nerves. Hemicholinium prevents the uptake of choline into both preganglionic and postganglionic cholinergic neurons, but does not enter brain and has no central effects. Hemicho-

linium also acts on motor neurons to striate muscle and in sufficient doses can cause respiratory arrest through paralysis of cholinergic transmission. Botulinus toxin inhibits the release of ACh from storage vesicles and has pharmacological effects similar to those of hemicholinium.

3. *Drugs That Block Inactivation.* Acetylcholinesterase is inhibited by several drugs including physostigmine and diisopropylfluorophosphate (DFP). Since acetylcholine has a very high turnover rate, the effects of inhibiting acetylcholinesterase are striking and often somewhat similar to the effects of the parasympathomimetic agents (see above). Empirically, different inhibitors of cholinesterase have stronger effects on one system than on another. For further details of the strongest effect on any given system, one should consult a pharmacology textbook (Goldstein *et al.*, 1974; Goodman and Gilman, 1970). In general, these agents augment activity in the small and large intestine. They cause pupillary constriction and spasms of accommodation along with a decrease in the intraocular pressure in the eye as a result of the miosis. Secretions of various glands are generally increased. These include bronchial glands, endocrine glands, sweat glands and the intestinal and pancreatic glands. These agents also tend to relax smooth muscles of bronchial tubes and the uterus. In the heart, bradycardia occurs along with decreased force of contraction.

4. *Receptor Blockers:*

(a) *Muscarinic blockers.* Muscarinic blockers inhibit the action of acetylcholine in structures innervated by *postganglionic parasympathetic* nerves. They are classified as antimuscarinic compounds. The prototypic compound in this class is atropine, a very old compound, extracted from *Atropa belladonna*, the deadly nightshade. Scopolamine is another cholinergic blocker, having much the same properties as atropine. Atropine blocks the response of the ciliary muscle of the lens and the sphincter muscle of the iris to stimulation by acetylcholine; this effect leads to pupillary dilation. In the GI tract, atropine inhibits contractions. It also inhibits secretions of the nose, pharynx, mouth and bronchial tubes and is a bronchial dilator. Atropine causes an initial rise in heart rate because of the blockade of acetylcholine released from the vagus. The dual effect of acetylcholine as a muscarinic and a nicotinic stimulator has been nicely illustrated using atropine as a pharmacological tool (Fig. 3-4).

(b) *Nicotinic blockers.* There are a number of compounds that block transmission in autonomic ganglia and therefore are presumed to be nicotinic blockers. Hexamethonium, tetraethylammonium and mecamylamine are a few of the nicotinic blocking drugs. We will consider the general effects of these compounds in the autonomic system. Since only mecamylamine enters the brain readily, we will consider its use in studying cholinergic systems in the CNS.

The effect of administration of a ganglionic blocker depends on the prevailing autonomic tone in a given organ. For example, if the prevailing tone in arterioles is sympathetic, then administration of hexamethonium would lead to vasodilation, increased peripheral blood flow and hypotension. In general, with nicotinic blockers there is a pooling of blood in veins and decreased venous return, reduced GI motility, mild tachycardia, decreased sweating and paralysis of the ciliary muscle in the eye. Notice that some of these effects are similar to those of muscarinic blockers. This is the case when sympathetic tone predominates prior to drug administration. When the ganglionic blocker is given, it blocks transmission through both sympathetic and parasympathetic ganglia. The end organ response is determined by which division of the ANS is exerting the greater control prior to administration of the drug. Thus, tissues predominantly under parasympathetic control will show "antimuscarinic" responses with ganglionic blockade, while those predominantly under sympathetic control will show "antinoradrenergic" responses with ganglionic blockade.

SUMMARY

The autonomic nervous system was reviewed with regard to its basic anatomical and physiological properties with an emphasis on chemical transmission. Basic pharmacological principles and prototypic drugs were discussed with a view toward understanding the mechanism of action of these drugs in both the autonomic and the central nervous systems. Models of both the noradrenergic and the cholinergic neuron were presented.

REFERENCES

Ahlquist, R. P. 1948. A study of the adrenotropic receptors. *Am. J. Physiol.* **153**: 586–600.

Albers, R., G. Siegel, R. Katzman and B. Agranoff (eds.). 1972. *Basic Neurochemistry*. Little, Brown & Co., Boston.

Axelrod, J., L. G. Whitby and G. Hertting. 1961. Effect of psychotropic drugs on the uptake of ^{3}H-Norepinephrine by tissues. *Science* **133**: 383–384.

Blaschko, H. 1939. The specific action of L-dopa decarboxylase. *Proc. Physiol. Society (London)* **96**: 50_p–51_p.

Burn, J. H. 1968. *The Autonomic Nervous System*. Blackwell Scientific Publications, Oxford.

Cannon, W. B. 1927. The James-Lange theory of emotions: A critical examination and an alternative theory. *Am. J. Psychol.* **39**: 106–124.

Carlsson, A. 1966. Drugs which block the storage of 5-HT and related amines. *Handbook of Experimental Pharmacology*, Vol. XIX 5-Hydroxytryptamine and Related Indolalkylamines. Springer-Verlag, New York, pp. 529–592.

Cooper, J. R., F. E. Bloom and R. H. Roth. 1974. *The Biochemical Basis of Neuropharmacology*. Oxford University Press, New York.

Gellhorn, E. 1968. *Biological Foundations of Emotion*. Scott, Foresman and Co., Glenview, Ill.

Goldstein, A., L. Aronow and S. M. Kalman. 1974. *Principles of Drug Action*. Wiley, New York.

Goodman, L. S. and A. Gilman. 1970. *The Pharmacological Basis of Therapeutics*. Macmillan Company, New York.

Harris, A. H. and J. V. Brady. 1974. Animal learning—visceral and autonomic conditioning. *Ann. Rev. Psychol.* **25**: 107–133.

Harris, A. H. and J. V. Brady. 1973. Instrumental (operant) conditioning of visceral and autonomic functions. *Seminars Psychiat.* **5**: 369–376.

Holtz, P., R. Heise and K. Lüdtke. 1938. Fermentativer abbau von 1-dioxyphenylalanine (Dopa) durch niere. *Naunyn-Schmeidebergs Arch. Pharmakol.* **191**: 87–118.

Iversen, L. L. 1967. *The Uptake and Storage of Noradrenaline in Sympathetic Nerves*. Cambridge University Press, Cambridge.

James, W. 1950. *Principles of Psychology*. Dover, New York.

Miller, N. E. 1969. Learning of visceral and glandular responses. *Science* **163**: 434–445.

Von Euler, U. S. 1946. A specific sympathomimetic ergone in adrenergic nerve fibers (sympathin) and its relation to adrenaline and noradrenaline. *Acta Physiol. Scand.* **12**: 73–97.

4
Serotonin and Behavior

The investigation of serotonin function in the central nervous system began with three fundamental discoveries (also see the introduction to this section): (1) serotonin, as well as many compounds which have hallucinogenic properties, was found to contain the indole nucleus; (2) serotonin was found to produce contractions in smooth muscle which could be antagonized by many of the hallucinogens; (3) serotonin was shown to be depleted from brain and from other tissues in which it occurred by reserpine, a drug that has profound effects on behavior in man and animal. Moreover, recent research suggests that serotonin plays a role in reactivity to painful stimuli such as shock and in the control of sleep, aggressive behavior, sexual behavior and seizures (see the review by Chase and Murphy, 1973). The investigation of serotonin and its functional role in behavior is rapidly expanding as interest is generated by current findings and the availability of new pharmacological agents that affect the serotonin system. While there is some disagreement over data and interpretations, tentative generalizations can be made from available data.

BIOCHEMISTRY AND PHARMACOLOGY OF SEROTONIN

Distribution in the Central Nervous System

The localization of serotonin (5-hydroxytryptamine or 5-HT) within nerve cells and the anatomical distribution of these cells within the central nervous system involves techniques drawn from pharmacology, histochemistry, neuroanatomy and biochemistry. While the description presented in the following paragraphs has general acceptance among scientists working in this area, there are points of disagreement. As techniques for localization of compounds in the central nervous system become more sensitive, however, portions of the 5-HT map may be added or revised.

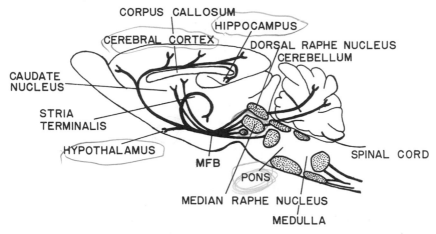

CORPUS CALLOSUM
HIPPOCAMPUS
CEREBRAL CORTEX
DORSAL RAPHE NUCLEUS
CEREBELLUM
CAUDATE NUCLEUS
STRIA TERMINALIS
HYPOTHALAMUS
SPINAL CORD
MFB
PONS
MEDIAN RAPHE NUCLEUS
MEDULLA

Fig. 4-1. Diagrammatic representation of serotonergic pathways: the ascending pathways which send fibers to the cortex, caudate and hippocampus as well as other areas of the forebrain not shown in this diagram have cell bodies that lie in the dorsal and medial raphé nuclei. MFB: medial forebrain bundle.

Heller *et al.* (1962) were the first to present evidence that 5-HT was found in nerve cells. They made lesions in the lateral hypothalamus and observed a decline in 5-HT levels in brain over a period of several days. These data suggested that serotonergic axons had been destroyed as a result of the lesion. Subsequently Anden *et al.* (1966) showed with fluorescence microscopy that 5-HT is located within certain neurons. With the aid of lesion and drug studies, they mapped the distribution of the 5-HT system. In addition, Jouvet (1969) demonstrated that it was possible to reduce brain serotonin to 10% of its normal content by destroying a small part of the pons known as the raphé system. Since the raphé nuclei project to many areas, Jouvet concluded that the serotonergic system is diffuse in its projections.

Most of the 5-HT cell bodies are located in the raphé region (Fig. 4-1), but there are many cell bodies in the raphé that are not serotonergic (Fuxe and Jonsson, 1974). 5-HT terminals are widely distributed in the telencephalon and diencephalon. As can be seen from Fig. 4-1, areas particularly rich in 5-HT nerve terminals include cerebral cortex, hippocampus, hypothalamus, caudate nucleus and anterior colliculus. In addition there seems to be cerebellar and spinal projections containing 5-HT. Figure 1 presents a rough schematic representation of the 5-HT system.

Metabolism and Storage

In mammals, 5-HT is derived from the essential amino acid, tryptophan. Tryptophan is used primarily in protein synthesis, but a very small portion of it is also metabolized by the 5-HT system. The first step (Fig. 4-2) in the synthesis of 5-hydroxytryptamine is hydroxylation of tryptophan to form 5-HTP (i.e., 5-hydroxytryptophan). The enzyme that catalyzes this reaction is tryptophan hydroxylase. This is the rate-limiting step in the synthesis of 5-HT. The hydroxylase is specific for tryptophan and is found in brain and other serotonin-containing tissues. 5-HTP is decarboxylated through the action of aromatic-L-amino acid decarboxylase to form 5-hydroxytryptamine. Since 5-HT passes from the blood to the CNS with great difficulty, 5-HT levels in brain are usually raised with a precursor such as 5-HTP. Both tryptophan and 5-HTP can penetrate the blood-brain barrier and elevate the serotonin content of the CNS.

The enzyme primarily responsible for the degradation of 5-HT in nerve is MAO. The action of MAO on 5-HT results in the formation of 5-HIAA. A second metabolic pathway for serotonin exists in mammals; the enzymes in this pathway are present in high concentrations in the pineal gland; in addition, there is evidence suggesting that these enzymes may be present in much lower concentrations in some serotonergic nerves (Björklund *et al.*, 1971; Koslow and Green, 1973). Serotonin is acetylated by serotonin N-acetylase to form N-acetyl serotonin which is methylated by 5-hydroxyindole-O-methyl transferase to form melatonin. Melatonin has been implicated in the maintenance of biological and behavioral rhythms (primarily sexual in nature); a discussion of these implications is beyond the scope of this text. 5-HT can also be deactivated by reuptake into the presynaptic nerve ending. This is similar to the reuptake process for norepinephrine outlined in Chapter 3.

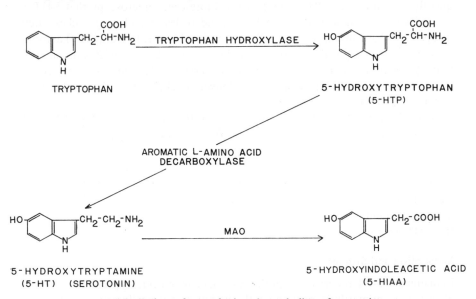

Fig. 4-2. Pathway for synthesis and metabolism of serotonin.

Electron photomicrographs have revealed dense core serotonin granules that disappear with the administration of reserpine. Based on this evidence, as well as certain other considerations, it is believed that 5-HT is bound to granules located within the cell. Evidence suggests that these granules are synthesized in the cell body, and migrate along the axon to the synaptic ending. Serotonin synthesis occurs both in the cell body and in nerve endings of serotonergic neurons. Serotonin that is synthesized in nerve terminals can be taken up into granules located at the terminal.

Synaptic Transmission in the Central Nervous System

It is widely accepted that serotonin functions as an excitatory and/or inhibitory transmitter in the CNS (Fig. 4-3); it is therefore included in the category of "putative" transmitters. The criteria for establishing a compound as a transmitter substance have been reviewed in the autonomic nervous system chapter (see Chapter 3). Briefly, they are the following: (1) The enzymes for synthesis of the transmitter, as well as the transmitter itself, must be present in the nerve cell. (2) The substance must be shown to be released into the synapse when the presynaptic fiber is stimulated. (3) Local administration of the compound to the synapse should mimic the effects of presynaptic stimulation. (4) Interfering with the synthesis, degradation, storage or pharmacological action of the substance should have an effect on transmission. 5-HT has met several of these criteria. First, it has been demonstrated that 5-HT and the enzymes responsible for its synthesis and degradation, exist in the nerve cell. Second, it has been shown that stimulation of serotonin-containing tracts in the CNS causes the re-

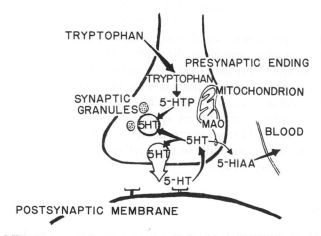

Fig. 4-3. A 5-HT synapse. Abbreviations: 5-HT, 5-hydroxytryptamine; 5-HTP, 5-hydroxytryptophan; 5-HIAA, 5-hydroxyindoleacetic acid; MAO, monoamine oxidase.

lease of 5-HT, since an increased amount of 5-HIAA (a 5-HT metabolite) is present at points distal to the stimulating electrode following stimulation. Third, the effects of topical application of 5-HT on nerve discharge and firing rate in the CNS have been observed in a variety of studies. For example, it has been shown that an intra-arterial injection of 5-HT will attenuate evoked potentials in the optic cortex. These effects are mimicked by mescaline and LSD but not by norepinephrine, thereby reinforcing the idea that mescaline and LSD act via a serotonergic mechanism. There is some question, however, whether small doses of 5-HT injected intra-arterially reach the optic cortex because of the relative impermeability of the blood-brain barrier to serotonin. Furthermore, if the nerve cell from which the recordings are made does not contain a serotoninergic input, it is possible that the attenuation may be a pharmacological effect of 5-HT (i.e., acting as a drug) rather than a physiological effect.

It has also been shown that an injection of the serotonin precursor 5-HTP which readily crosses the blood-brain barrier produces a slowing of the EEG. It should be pointed out that data based on 5-HTP injections are confounded by the fact that the enzyme which catalyzes the decarboxylation of 5-HTP to 5-HT also exists in neurons not containing 5-HT; therefore, when 5-HTP is injected, 5-HT is also formed in nerves not normally containing 5-HT (Macchitelli et al., 1966). More detailed work in this area has been accomplished using both single cell recording and application of 5-HT to single cells. Taken together, these studies have shown that some cells in both the spinal cord and the diencephalon are responsive to the application of 5-HT, and that the response to 5-HT closely mimics stimulation of axons having projections to the area on which the 5-HT is applied.

The fourth method for establishing a transmitter substance (i.e., interference with the synthesis or degradation of the substance) has also been investigated with 5-HT. It has been shown that MAO inhibitors (which should increase free 5-HT by interfering with its degradation) cause a depression of the rate of firing of serotonin-containing neurons in the raphé. Moreover, it has been inferred from this observation that the excess 5-HT causes a decrease in the firing rate of the raphé unit. The decrease in firing rate can be blocked by depletion of 5-HT prior to the administration of MAO inhibitors. Therefore, data from pharmacological, electrophysiological, direct application, enzymatic and distributional studies suggest that 5-HT serves as a transmitter. Moreover, it appears that 5-HT serves as an inhibitory transmitter in some cells and as an excitatory transmitter in others (see Krnjevic, 1974).

Drug Effects

By virtue of its proposed function as a neurotransmitter, a model of the serotonergic neuron (Fig. 4-3) has evolved that is very similar to the model of the

**TABLE 4-1. Prototypic drugs affecting processes within
the serotonergic neuron**

Process	Drug
Receptor stimulation	serotonin (5-HT)
Synthesis inhibition	
Tryptophan hydroxylase	parachlorophenylalanine (PCPA)
	parachloroamphetamine (PCA)
Aromatic-L-amino acid-decarboxylase	Ro 4-4602-1
MAO inhibition	nialamide
	pargyline
	iproniazid
Reuptake blockade	chlorimipramine
	imipramine
Receptor blockade	lysergic acid diethylamide
	methysergide
	chlorpromazine
Storage	reserpine
	tetrabenazine
Neurotoxin	5,6-dihydroxytryptamine (5,6-DHT)

adrenergic neuron which was detailed in Chapter 3 (Fig. 3-5). As with the noradrenergic neuron, synthesis, storage, uptake, degradation and action on the receptor are important considerations (Table 4-1).

Receptor Agonists. Serotonin is a naturally occurring compound found in pre-synaptic neurons which, when released by nerve impulses, affects the firing rate of postsynaptic neurons. It is the only compound that stimulates serotonin receptors. Receptor stimulation can be induced pharmacologically in the CNS by administration of 5-HTP, which is converted to 5-HT in the CNS.

Synthesis Inhibitors. Parachlorophenylalanine (PCPA) is an inhibitor of the enzyme tryptophan hydroxylase, the rate-limiting enzyme in 5-HT synthesis. While PCPA is an effective and relatively specific inhibitor of tryptophan hydroxylase, PCPA also depletes NE and DA. For example, after a single administration of PCPA (316 mg/kg), rat brain 5-HT is depleted to less than 20% of normal for a period of five days, reaching a low point of less than 10% of normal three days after administration. Levels of 5-HT return to normal after 16 days. Catecholamine levels are depleted to only 80% of normal and return to normal five to six days after administration (Koe and Weissman, 1966). There are reports that catecholamine depletion is less than 80% a few hours after PCPA administration (Miller *et al.*, 1970). Since the effects of PCPA are usually measured more than 24 hours after administration, the depletion of catecholamines is probably not a significant factor in its pharmacological actions; however, as with all drugs, it must be remembered that a single mode of action cannot be assumed (Weissman, 1973).

Parachloroamphetamine (PCA) also acts by inhibiting tryptophan hydroxylase (Sanders-Bush and Sulser, 1970). It differs from PCPA, however, in having a longer duration of action on tryptophan hydroxylase; it has been suggested that this inhibition is irreversible. PCA also has several transitory effects which occur soon after administration. These effects include reuptake blockade and 5-HT release. PCA does not deplete brain catecholamines; but it does increase catecholamine metabolites, suggesting that PCA stimulates catecholamine turnover rates (Sanders-Bush *et al.*, 1974; Miller *et al.*, 1970).

Ro 4-4602 also inhibits the synthesis of serotonin. It does so by inhibiting the enzyme that decarboxylates 5-HTP to serotonin. This enzyme is present in excess; therefore, its partial inhibition does not dramatically alter 5-HT content in brain. In spite of this problem, the decarboxylase inhibitor has served as a useful tool for differentiating the effects of the precursor 5-HTP from its product, 5-HT. An important feature of Ro 4-4602 is that it does not cross the blood-brain barrier at a dose of less than about 100 mg/kg. Therefore, a low dose of Ro 4-4602 can be used in combination with 5-HTP to examine the effects of 5-HT in brain since a low dose of Ro 4-4602 will block the conversion of 5-HTP to 5-HT in extracerebral tissues.

MAO Inhibitors. MAO inhibitors, such as iproniazid, pargyline and nialamide, alter the degradation of serotonin by interfering with the enzyme responsible for its destruction.

Reuptake Blockers. Carlsson *et al.* (1969) have shown that some tricyclic antidepressants may block serotonin uptake (and/or reuptake). As with many other drugs, the tricyclics are not specific to serotonergic systems, but block uptake in catecholaminergic systems as well.

Receptor Blockers. There are at present no confirmed release or receptor blockers of serotonin although chlorpromazine, LSD and methysergide have been proposed as blockers of 5-HT receptors.

Drugs That Interfere With Storage. Brodie and his colleagues (see Brodie and Shore, 1957) discovered that reserpine administration caused the depletion of serotonin from brain and other tissues in which it occurred. They also showed that reserpine did not inhibit the synthesis of 5-HT, and postulated that reserpine caused the release of serotonin from its storage sites by interfering with storage.

Furthermore, they were able to show by using isotopically labeled reserpine that reserpine itself was not responsible for the long-lasting effects. While the labeled reserpine disappeared from the brain within an hour, some of the effects of reserpine treatment, including 5-HT depletion, could be observed for several days. Injection of 5-HTP caused a transient increase in serotonin levels in brain and mimicked many effects of reserpine. On the basis of these facts, it was postulated that reserpine causes an increase in the amount of *free* 5-HT in brain by interfering with granular storage, even though it decreases the *total amount* of 5-HT present.

An understanding of the biochemical mediation of reserpine effects was complicated, however, by the independent discovery in two laboratories (Holzbauer and Vogt, 1956; Carlsson *et al.*, 1957a,b) that reserpine also depleted both norepinephrine and dopamine from brain and other tissues (see Chapter 5 for a discussion of this work). It is important to note here that reserpine, like many drugs, has effects on several endogenous chemicals. Its behavioral effects may be mediated by one or all of those chemicals. All of these endogenous systems must therefore be considered in an investigation of the biochemical mediation of reserpine effects.

Neurotoxin. 5,6-Dihydroxytryptamine (5,6-DHT) injected into the lateral ventricle in rats causes a long-lasting and relatively selective diminution of cerebral 5-HT (Baumgarten *et al.*, 1971). The decrease is thought to be due to selective degeneration of serotonin-containing nerves. Subsequent recovery of 5-HT has been attributed to regeneration of axons which derive from serotonergic cell bodies not destroyed by 5,6-DHT. Other investigators have confirmed that 5,6-DHT causes a long-lasting depletion of 5-HT in brain after intracisternal administration (Costa *et al.*, 1972; Breese *et al.*, 1974; Longo *et al.*, 1974). Although the 5,6-DHT-induced reduction in 5-HT is long-lasting, it does not appear to be permanent except in the spinal cord.

The extent and the duration of 5-HT depletion and the amount of recovery following 5,6-DHT differ between areas in the central nervous system. Björklund *et al.* (1974) injected 75 μg of 5,6-DHT intraventricularly and examined 5-HT levels in a number of central nervous system structures at various times, ranging from three hours to six months postinjection. In the spinal cord, 5-HT was depleted by 90% within one day after 5,6-DHT administration and remained at this low level up to six months. In the hypothalamus, 5-HT was depleted by 60% one day after 5,6-DHT. At six months 5-HT had recovered to 130% of normal. In the mesencephalon, 5-HT was depleted by 50% one day after injection, which recovered to 90% of normal six months later. In the septum 5-HT was also depleted by 50% one day after 5,6-DHT, with only a small amount of recovery within 30 days after injection. After six months, 5-HT levels in the septal area were 160% of control levels. In the striatum, 5-HT was depleted by

20% at 1 to 30 days after administration of 5,6-DHT. By six months, 5-HT in the striatum had recovered to normal levels. 5,6-DHT also produced a small elevation in norepinephrine which occurred 10 days postinjection, but returned to normal by 30 days; there was no effect on dopamine. Although reserpine, PCPA, PCA and 5,6-DHT all cause a diminution of 5-HT in the CNS, they each have different selectivities which depend in part upon dose and pretreatment times.

Other Drugs. Amphetamine, cocaine and morphine have also been linked to 5-HT mechanisms, but the nature of their effects is not well understood (see Chapter 6).

SEROTONIN AND BEHAVIOR

General Approach

In order to infer a causal relationship between serotonin and behavior, one must observe more than a concomitant alteration of the two. Additional evidence is frequently necessary to show that the two events are dependent upon one another. For example, if PCPA causes a change in behavior as well as a change in the levels of serotonin in brain, the biochemical mechanism underlying that effect might be investigated by replacing serotonin, and observing whether or not the behavior returns to normal.

Since no single approach is adequate to investigate the function of endogenous chemicals in the mediation of behavior, a variety of approaches are used. In this chapter, we will examine the approaches used to investigate relationships between serotonin and behavior.

Three basic approaches are used in this research. These include: (1) reduction of serotonin levels; (2) elevation of serotonin levels; (3) agonism/antagonism of 5-HT sites in the CNS. The first two approaches will be emphasized in this chapter, as most of the research relating the functions of serotonin to behavior has employed these first two approaches.

Reduction of 5-HT Levels. A number of drugs cause the depletion of 5-HT (as well as the depletion of catecholamines) from brain:

1. Reserpine and tetrabenazine deplete 5-HT as well as NE and DA from brain by interfering with storage in granules.
2. Parachlorophenylalanine and *p*-chloroamphetamine interfere with 5-HT synthesis.
3. Certain toxins destroy serotonergic nerves, and this destruction causes relatively long-lasting changes in serotonin levels in brain.
4. Stereotaxically placed electrolytic lesions in the brain often reduce 5-HT concentrations in specific brain regions. These lesions are placed by im-

planting an electrode into the animal's brain using a predetermined set of coordinates for the location of the electrode tip. When the electrode is in the proper place, current is passed through the electrode and results in destruction of nerve cells around the tip of the electrode. The size of the lesion can be controlled by the level (amount of current) and duration of current.

Elevation of 5-HT Levels. Serotonin can be elevated or replaced with adminis-tration of its metabolic precursor 5-hydroxytryptophan, which, unlike serotonin, can cross the blood-brain barrier. Replacement sometimes can also be achieved by intraventricular-intracerebral infusion of serotonin. The latter technique in-volves placing a small needle or cannula into the proper area of brain and another needle into some other more remote brain area and passing fluid through the system. The needles (or cannula) both deliver fluid to, and withdraw fluid from, the system.

Problems can arise with both techniques. 5-HTP can be taken up and de-carboxylated in cells that normally do not contain serotonin. For example, cells containing catecholamines also contain aromatic-L-amino acid decarboxylase. In addition, 5-HT introduced directly into the brain by intracerebral or intraven-tricular infusion may be taken up by nerve terminals not normally containing 5-HT. Therefore, caution must be exercised in interpreting results from these techniques.

In the rest of this chapter, the role of 5-HT in behavior will be examined along with the theories that have been generated from this work. In this work, it must be remembered that there are difficulties in using drugs as tools to investigate the function of an endogenous compound, i.e., *no drug has a single effect*. Most drugs have at least two or three known effects, and there may be others. More-over, it is usually impossible to attribute a behavioral effect to one endogenous compound.

Sensitivity to Painful Stimuli

In this section, the words "pain" and "analgesia" will be used frequently. Sev-eral different behavioral techniques have been used to measure pain or analgesia. All involve the animal's response to some stimulus that is thought to be painful. An animal's response to these stimuli might not be attributable to a change in pain perception or analgesia, and so care must be taken in using these terms.

Lesions of the medial forebrain bundle (MFB) lead to a decrease in serotonin and norepinephrine in brain areas rostral to the lesion, including limbic structures and the cerebral cortex. Lints and Harvey (1969) showed that rats with bilateral MFB lesions exhibited an increased sensitivity to electric shock as evidenced by a lowered jump threshold in a flinch-jump procedure (see Chapter 1). Control animals with lesions in the medial hypothalamus did not show changes in amines or altered shock sensitivity. Amine depletion in the MFB group had a delayed onset which corresponded to the time that would be expected for nerve degeneration to occur; there was a corresponding delay in the development of increased sensitivity to the electrical shock. These results suggested that the amine deficit was responsible for increased sensitivity to the electric shock. Administration of *l*-5-HTP, the isomer metabolized to 5-HT, reversed both the biochemical and behavioral effects of the lesion (i.e., there was a rise in brain 5-HT and a decrease in pain sensitivity), whereas neither *d*-5-HTP (a nonmetabolized isomer of 5-HTP), nor *l*-dihydroxyphenylalanine (L-dopa) had an effect. Measurement of telencephalic 5-HT content in rats with lesions in the medial forebrain bundle and subsequently treated with varying doses of 5-HTP revealed a dose-dependent increase in telencephalic 5-HT. The correlation between jump threshold and the telencephalic content of serotonin in the animals with the MFB lesion was 0.80 (Fig. 4-4). The medial forebrain bundle lesion also caused a decrease in the latency on a hot plate (Chapter 1). Since the medial forebrain bundle lesion did not cause an increase in a noise-induced startle response, it was concluded that the lesion did not produce general hyperresponsiveness (Harvey and Yunger, 1973). When other areas were lesioned, a decrease in brain 5-HT was produced which was accompanied by an increased sensitivity to electric

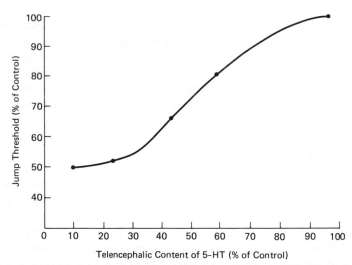

Fig. 4-4. Relationship between telencephalic content of 5-HT and jump threshold. Note that as the amount of telencephalic 5-HT increases the jump threshold goes toward normal. These rats had MFB lesions and 5-HTP treatment. The rats were killed immediately after testing, and the telencephalon in each rat was assayed for 5-HT. (From Harvey and Yunger, 1973.)

shock; these areas included the septal area, dorsal medial tegmentum and the medial raphé nucleus.

In further studies (Harvey *et al.*, 1974), lesions in other brain areas were also found to cause a depletion of 5-HT in the telencephalon; however, decreased latencies in the hot plate technique were not observed with all lesions which produced decreases in brain 5-HT. Indeed, some of the lesions increased the rats' paw-lick latencies. For example, lesions in the central grey raphé nucleus, and the dorsal medial tegmentum, produced a decrease in telencephalic 5-HT and either increased or had no effect on hot plate latencies. On the other hand, lesions in the nigrostriatal bundle, the septal area and the medial forebrain bundle caused a loss of telencephalic 5-HT, but decreased hot plate latencies. The lesions that did not affect or decrease hot plate latencies all destroyed a portion of the central grey area in the rat brain. The central grey area is believed to contain a pathway that mediates an animal's response to painful stimuli. Therefore, failure to observe an increase in sensitivity to heat may be due to the fact that the decrease in 5-HT was "cancelled out" by destruction of the central grey area. Harvey *et al.* (1974) also observed day/night changes on the hot plate test which corresponded to day/night changes in 5-HT levels in various telencephalic structures. While this evidence suggests that there is a correlation between 5-HT levels and shock sensitivity, Hole and Lorens (1975) have failed to find changes in shock sensitivity with midbrain raphé lesions in a flinch-jump technique.

Since morphine produces a decrease in pain sensitivity in several procedures, including the flinch-jump technique and the hot plate, it has been suggested that morphine's effects might be mediated by the 5-HT system. Tenen (1968) found that pretreatment with parachlorophenylalanine (PCPA), a serotonin (5-HT) depletor, blocked the effect of morphine on the flinch-jump test. Tenen speculated that the PCPA antagonism of the morphine analgesia was a result of deficient brain 5-HT. In support of Tenen's results, Samanin *et al.* (1970) reported that lesions of the raphé nuclei blocked morphine analgesia as measured on a hot plate test. On the other hand, others have not observed changes in morphine analgesia using PCPA or serotonin reducing lesions (Lorens and Yunger, 1974; Harvey *et al.*, 1974), in either flinch-jump or hot plate techniques. The reason for the differences in these results has not been resolved.

Although isolated reports to the contrary exist, it has been found that neither chronic nor acute administration of morphine changes the levels of serotonin within the brain. Way and his colleagues (1972), however, have found changes in 5-HT turnover following the development of tolerance (see Chapter 6, p. 203) to morphine. Way measured serotonin turnover in tolerant and nontolerant animals by administering an MAO inhibitor (pargyline) and measuring the rate of 5-HT accumulation. It was found that the rate of 5-HT accumulation after tolerance development was nearly twice that of the nontolerant controls (see Fig. 4-5), suggesting that morphine tolerance produces an increase in sero-

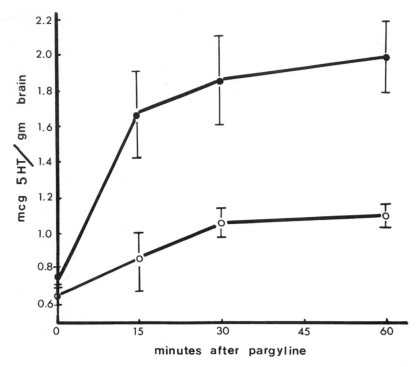

Fig. 4-5. Brain 5-HT levels at various intervals after pargyline in tolerant (●——●) and non-tolerant (○——○) mice. Each point represents 20 determinations, and the bar indicates S.E. (From Shen *et al.*, 1970.)

tonin turnover. Moreover, the fact that cycloheximide, an inhibitor of protein synthesis, blocked the increased rate of serotonin synthesis induced by morphine suggests that morphine alters the enzymes for 5-HT synthesis. Other workers (Cheney *et al.*, 1971), using a radiochemical tracer technique to measure the turnover rate of 5-HT in brain, have found no differences between mice tolerant to morphine and nontolerant controls. The reason for this difference in results is not clear; Cheney *et al.* suggest that the difference may be related to the fact that Way and his colleagues used an MAO inhibitor to estimate turnover. Since it is generally agreed that turnover estimation with either the MAO-inhibition method or the tracer method give similar results, this is not a satisfactory explanation. In addition, a number of other investigators have failed to observe changes in 5-HT levels (Segal *et al.*, 1972) or turnover using different methods (see Algeri and Costa, 1971; Marshall and Grahame-Smith, 1970; Schecter *et al.*, 1972). Further studies will be needed to account for discrepant data. Since other transmitters are involved in morphine effects, a complex relationship between these compounds and drug action is likely. (See Chapter 6 for further details.)

Schedule-Controlled Behavior

In this section we will discuss the role of 5-HT in behavior that is maintained by either positive or negative reinforcement. The relative stability of schedule-controlled behavior makes it a very useful baseline for examining interactions between behavior and endogenous chemicals.

Positive Reinforcement. Aprison and colleagues (1965) observed the effects of serotonin elevation on behavior maintained by a multiple schedule of food presentation. Food-deprived pigeons were trained to peck a key for food presentation on a multiple FR 50 FI 10-min schedule. Sessions lasted either until the pigeons received 55 food presentations or until a six-hour period had passed. After repeated experience on this schedule, the distribution of responding characteristic of these schedules of reinforcement emerged. Because of the long FI requirement of the schedule, sessions lasted between three and four hours. Injections of 5-HTP (25–75 mg/kg) completely suppressed key pecking for a period of time called the "period of atypical responding" (see Fig. 4-6). The length of this period of atypical responding was related to the dose of 5-HTP. When pecking behavior returned later in the session, the rate and pattern of responding were normal.*

The suppression of key pecking by 5-HTP could be potentiated by pretreating the pigeons with an MAO inhibitor (iproniazid) which had no effect on the behavior when given alone. When MAO activity was reduced by iproniazid (which presumably increases serotonin content), a smaller dose of 5-HTP produced the same amount of behavioral suppression as when MAO activity was normal. This suggests that serotonin (i.e., the amine substrate of MAO) rather than 5-HTP itself (Fig. 4-7a) was responsible for the response suppression. The behavioral effects of 5-HTP were closely correlated with the degree of brain MAO inhibition (Fig. 4-7b).

These observations are consistent with the notion that free serotonin action on central receptor sites caused a depression of key pecking. Moreover, the time course of elevation of brain serotonin as a result of the 5-HTP treatment corresponded closely with the period of atypical behavior.

Negative Reinforcement. In the preceding pages evidence was presented that 5-HT plays a role in mediating responses to painful stimuli. Therefore, it is in-

---

*It is of interest that this same biphasic response pattern (i.e., suppression for a period of time followed by normal responding has been observed with LSD on an FR 30 schedule of reinforcement (Appel and Freedman, 1965).

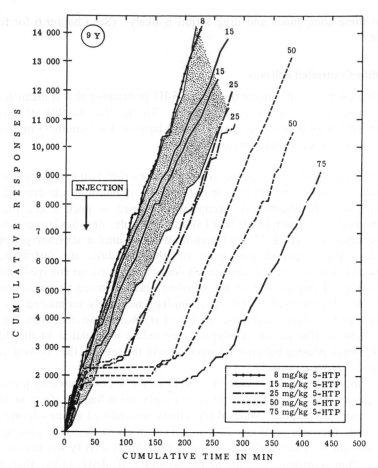

Fig. 4-6. Bird 9Y, a reduced plot of periods of a typical responding. Each curve is a reduced plot of responses cumulating against time for a single experimental session. The range of the control session is given by the stippled area, and the doses of the experimental sessions are marked on the curve (Aprison, 1965).

teresting to examine the role of 5-HT in behavior that is maintained by negative reinforcement, since shock is generally used as the negative reinforcing stimulus.

It has been shown that when PCPA was administered to rats 72, 48 and 24 hours prior to training, the rats learned to jump to a platform to avoid electrical shock in fewer trials than controls (Tenen, 1967). The facilitation of avoidance acquisition has been correlated with serotonin depletion. The effects could be antagonized by 5-HTP, but not by 5-HT, indicating that the effect was central rather than peripheral. Since serotonin has been implicated in sensitivity to

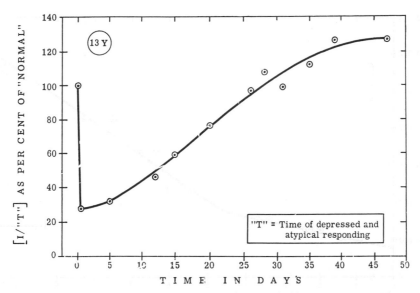

Fig. 4-7a. Potentiation of the effect of 5-HTP by iproniazid pretreatment. The curve expresses the behavioral effect, 1/"T", of a constant 5-HTP injection periodically given during 47 days following iproniazid treatment (Aprison, 1965).

stimuli such as shock (see pp. 95–98), it is important to examine the extent to which a facilitation in acquisition of an avoidance response might be due to increased sensitivity to shock. In addition, decreased emotional reactivity, increased general motor activity or increased learning ability,* might also account for the facilitation. Tenen examined each of these possibilities.

If increased sensitivity to shock were responsible for the more rapid acquisition of avoidance responding produced by PCPA, the use of a higher shock intensity should eliminate the differences between the animals treated with PCPA and the control animals. In the original experiment, the PCPA group took an average of 4.5 trials to acquire the avoidance response, while the controls took about 23 trials. Tenen repeated the experiment using a high level of shock intensity for both groups. With the higher shock level, both PCPA and control groups acquired the avoidance response in less than 5 trials. These data are consistent with the idea that increased sensitivity to shock leads to more rapid acquisition of avoidance responding and that PCPA depletion of serotonin is responsible for increased sensitivity to shock.

Tenen also argued that it was possible that changes in avoidance acquisition were a result of changes in emotional reactivity. Operationally, emotional re-

*Learning is defined as the ability to make a "meaningful association" between two discrete events, realizing that this ability is intimately tied to other factors (Tenen, 1967).

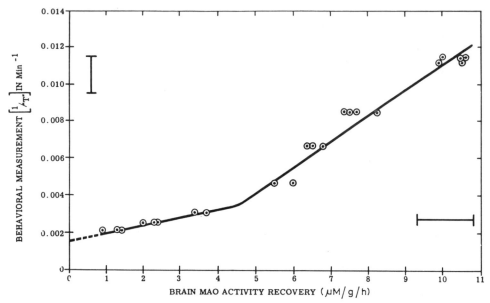

Fig. 4-7b. Correlation of the behavioral effect of 50 mg/kg of 5-HTP with the brain MAO activity current at the time of injection. The range of the behavioral measurement and brain MAO activity are given in the upper left- and lower right-hand part of the figure respectively. The behavioral measurement was expressed as $1/"T"$, the reciprocal of the time during which the bird's performance was depressed or atypical. Brain MAO activity was expressed as μmoles of $NH_3/gm/hr$ (Aprison, 1965).

activity may be defined as a response pattern consisting of crouching, freezing, defecating and urinating. Such responses might compete with the acquisition of the jumping response required in this avoidance paradigm. In order to determine whether the PCPA animals were less emotional than the control animals, Tenen used a modification of the conditioned suppression procedure (see Chapter 1, p. 22); a light was paired repeatedly with an unavoidable shock while rats were drinking. The suppression of drinking behavior during the light was used as the measure of emotionality. The PCPA animals exhibited a smaller decrease in drinking behavior during the conditioned suppression session than the control animals. Animals treated with PCPA *plus* 5-HTP also exhibited a smaller decrease in drinking than controls, however. Thus, while it appears that PCPA reduces emotionality as measured by this procedure, the fact that this reduction could not be antagonized by 5-HTP suggests that this particular effect may not be related to 5-HT.

Measurements of spontaneous motor activity in a jiggle cage revealed that the PCPA-treated animals were less active than control animals, thus tending to rule out increased motor activity as a factor in the facilitation of avoidance acquisition. Nevertheless, others (Brody, 1970; Jacobs *et al.*, 1974; Steranka and Barrett, 1974) have reported that rats with lesions of the median raphé nuclei which reduced telencephalic 5-HT had an increase in locomotor activity. Similarly, reduction in brain 5-HT by intraventricular injection of 5,6-dihydroxy-tryptamine was reported to increase the number of intertrial responses made by rats and to facilitate the acquisition of an avoidance response (Breese *et al.*, 1974). While the facilitated acquisition of the avoidance response is consistent with Tenen's results (1967), the Breese *et al.* study leaves open the possibility that the facilitated avoidance acquisition is related to increases in motor activity. These differences may stem from the different procedures used to reduce 5-HT or to measure locomotor activity. For example, 5-HT was reduced by either PCPA, raphé lesions or 5,6-DHT; and motor activity was measured in jiggle cages, a tilt cage or a two-way avoidance chamber.

Tenen also found that administration of PCPA did not facilitate learning to go to one side of a t-maze for food reinforcement. Therefore, it would appear that PCPA does not have direct effects on the ability to form associations. From these results, Tenen concluded that PCPA administration and the consequent depletion of serotonin produced an increase in sensitivity to electric shock which may partially explain the animal's more rapid acquisition of a discrete trial avoidance task. PCPA also decreased emotional reactivity, which may also help account for the effects of PCPA on the acquisition of an avoidance response.

Other investigators have also found that decreased levels of serotonin in brain facilitate the acquisition or maintenance of an avoidance response. Brody (1970) found increased acquisition of both one-way and two-way avoidance responding using PCPA to reduce 5-HT levels. Similarly, depletion of 5-HT by 5,6-DHT facilitated the acquisition of an avoidance task (Breese *et al.*, 1974), and administration of PCPA markedly increased the response rate in rats trained on a continuous avoidance paradigm (Tanaka *et al.*, 1972). Lesions in the raphé nucleus which reduce telencephalic 5-HT have also been reported to increase the rate of acquisition of an avoidance response (Lorens and Yunger, 1974; Steranka and Barrett, 1974). Hole and Lorens (1975), however, found a decreased rate of acquisition with somewhat more discrete lesions in the raphé which also caused 5-HT reductions. Generally, reduction in brain 5-HT leads to facilitated acquisition of avoidance responding. Whether or not the effect is mediated through a change in reactivity to shock, increased locomotor behavior, a combination of these two or another effect, is still not resolved.

Sleep

Recall from Chapter 1 (see pp. 8–9) that sleep is thought to consist of four stages which can be differentiated using an electroencephalograph and an electromyograph. These four stages are: (1) waking, which consists of a low voltage,

TABLE 4-2. Electroencephalographic and electromyographic correlates of sleep

Behavior	EEG	EMG
Waking	Low voltage, fast	Active
Slow wave sleep	High voltage, slow	Relaxed
Pre- and Postparadoxical sleep	High voltage, slow; PGO spike	Some activity
Paradoxical sleep	Low voltage, fast	Relaxed, REM

fast cortical EEG accompanied by an active electromyogram (EMG); (2) slow wave sleep, which consists of high voltage cortical and subcortical spindles with slow waves accompanied by a relaxed EMG; (3) pre- and postparadoxical sleep, which consists of slow wave sleep as in (2), accompanied by ponto-geniculo-occipital (PGO) spikes with a more active EMG; and (4) paradoxical sleep, which consists of a tonic component characterized by fast, low voltage activity and a phasic component consisting of rapid eye movements (50–60 per minute) and bursts of PGO spikes (Table 4-2). In most species, PGO activity almost invariably precedes paradoxical sleep for a period of 30–60 seconds.

For some time, sleep was considered to be a passive relaxation of the reticular formation, since stimulation of the reticular activating system (RAS) located in the medullary and pontine reticular formation was found to lead to the electrocortical features of wakefulness and behavioral arousal. Later work indicated that sleep was in part the result of active influence originating from discrete neuroanatomical structures located in the raphé system. Sleep can be triggered by central stimulation; moreover, certain limited brain-stem lesions can produce total insomnia.

Jouvet and his colleagues (1969, 1973) investigated the involvement of serotonin in the underlying mechanisms leading to the active processes involved in both slow wave sleep (SS) and paradoxical sleep (PS) in cats. Jouvet evolved the following theory about the pathways and neurochemicals important in the mediation of paradoxical and slow wave sleep. He proposed that the transition from wakefulness to slow wave sleep is dependent on the serotonin-containing cells of the raphé system and that the initiation of paradoxical sleep is dependent on several neurochemicals including 5-hydroxyindoleacetic acid (5-HIAA), acetylcholine (ACh) and norepinephrine. Jouvet drew on several lines of evidence to support the idea that serotonin is involved in the elaboration of slow wave sleep (see Table 4-3 for a summary of this evidence). Chicks whose blood-brain barrier is permeable to serotonin show signs of slow wave sleep when injected with 0.1–2.0 mg/kg of serotonin (Spooner and Winters, 1966, 1967). 5-HTP can induce some of the EEG characteristics of slow wave sleep in mammals whose blood-brain barrier is not permeable to serotonin; high voltage slow waves are seen, but the subject does not appear to be asleep. Moreover, MAO

TABLE 4-3. Evidence for serotonin (5-HT) involvement in sleep

Manipulation	Biochemical effect	Behavior
5-HTP administration	Increase 5-HT	High voltage, slow wave EEG, subject awake
MAO inhibitor administration	Increase 5-HT	Increase slow wave sleep, suppress paradoxical sleep
Reserpine administration	Decrease 5-HT	Suppress slow wave sleep, suppress paradoxical sleep, trigger PGO activity
Replacement with:		
a. 5-HTP	Increase 5-HT	Slow wave sleep returns
b. L-dopa	Increase CA	Slow wave sleep returns, paradoxical sleep returns
PCPA administration	Decrease 5-HT	Insomnia
Raphé lesion	Decrease 5-HT	Insomnia

inhibitors often cause an increase in slow wave sleep, but suppress paradoxical sleep in the cat for several weeks; following termination of MAO inhibition, there is a rebound of paradoxical sleep, and slow wave sleep is decreased.

Furthermore, drugs such as reserpine which deplete serotonin cause a decrease in the amount of slow wave sleep in cats. Twenty-four hours after reserpine administration, a low voltage fast EEG with continuous bursts of PGO spikes is seen; no paradoxical sleep is apparent when slow wave sleep has been suppressed, in spite of the fact that the animal looks sedated and often appears asleep. Interestingly, the EMG does not show relaxation even during periods of PGO activity. Slow wave sleep is suppressed for 12 to 14 hours, and paradoxical sleep is suppressed completely for 22 to 24 hours; PGO spikes are prominent for 50 to 60 hours; control levels of PGO activity are reached only after five to six days. This indicates that reserpine selectively induces PGO activity which becomes dissociated from paradoxical sleep. Replacement of serotonin through the administration of 5-HTP produces the signs of slow wave sleep (both EEG and EMG); this is a temporary phenomenon, however, lasting four to six hours after 5-HTP administration. In addition, 5-HTP suppresses reserpine-induced PGO activity for a duration of about four to six hours. Replacement of depleted catecholamines by L-dopa induces both slow wave sleep and paradoxical sleep. As with 5-HTP, the effects of L-dopa are temporary and last between five and six hours. Depletion of serotonin by PCPA leads to total insomnia beginning 30 hours after the injection of PCPA, suggesting that the effect is due to the depletion of 5-HT rather than a direct effect of PCPA. Furthermore, the insomnia induced by serotonin depletion can be antagonized by replacement of 5-HT. A similar correlation between slow wave sleep and the decrease in cerebral 5-HT has been reported by others (Koella *et al.*, 1968; Pujol *et al.*, 1971).

Additional evidence (Jouvet 1969, 1973) for a role of serotonin in the elaboration of slow wave sleep comes from studies in which the raphé system of cats was selectively lesioned. Neurochemical assays and histological reconstruction of raphé lesions in the same animal demonstrated an excellent correlation between the extent of the raphé lesion and the amount of serotonin depleted from brain. Further, there was a correlation between the percentage of waking time (i.e., insomnia) and the amount of 5-HT depletion. The role for serotonin in the elaboration of sleep is therefore probably best supported by three lines of evidence: (1) reserpine produces changes in both slow wave sleep and paradoxical sleep which are antagonized by 5-HTP; (2) PCPA produces insomnia which is antagonized by 5-HTP; and (3) raphé lesions produce a concomitant depletion of serotonin and induction of insomnia.

Jouvet and his colleagues have also presented evidence that catecholamine neurons play a role in general arousal. Furthermore, Jouvet concluded that norepinephrine (NE) and not dopamine (DA) is the important transmitter in arousal, since lesions which selectively decrease DA levels in brain do not interfere with arousal, but lesions which reduce NE content decrease central arousal and lead to hypersomnia (Jouvet, 1972). The hypersomnia (increase in both slow wave sleep and paradoxical sleep) is accompanied by an increase in the turnover rate of 5-HT (Petitjean and Jouvet, 1970). As a result of several studies with different lesions which reduce DA or 5-HT in brain, Jouvet (1973) has concluded that the sleep-waking cycle is regulated by two opposing systems of neurons (Jouvet and Pujol, 1974): the 5-HT neurons for inducing slow wave sleep and priming paradoxical sleep and the noradrenergic system for waking and paradoxical sleep.

Several attempts have been made to replicate Jouvet's findings. Mouret *et al.* (1968) found that a large single dose of PCPA produced a 70% decrease in total sleep time in rats; however, Rechtschaffen *et al.* (1969, 1973) did not replicate this effect in rats. While both groups of investigators found that PCPA had a similar effect on brain serotonin, each reported different effects on sleep. Rechtschaffen and his colleagues (1973) explored several variables such as prior sleep deprivation, dose of PCPA, environmental noise and the time of day at which the effects on sleep were measured. None of these variables could adequately account for the differences in PCPA effects on sleep observed in the two laboratories. Since these conflicting results remain unexplained, the generality of these findings is limited, at least in rats.

Jouvet's work has been replicated and extended by others in cats (Dement *et al.*, 1973; Henriksen *et al.*, 1974). In these experiments, PCPA was administered daily and the amount of slow wave sleep was dramatically reduced between days 2 and 6 after PCPA administration. By day 8 slow wave sleep returned to normal in spite of the fact that 5-HT was still 90% depleted. The primary effect of 5-HT reduction in these studies was on the regulation of PGO spikes. Under normal circumstances, PGO spikes occur before and sometimes during paradoxical sleep; but after 5-HT depletion, the PGO spikes were found to occur during all EEG states, with the exception of very strong behavioral arousal. The changes in PGO spike activity more directly parallel 5-HT alterations than do changes in any other sleep state measured.

The data reviewed in this section concerning the role of 5-HT in sleep indicate that 5-HT plays a role in the various stages of sleep. The data also indicate that the role of 5-HT in the production of sleep in the rat is currently contradictory, which limits conclusions about the general role of 5-HT in sleep in all species. The data also indicate that other important neurochemical factors may also be important determinants of sleep. (See also Jouvet, 1972; King, 1974.)

Aggressive Behavior

In this section, we will discuss the relationship of 5-HT to a limited range of aggressive behaviors in mice or rats under controlled experimental conditions. As we shall see, even with the limited studies in rodents, there is no clear-cut role for brain 5-HT in agression, although existing data clearly point to involvement of 5-HT (Eichelman and Thoa, 1973; Reis, 1974).

Prolonged isolation produces an increase in aggressiveness in male mice. Therefore, attempts have been made to correlate changes in 5-HT metabolism with changes in aggressive behavior in isolated mice. In one experiment (Giacalone et al., 1968) mice were housed alone or in groups of 5, 10 or 20 for 1, 5, 10, 20 or 28 days. Aggression was measured by the frequency of approaches, attacks and biting. Following 28 days of isolation, brain levels of serotonin and catecholamines were within normal limits; however, 5-HIAA levels were consistently lower in isolated mice, suggesting that 5-HT turnover rates were decreased as a result of isolation. MAO levels were also lower in the isolated animals. Metabolic studies indicated that the rate of synthesis and turnover of 5-HT were decreased as a result of isolation. It is important to note that while isolation-induced aggression does not appear in all mice (Goldberg et al., 1973), the decrease in 5-HT turnover appeared only in those mice which showed isolation-induced aggression (Valzelli, 1974). Isolation-induced aggression can be decreased by administration of PCPA (Welch and Welch, 1968), or by a lesion of the raphé (Kostowski and Valzelli, 1974), both of which deplete serotonin. Thus it appears that while a decrease in 5-HT turnover is correlated with an increase in aggression, blockade of serotonin synthesis by PCPA or reduction in serotonin levels by raphé lesions blocks isolation-induced aggressiveness. These two contradictory results are not readily explainable.

The role of 5-HT in aggressive behavior in rats has also been explored with drugs and lesions which affect brain 5-HT. The two procedures most commonly used to examine aggressive behavior in rats are muricide and shock-induced fighting. Recall from Chapter 1 that the muricide procedure consists of placing a mouse in a cage with a rat and observing the incidence of mouse killing. In the shock-induced fighting procedure, two rats are placed together in a small compartment, and they are shocked repeatedly. This situation usually elicits fighting between the two rats, which is measured by observing: (1) typical "pre-fight" postures that the rats exhibit toward one another, (2) the number of physical contacts made by the rats in this pre-fight posture and (3) the amount of biting that occurs between the two rats (see Moyer, 1968; Eichelman and Thoa, 1973).

Muricide has been shown to increase in several situations. For example, PCPA has been found to dramatically increase the frequency of muricide in rats (Sheard, 1969; DiChiara et al., 1971). Rats with septal lesions that cause a small decrease in brain 5-HT levels also show muricidal behavior, which can be blocked by PCPA administration (Dominguez and Longo, 1969). Moreover, muricide is also increased by the administration of 5,6-DHT either in the raphé region of the brain or intracisternally, which causes a marked reduction of 5-HT content in brain (Breese et al., 1974). Prolonged isolation can also produce an increase in muricidal behavior in rats, but the effects are variable (Valzelli, 1974).

While shock-induced fighting in rats has been reported following electrolytic lesions of the raphé which reduce 5-HT content in brain, PCPA has no effect on shock-induced fighting in rats (Conner et al., 1973). It might also be noted that increased attack behavior, especially toward handlers, has been reported in cats after PCPA administration (Ferguson et al., 1970), but this observation is not always confirmed (Zitrin et al., 1970).

It would be difficult, to make any consistent generalizations about the role of 5-HT in aggression from these data. Since different species, behavioral procedures and means of producing changes in 5-HT content have been used in these experiments, further detailed research into this question is necessary to ascertain the precise role of 5-HT in the various types of behavior labeled aggressive.

Sexual Behavior

There is considerable evidence to support the view that brain 5-HT partly mediates copulatory behavior in male and female rat and cat. Administration of PCPA arouses sexual activity in male rats (Sheard, 1969). For example, when isolated male rats were given PCPA (100mg/kg) for a period of four days and then placed together, the frequency of male mounting behavior increased dramatically over that of rats which received control injections (Tagliamonte et al., 1969). Rats treated with PCPA exhibited other signs of sexual behavior, such as increased grooming, scratching and mutual smelling of the genitalia.

The sexual excitation induced by PCPA was blocked by 5-hydroxytryptophan (5-HTP) but potentiated by the MAO inhibitor pargyline (Ahlenius *et al.*, 1971). Therefore, when 5-HT levels were reduced by PCPA and CA levels were increased by pargyline, sexual behavior increased. The authors suggested that expression of sexual behavior is under the control of both the catecholaminergic and the serotonergic systems; the former being excitatory and the latter inhibitory (Gessa and Tagliamonte, 1974). Similar increases in sexual behavior caused by depletion of 5-HT and an increase in CAs were reported in a heterosexual situation where the frequency of copulation and ejaculation were measured (Tagliamonte *et al.*, 1971). Reduction of 5-HT by 5,6-DHT has also been shown to lead to an increase in mounting behavior (Da Prada *et al.*, 1972; Breese *et al.*, 1974).

The increases in sexual behavior seen following PCPA can be blocked by castration; however, they are restored when testosterone is given (Gessa *et al.*, 1970). While these results suggest that the effects of PCPA on sexual behavior are dependent on testosterone in male rats, Bond *et al.* (1972) reported increased sexual behavior in castrated male rats following PCPA. Factors such as age, time of testing, drug dose and different measures of sexual behavior may account for these differences.

The lordosis response in female rats is inhibited by 5-HT, although there also seem to be other transmitters of importance in the lordosis response (see Meyerson *et al.*, 1973; Meyerson *et al.*, 1974). There is some evidence to suggest that progesterone may act to suppress 5-HT in brain, but this has not been clearly demonstrated (see also Södersten and Ahlenius, 1972).

Ferguson *et al.* (1970) reported hypersexuality after daily administration of PCPA to normal male cats. Hypersexuality was defined as the tendency of one male cat to attempt intercourse with another male cat. These changes appeared three to five days after the beginning of PCPA treatment and were presumed to be mediated by either lack of sleep caused by the PCPA and/or depletion of serotonin. Administration of 5-HTP caused a reduction in the abnormal behavior for about eight hours. The mounting of male cats suggested changes in perception induced by PCPA; observation of abnormal rapid eye movements, staring at fixed points and inappropriate hissing responses were consistent with this interpretation. In a later study, Whalen and Luttge (1970) found that PCPA increased the frequency of homosexual, but not of heterosexual mounting behavior in cats. Frequency of intromission was not changed by PCPA treatment. On the other hand, Zitrin *et al.* (1970) observed no changes in heterosexual or aggressive behavior in cats following PCPA administration. The reasons for these discrepancies are not apparent. It should be noted that each study used different methods to quantify sexual behavior. The dose of PCPA used also differed, as well as the number of times the drug was administered during testing. Moreover, PCPA also depletes NE (Koe and Weissman, 1966). The extent and duration of this depletion depends on both the dose and the frequency of PCPA administration. In the absence of 5-HT and NE measurements, one cannot assess the relative importance of any one amine in this effect.

Seizure Susceptibility

The incidence of spontaneous seizures and seizure characteristics vary widely between animal species; in vertebrates, a seizure pattern is characterized by two distinct motor components: clonic and tonic. A clonic seizure involves persistent involuntary jerking movements of the limbs and neck (flexor-extensor alteration). The movements are uncoordinated and rapid enough to resemble tremor. The tonic phase consists of a coordinated movement where extensor muscles take over completely. Clonic-tonic seizures in humans are referred to as grand mal seizures and do not occur frequently in animals. However, clonic-tonic seizures can be triggered in various animals by loud sounds, flashing lights, strong electrical shock or chemicals. Seizures induced by these stimuli have been used as an animal model for studying the biochemical basis of seizures. They are also used as screening procedures for antiepileptic drugs. It must be borne in mind that susceptibility to seizures produced by these techniques varies widely with species and age. However, in spite of the qualifications and difficulties involved, it seems fair to say that there is a possible role for serotonin as well as other endogenous neurochemicals in seizure susceptibility.

Reserpine causes increased susceptibility to induced seizures both in mice and rats. Koe and Weissman (1968) have found that PCPA reduces the shock threshold for seizures in rats. In mice, audiogenic seizures facilitated by reserpine can be prevented by administration of 5-HTP (Boggan, 1973; Koe and Weissman, 1968). Further evidence for an involvement of 5-HT in seizure activity derives from two inbred strains of mice which differentially display audiogenic seizures. At 21 days of age, one strain shows high susceptibility to seizure while the other does not. Furthermore, the F_1 hybrid of these two strains shows seizure susceptibility intermediate between the two strains (Schlesinger et al., 1965). Brain levels of 5-HT and NE were determined in all three strains and an inverse correlation was found between seizure susceptibility and 5-HT and NE levels. These differences in amine levels were found only at the time of maximum seizure susceptibility (see also Kellogg, 1971; Boggan, 1973; Schreiber and Schlesinger, 1971; Wada et al., 1972).

SUMMARY

Although there is not complete agreement about the data or their interpretation, the weight of the evidence from the studies cited in this chapter indicates that a decrease in the brain content of 5-HT results in the following:

1. Increased sensitivity to stimuli such as heat and shock
2. Increased wakefulness, i.e., loss of sleep
3. Increased aggressive behavior
4. Increased sexual behavior
5. Increased susceptibility to seizures

In addition, studies have demonstrated that animals acquire an avoidance response more quickly when brain 5-HT levels are lowered, although there is no agreement as to whether or not the increased rate of avoidance acquisition can be related to changes in sensitivity to shock or increased motor activity, or both.

If a decrease in brain 5-HT content causes an increase in the types of behaviors noted above, then it is reasonable to infer that these behaviors are decreased when 5-HT content in brain is normal. One might conceive of a given behavior as under the control of both excitatory and inhibitory influences. For example, in the ANS, contraction of the stomach is under the control of both the parasympathetic (excitation) and sympathetic (inhibition) branches of the ANS. Similarly, the 5-HT system in brain might play an inhibitory role in the regulation of several behaviors.

REFERENCES

Ahlenius, S., H. Eriksson, K. Larsson, K. Modigh and P. Södersten. 1971. Mating behavior in the male rat treated with p-chlorophenylalanine methyl ester alone and in combination with pargyline. *Psychopharmacologia* 20: 383–388.

Algeri, S. and E. Costa. 1971. Physical dependence on morphine fails to increase serotonin turnover rate in rat brain. *Biochem. Pharmacol.* 20: 877–884.

Anden, N. E., K. Fuxe and K. Larsson. 1966. Effect of large mesencephalic-diencephalic lesions on the noradrenalin, dopamine and 5-hydroxytryptamine neurons of the central nervous system. *Experientia* 22: 842–843.

Appel, J. B. and D. X. Freedman. 1965. The relative potencies of psychotomimetic drugs. *Life Sci.* 4: 2181–2186.

Aprison, M. H. 1965. Research approaches to problems in mental illness: Brain neurohumor-enzyme systems and behavior. *Prog. Brain Res.* 16: 48–80.

Baumgarten, H. G., A. Björklund, L. Lachenmayer, A. Nobin and U. Stenevi. 1971. Long-lasting selective depletion of brain serotonin by 5,6-dihydroxytryptamine. *Acta Physiol. Scand.* Suppl. 373: 1–15.

Björklund, A., H. G. Baumgarten and A. Nobin. 1974. Chemical lesioning of central monoamine axons by means of 5,6-dihydroxytryptamine and 5,7-dihydroxytryptamine. *Advances in Biochemical Psychopharmacology* 10: 13–33.

Björklund, A., B. Falck and U. Stenevi. 1971. Classification of monoamine neurons in the rat mesencephalon: distribution of new monoamine neuron system. *Brain Res.* 23: 269–285.

Boggan, W. O. 1973. Serotonin and convulsions. *In* J. Barchas and E. Usdin (eds.), *Serotonin and Behavior*. Academic Press, New York and London, pp. 167–172.

Bond, V. J., E. E. Shillito and M. Vogt. 1972. Influence of age and of testosterone on the response of male rats to parachlorophenylalanine. *Brit. J. Pharmacol.* 46:46–55.

Breese, G. R., B. R. Cooper, L. D. Grant and R. D. Smith. 1974. Biochemical and behavioural alterations following 5,6-dihydroxytryptamine administration into brain.
Neuropharmacology **13**: 177–187.

Brodie, B. B. and P. A. Shore. 1957. A concept for a role of serotonin and norepinephrine
as chemical mediators in the brain. *Ann. N.Y. Acad. Sci.* **66**: 631–642.

Brody, J. F., Jr. 1970. Behavioral effects of serotonin depletion and of parachlorophenylalanine (a serotonin depleter) in rats. *Psychopharmacologia* **17**: 14–33.

Carlsson, A., J. Jonason, M. Lindqvist and K. Fuxe. 1969. Demonstration of extraneuronal
5-hydroxytryptamine accumulation in brain following membrane-pump blockade by
chlorimipramine. *Brain Res.* **12**: 456–460.

Carlsson, A., M. Lindqvist, and T. Magnusson. 1957a. 3,4-dihydroxyphenylalanine and
5-hydroxytryptophan as reserpine antagonists. *Nature* **180**:1200.

Carlsson, A., E. Rosengren, A. Bertler and J. Nilsson. 1957b. Effect of reserpine on the
metabolism of the catecholamines. *In* S. Garattini and V. Ghetti (eds.), *Psychotropic
Drugs*. Elsevier Press, Amsterdam, pp. 363–372.

Chase, T. N. and D. L. Murphy. 1973. Serotonin and central nervous system function.
Ann. Rev. Pharmacol. **13**: 181–197.

Cheney, D. L., A. Goldstein, S. Algeri and E. Costa. 1971. Narcotic tolerance and dependence: Lack of relationship with serotonin turnover in the brain. *Science* **171**:1169–1170.

Conner, R. L., J. M. Stolk and S. Levine. 1973. Effects of PCPA on fighting behavior
and habituation of the startle response in rats. *In* J. Barchas and E. Usdin (eds.),
Serotonin and Behavior. Academic Press, New York and London, pp. 325–333.

Costa, E., J. Daly, H. LeFevre, J. Meek, A. Revuelta, F. Spano and S. Strada. 1972. Serotonin and catecholamine concentrations in brain of rats injected intracerebrally with
5,6-dihydroxytryptamine. *Brain Res.* **44**: 304–308.

Da Prada, M., M. Carruba, R. A. O'Brien, A. Saner and A. Pletscher. 1972. The effect
of 5,6-dihydroxytryptamine on sexual behaviour of male rats. *Eur. J. Pharmacol.* **19**:
288–290.

Dement, W. C., S. Henriksen and J. Ferguson. 1973. The effect of the chronic administration of *para*chlorophenylanine (PCPA) on sleep parameters in the cat. *In* J. Barchas and
E. Usdin (eds.), *Serotonin and Behavior*. Academic Press, New York and London, pp.
419–424.

DiChiara, G., R. Cambra and P. F. Spano. 1971. Evidence for inhibition by brain serotonin of mouse killing behaviour in rats. *Nature* **233**:272–273.

Dominguez, M. and V. G. Longo. 1969. Taming effects of para-chlorophenylalanine on
septal rats. *Physiol. Behav.* **4**:1031–1033.

Eichelman, B. S., Jr. and N. B. Thoa. 1973. The aggressive monoamines. *Biol. Psychiat.*
6:143–164.

Ferguson, J., S. Henriksen, H. Cohen, G. Mitchell, T. Barcas and W. Dement. 1970. Hypersexuality and behavioral changes in cats caused by administration of *p*-chlorophenylal-
anine. *Science* **168**:499–501.

Fuxe, K. and G. Jonsson. 1974. Further mapping of central 5-hydroxytryptamine neurons:
Studies with the neurotoxic dihydroxytryptamines. *Advances in Biochemical Psychopharmacology* **10**:1–12.

Gessa, G. L. and A. Tagliamonte. 1974. Possible role of brain serotonin and dopamine in
controlling male sexual behavior. *Advances in Biochemical Psychopharmacology* **11**:
217–228.

Gessa, G. L., A. Tagliamonte, P. Tagliamonte and B. B. Brodie. 1970. Essential role of
testosterone in the sexual stimulation induced by *p*-chlorophenylalanine in male
animals. *Nature* **227**: 616–617.

Giacalone, E., M. Tensella, L. Valzelli and S. Garattini. 1968. Brain serotonin metabolism in isolated aggressive mice. *Biochem. Pharmacol.* **17**: 1315-1327.

Goldberg, M. E., B. Dubnick, M. Hefner and A. Salama. 1973. Influence of chlorpromazine on brain serotonin turnover and body temperature in isolated aggressive mice. *Neuropharmacology* **12**: 249-260.

Harvey, J. A. and L. M. Yunger. 1973. Relationship between telencephalic content of serotonin and pain sensitivity. *In* J. Barchas and E. Usdin (eds.), *Serotonin and Behavior.* Academic Press, New York and London, pp. 179-189.

Harvey, J. A., A. J. Schlosberg and L. M. Yunger. 1974. Effect of *p*-chlorophenylalanine and brain lesions on pain sensitivity and morphine analgesia in the rat. *Advances in Biochemical Psychopharmacology* **10**: 233-245.

Heller, A., J. A. Harvey and R. Y. Moore. 1962. A demonstration of a fall in brain serotonin following central nervous system lesions in the rat. *Biochem. Pharmacol.* **11**:859-866.

Henriksen, S., W. Dement and J. Barchas. 1974. The role of serotonin in the regulation of a phasic event of rapid eye movement sleep: The ponto-geniculo-occipital wave. *Advances in Biochemical Psychopharmacology* **11**: 169-179.

Hole, K. and S. A. Lorens. 1975. Response to electric shock in rats: Effects of selective midbrain raphe lesions. *Pharmacol. Biochem. Behav.* **3**:95-102.

Holzbauer, M. and M. Vogt. 1956. Depression by reserpine of the noradrenaline concentration of the hypothalamus of the cat. *J. Neurochem.* **1**:8-11.

Jacobs, B. L., W. D. Wise and K. M. Taylor. 1974. Differential behavioral and neurochemical effects following lesions of the dorsal or median raphe nuclei in rats. *Brain Res.* **79**:353-361.

Jouvet, M. 1969. Biogenic amines and the states of sleep. *Science* **163**:32-41.

Jouvet, M. 1972. The role of monoamines and acetylcholine containing neurons in the regulation of the sleep-waking cycle. *Ergebn. Physiol.* **64**:166-307.

Jouvet, M. 1973. Serotonin and sleep in the cat. *In* J. Barchas and E. Usdin (eds.), *Serotonin and Behavior.* Academic Press, New York and London, pp. 385-400.

Jouvet, M. and J. F. Pujol. 1974. Effects of central alterations of serotoninergic neurons upon the sleep waking cycle. *Advances in Biochemical Psychopharmacology* **11**:199-209.

Kellogg, C. 1971. Serotonin metabolism in the brains of mice sensitive or resistant to audiogenic seizures. *J. Neurobiol.* **2**:209-219.

King, C. D. 1974. 5-hydroxytryptamine and sleep in the cat: A brief overview. *Advances in Biochemical Psychopharmacology* **11**:211-216.

Koe, B. K. and A. Weissman. 1966. *p*-Chlorophenylalanine: A specific depletor of brain serotonin. *J. Pharmacol. Exp. Ther.* **154**:499-516.

Koe, B. K. and A. Weissman. 1968. The pharmacology of *p*-chlorophenylalanine, a selective depletor of serotonin stores. *Adv. Pharm.* **6B**: 29-48.

Koella, W. P., A. Feldstein and J. S. Czicman. 1968. The effect of para-chlorophenylalanine on the sleep of cats. *EEG Clin. Neurophysiol.* **25**:481-490.

Koslow, S. H. and A. R. Green. 1973. Analysis of pineal and brain indole alkyl-amines by gas chromatography-mass spectrometry. *Adv. Biochem. Psychopharmacol.* **7**:33-43.

Kostowski, W. and L. Valzelli. 1974. Biochemical and behavioral effects of lesions of raphe nuclei in aggressive mice. *Pharmacol. Biochem. Behav.* **2**:277-280.

Krnjevic, K. 1974. Chemical nature of synaptic transmission in vertebrates. *Physiol. Rev.* **54**:418-540.

Lints, C. E. and J. A. Harvey. 1969. Altered sensitivity to footshock and decreased brain content of serotonin following brain lesions in the rat. *J. Comp. Physiol. Psychol.* **67**:23-32.

Longo, V. G., A. Scotti de Carolis, A. Liuzzi and M. Massotti. 1974. A study of the central effects of 5,6-dihydroxytryptamine. *Advances in Biochemical Psychopharmacology* **10**:109–120.

Lorens, S. A. and L. M. Yunger. 1974. Morphine analgesia, two-way avoidance and consummatory behavior following lesions in the midbrain raphe nuclei of the rat. *Pharmac. Biochem. Behav.* **2**:215–221.

Macchitelli, F. J., D. Fischetti and N. Jr. Montanerelli. 1966. Changes in behavior and electrocortical activity in the monkey following administration of 5-hydroxytryptophan. *Psychopharmacologia* **9**:447–456.

Marshall, I. and D. G. Grahame-Smith. 1970. Unchanged rate of brain serotonin synthesis during chronic morphine treatment and failure of parachlorophenylalanine to attenuate withdrawal syndrome in mice. *Nature* **228**:1206–1208.

Meyerson, B. J., H. Carrer and M. Eliasson. 1974. 5-hydroxytryptamine and sexual behavior in the female rat. *Advances in Biochemical Psychopharmacology* **11**:229–242.

Meyerson, B. J., M. Eliasson, L. Lindstrom, A. Michanek and A. C. Soderlund. 1973. Monoamines and female sexual behavior. *In* T. A. Ban, J. R. Boisser, G. J. Gessa, H. Heimann, L. Hollister, H. E. Lehmann, I. Munkvad, H. Steinberg, F. Sulser, A. Sundwall, and O. Vinar (eds.), *Psychopharmacology, Sexual Disorders and Drug Abuse.* North Holland Publ. Co., Amsterdam, Holland, pp. 463–472.

Miller, F. P., R. H. Cox Jr., W. R. Snodgrass and R. P. Maickel. 1970. Comparative effects of *p*-chlorophenylalanine, *p*-chloroamphetamine, and *p*-chloro-N-methylamphetamine on rat brain norepinephrine, serotonin and 5-hydroxyindole-3-acetic acid. *Biochem. Pharmacol.* **19**:435–442.

Mouret, J., P. Bobillier and M. Jouvet. 1968. Insomnia following *p*-chlorophenylalanine in the rat. *Eur. J. Pharmacol.* **5**:17–22.

Moyer, K. E. 1968. Kinds of aggression and their physiological basis. *Commun. Behav. Biol. Part A* **2**:65–87.

Petitjean, F. and M. Jouvet. 1970. Hypersomnie et augmentation de l'acide 5-hydroxyindolacetique cerebral par lesion isthmique chez le chat. *Comptes Rendus de la Société de Biologie* **164**:2288–2293.

Pujol, J. F., A. Buguet, J. L. Froment, B. Jones and M. Jouvet. 1971. The central metabolism of serotonin in the cat during insomnia: A neurophysiological and biochemical study after *p*-chlorophenylalanine or destruction of the raphé system. *Brain Res.* **29**:195–212.

Rechtschaffen, A., R. A. Lovell, D. X. Freedman, P. K. Whitehead and M. Aldrich. 1969. Effect of parachlorophenylalanine on sleep in rats. *Psychophysiology* **6**:223.

Rechtschaffen, A., R. A. Lovell, D. X. Freedman, W. E. Whitehead and M. Aldrich. 1973. The effect of parachlorophenylalanine on sleep in the rat: Some implications for the serotonin sleep-hypothesis. *In* J. Barchas and E. Usdin (eds.), *Serotonin and Behavior.* Academic Press, New York and London, pp. 401–418.

Reis, D. J. 1974. Central neurotransmitters in aggression. *Res. Publ. Assoc. Res. Nerv. Ment. Dis.* **52**:119–148.

Samanin, R., W. Gumulka and L. Valzelli. 1970. Reduced effect of morphine in mid-brain raphé lesioned rats. *Eur. J. Pharmacol.* **10**:339–343.

Sanders-Bush, E. and F. Sulser. 1970. Biochemical considerations in the mode of action of *p*-chloroamphetamine. *In* E. Costa and S. Garatinni (eds.), *Amphetamines and Related Compounds.* Raven Press, New York, pp. 349–355.

Sanders-Bush, E., D. A. Gallager and F. Sulser. 1974. On the mechanism of brain 5-hydroxytryptamine depletion by *p*-chloroamphetamine and related drugs and the specificity of their action. *Advances in Biochemical Psychopharmacology* **10**:185–194.

Schechter, P. J., W. Lovenberg and A. Sjoerdsma. 1972. Dissociation of morphine tolerance and dependence from brain serotonin synthesis rate in mice. *Biochem. Pharmacol.* 21:751–753.

Schlesinger, K., W. O. Boggan and D. X. Freedman. 1965. Genetics of audiogenic seizures: I. Relation to brain serotonin and norepinephrine in mice. *Life Sci.* 4:2345–2351.

Schreiber, R. A. and K. Schlesinger. 1971. Circadian rhythms and seizure susceptibility: Relation to 5-hydroxytryptamine and norepinephrine in brain. *Physiol. Behav.* 6:635–640.

Segal, M., G. A. Deneau and M. H. Seevers. 1972. Levels and distribution of central nervous system amines in normal and morphine-dependent monkeys. *Neuropharmacology* 11:211–222.

Sheard, M. 1969. The effect of *p*-chlorophenylalanine on behavior in rats: Relation to brain serotonin and 5-hydroxyindoleacetic acid. *Brain Res.* 15:524–528.

Shen, F. H., H. H. Loh and E. L. Way. 1970. Brain serotonin turnover in morphine tolerant and dependent mice. *J. Pharmacol. Exp. Ther.* 175:427–434.

Södersten, P. and S. Ahlenius. 1972. Female lordosis behavior in estrogen-primed male rats treated with *p*-chlorophenylalanine or alpha-methyl-*p*-tyrosine. *Hormones Behav.* 3:181–189.

Spooner, C. E. and W. D. Winters. 1966. Neuropharmacological profile of the young chick. *Int. J. Neuropharmacol.* 5:217–236.

Spooner, C. E. and W. D. Winters. 1967. The influence of centrally active amine induced blood pressure changes on electroencephalogram and behavior. *Int. J. Neuropharmacol.* 6:109–118.

Steranka, L. R. and R. J. Barrett. 1974. Facilitation of avoidance acquisition by lesion of the median raphé nucleus: Evidence for serotonin as a mediator of shock-induced suppression. *Behav. Biol.* 11:205–213.

Tagliamonte, A., P. Tagliamonte, G. L. Gessa and B. B. Brodie. 1969. Compulsive sexual activity induced by *p*-chlorophenylalanine in normal and pinealectomized rats. *Science* 166:1433–1435.

Tagliamonte, A., P. Tagliamonte and G. L. Gessa. 1971. Reversal of pargyline-induced inhibition of sexual behaviour in male rats by *p*-chlorophenylalanine. *Nature* 230:244–245.

Tanaka, C., Y. Yoh and S. Takaori. 1972. Relationship between brain monoamine levels and Sidman avoidance behavior in rats treated with tyrosine and tryptophan hydroxylase inhibitors. *Brain Res.* 45:153–164.

Tenen, S. S. 1967. The effects of *p*-chlorophenylalanine, a serotonin depletor, on avoidance acquisition, pain sensitivity and related behavior in the rat. *Psychopharmacologia* 10:204–219.

Tenen, S. S. 1968. Antagonism of the analgesic effect of morphine and other drugs by *p*-chlorophenylalanine, a serotonin depletor. *Psychopharmacologia* 12:278–285.

Valzelli, L. 1974. 5-Hydroxytryptamine in aggressiveness. *Advances in Biochemical Psychopharmacology* 11:255–263.

Wada, J. A., E. Balzamo, B. S. Meldrum and R. Naquet. 1972. Behavioral and electrographic effects of L-5-hydroxytryptophan and D,L-para-chlorophenylalanine on epileptic senegalese baboon (*Papio papio*). *EEG Clin. Neurophysiol.* 33:520–526.

Way, E. L. 1972. Role of serotonin in morphine effects. *Fed. Proc.* 31:113–120.

Weissman, A. 1973. Behavioral pharmacology of parachlorophenylalanine (PCPA). *In* J. Barchas and E. Usdin (eds.), *Serotonin and Behavior*. Academic Press, New York and London, pp. 235–248.

Welch, A. S. and B. L. Welch. 1968. Effect of stress and para-chlorophenylalanine upon brain serotonin, 5-hydroxyindoleacetic acid and catecholamines in grouped and isolated mice. *Biochem. Pharmacol.* 17:699–708.

Whalen, R. E. and W. G. Luttge. 1970. *p*-Chlorophenylalanine methyl ester: an aphrodisiac? *Science* 169:1000–1001.

Zitrin, A., F. A. Beach, J. D. Barchas and W. C. Dement. 1970. Sexual behavior of male cats after administration of parachlorophenylalanine. *Science* 170:868–870.

5
Dopamine, Norepinephrine and Behavior

Brain catecholamines play an important role in the mediation of behavior. In addition, many behaviorally active drugs interact with catecholamines (CAs): i.e., dopamine (DA) and norepinephrine (NE). Some drugs affect the storage of the amines, others their synthesis or degradation, while still others act on catecholaminergic receptor sites (as agonists) or block receptor sites (as antagonists). Whether or not the interaction of drugs with catecholaminergic mechanisms is functionally related to their effect on behavior is a question that can only be answered through a variety of empirical, inferential and somewhat theoretical approaches. At the present state of development in this field, a large amount of the evidence is consistent with the notion that several drugs exert their behavioral effects through catecholaminergic mechanisms.

This chapter will review and explore three areas: (1) the pharmacology and biochemistry of catecholamines in the central nervous system (CNS), (2) the relationship of the CAs to the maintenance of different behaviors and (3) evidence which demonstrates that in addition to drugs, environmental and behavioral variables modify the distribution and metabolism of catecholamines.

PHARMACOLOGY AND BIOCHEMISTRY OF DOPAMINE AND NOREPINEPHRINE

Distribution of Catecholamines in the CNS

The neuroanatomical distribution and subcellular localization of the catecholamines in brain has been studied using a combination of fluorescence assay and histochemical fluorescence techniques. Specific CNS lesions have elucidated the main pathways by following anterograde and retrograde neuronal degeneration along with reduction of catecholamine levels in specific areas of the brain. These studies have revealed that both NE and DA are found in neurons and not glial cells. The concentration of NE and DA in nerve endings is high (1,000 to 10,000 µg/g) whereas the concentration in cell bodies is much lower (10 to 100 µg/g) (Cooper *et al.*, 1974; Iversen, 1967).

Dopamine. Brain concentrations (µg/g) of dopamine (DA) are highest in caudate nucleus, putamen, arcuate nucleus and olfactory tubercle. Dopamine is also found in terminals ending in the frontal neocortex, but the concentration (i.e., µg/g) in the neocortex is lower than in the striatal system (caudate nucleus, putamen) or the limbic structures (arcuate nucleus, olfactory tubercle).

Cell groups located in the mesencephalon give rise to most of the ascending dopamine-containing neurons. The DA neurons terminate in the striatum and limbic system structures, as well as in the neocortex (i.e., cerebral cortex). Most of the DA-containing cell bodies that give rise to axons innervating these structures, lie in the pars compacta of the substantia nigra or in the ventral tegmentum which is proximal to the pars compacta. DA fibers course through the ventral tegmentum and the medial forebrain bundle, and have endings in the caudate nucleus, putamen (part of the basal ganglia) and the amygdala. These mesencephalic cell bodies also send projections to the nucleus accumbens, the interstitial nucleus of the stria terminalis and the olfactory tubercle. In addition, a set of fibers with cell bodies located just anterior to the pars compacta send dopaminergic projections to the frontal cortex. There are also dopamine cell bodies located in the hypothalamus (arcuate nucleus) which send short fibers to the external layer of the median eminence. Figures 5-1a and 5-1b show a schematic drawing of the dopaminergic projection system (see Lindvall and Björklund, 1974; Ungerstedt, 1971b; Moore *et al.,* 1971).

Norepinephrine. Norepinephrine is found in several CNS areas including the medulla, pons, midbrain, septum, amygdala, hippocampus, cerebral cortex and cerebellum, as well as the spinal cord. The cell bodies of the norepinephrine-containing neurons are located mainly in the medulla, pons and midbrain. Cells that lie in the medulla give rise to fibers which terminate in the spinal cord. Ascending NE-containing fibers can be divided into two groups, a dorsal pathway and a ventral pathway. The *dorsal NE pathway* arises from a group of cells, the locus coeruleus, and fibers course through the ventral tegmentum and the medial forebrain bundle (in the lateral hypothalamus). The *dorsal pathway* innervates the cerebellum, thalamic nuclei, limbic structures (septum, hippocampus, amygdala), caudate-putamen and the entire neocortex, and sends some fibers to the hypothalamus. The *ventral NE pathway* has its cell bodies located in the medulla and pons and mainly innervates the medulla, pons, midbrain and hypothalamus (see Dahlström and Fuxe, 1964; Heller and Moore, 1968; Ungerstedt, 1971b, 1973; Lindvall and Björklund, 1974). The NE system in brain is diffuse

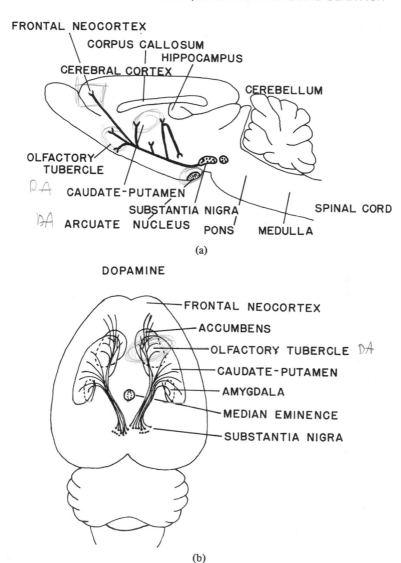

(a)

DOPAMINE

(b)

Fig. 5-1. (a) A schematic presentation of the *dopaminergic pathways* in brain in a sagittal projection. (b) Dopaminergic pathways from a horizontal projection.

in that it sends widespread projections from several prominent cell-body groups located in the brain-stem (Fig. 5-2). It is comparable to the serotonin system (see Chapter 4), the cell bodies of which lie in the medial raphé nucleus but send widespread ascending as well as descending projections.

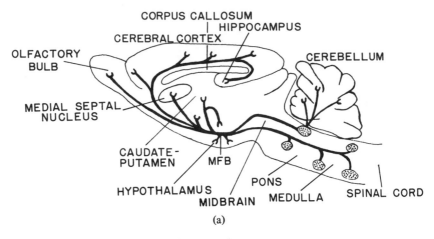

NOREPINEPHRINE

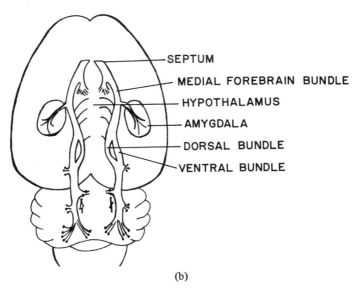

(b)

Fig. 5-2. (a) Sagittal projection of the noradrenergic pathways in the central nervous system. MFB: Medial forebrain bundle. (b) Noradrenergic pathways from a horizontal projection.

Metabolism and Storage

The metabolism and storage of CAs is extensively discussed in Chapter 3 (p. 72) in relationship to the peripheral nervous system. Metabolism, storage and degradation are the same in the CNS. Briefly, the synthesis is the following:

$$\text{Tyrosine} \longrightarrow \text{L-dopa} \longrightarrow \text{DA} \longrightarrow \text{NE}$$

Recall that the following enzymes are involved in synthesis: tyrosine hydroxylase catalyzes the conversion of tyrosine to L-dopa and is the rate-limiting enzyme in catecholamine synthesis. Aromatic-L-amino acid decarboxylase catalyzes the conversion of L-dopa to dopamine, and dopamine-beta-hydroxylase catalyzes the conversion of dopamine to norepinephrine. This enzyme is only present in cells containing norepinephrine. The degradative enzymes are the same as in the peripheral nervous system. Monoamine oxidase (MAO) catalyzes the oxidation of a catecholamine into an aldehyde, which in turn is oxidized to the corresponding acid. Catechol-O-methyltransferase (COMT) catalyzes the methylation of the catecholamine to the corresponding O-methylated catecholamine derivative (see Fig. 3-6, Chapter 3). Both MAO and COMT are found in specific localizations; MAO is located in mitochondria of the presynaptic nerve ending, and COMT is located on the postsynaptic membrance. Catecholamines can also be inactivated by the process of reuptake of the released compound back into the presynaptic nerve ending.

Synaptic Transmission

The criteria for identification of a compound as a transmitter are discussed in Chapters 3 and 4. Briefly, the criteria include: (1) that the transmitter be present within nerve cells along with the enzymes necessary for its synthesis and degradation; (2) that it be released upon nerve stimulation; (3) that it be capable of altering firing rate of the postsynaptic neuron; and (4) that interfering with synthesis, degradation and storage of the putative transmitter affect transmission. While it is difficult to demonstrate that norepinephrine and dopamine meet these criteria because of the inaccessibility of CNS synapses, some evidence exists that NE and DA function as transmitters in the CNS (Krnjevic, 1974).

The Central Dopaminergic Neuron. Dopamine satisfies several criteria for a synaptic transmitter. Dopamine is present in neurons along with the enzymes necessary for its synthesis and degradation (Fig. 5-3). In addition, DA storage granules are concentrated in nerve endings. Although evidence that DA is released upon nerve stimulation is tenuous, it seems that DA functions as an inhibitory transmitter in the striatum and hypothalamus. Pharmacological and biochemical data are consistent with this generalization, but electrophysiological evidence is not as convincing (see Cooper *et al.*, 1974; Krnjevic, 1974).

The Central Noradrenergic Neuron. The model (Fig. 5-4) of the noradrenergic neuron in the CNS is similar to the model of the noradrenergic neuron for the ANS described in Chapter 3, p. 71. In the ANS the junction is between nerve and muscle, whereas in the CNS the junction is between nerve and nerve. The

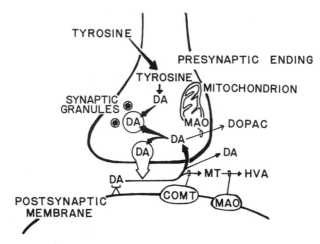

Fig. 5-3. Schematic model of a central dopaminergic neuron. Abbreviations–DOPAC: 3,4-dihydroxyphenylacetic acid; DA: dopamine; MT: methoxytyramine; HVA: homovanillic acid; COMT: catechol-O-methyltransferase; MAO: monoamine oxidase. Note that some of the monoamine oxidase is located on the postsynaptic membrane (see also Fig. 5-4).

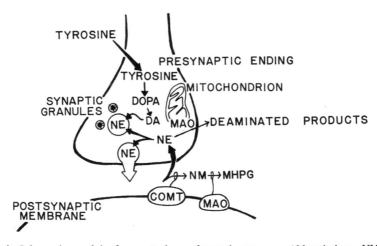

Fig. 5-4. Schematic model of a central noradrenergic neuron. Abbreviations–NM: normetanephrine; MHPG: 3-methoxy-4-hydroxyphenylglycol (note that this product is formed by the action of MAO on normetanephrine). In the peripheral nervous system, this reaction forms vanillyl-mandelic acid (see Chapter 3, p. 73) but in the central nervous system the acid is further released to the glycol, MHPG. COMT: catechol-O-methyltransferase; MAO: monoamine oxidase; DOPA: 3,4-dihydroxyphenylalanine; DA: dopamine; NE: norepinephrine.

noradrenergic neuron is similar to the dopaminergic neuron except that the enzyme dopamine-β-hydroxylase is present in the storage granules of NE-containing
cells. Recall that this enzyme converts DA to NE. Norepinephrine, like dopamine, appears to satisfy many of the same requirements for a synaptic transmitter in the CNS. Norepinephrine is present in neurons along with the enzymes
necessary for its synthesis and degradation. As with DA, the criteria of release
from presynaptic sites and action on postsynaptic neurons are more difficult to
establish within the CNS, but some evidence exists that NE acts as an inhibitory
transmitter within the central nervous system (Cooper *et al.*, 1974; Krnjevic,
1974).

Drug Effects

Many of the drugs that affect noradrenergic neurons also affect dopaminergic
neurons with certain exceptions. Therefore, drug effects on noradrenergic and
dopaminergic neurons will be discussed together and exceptions will be noted.
These drugs are listed in Table 5-1. As with the serotonergic neuron, synthesis,
storage, uptake, degradation and action on the receptor are important considerations. For a more thorough discussion of the noradrenergic neuron and drugs
affecting its function, see Chapter 3.

Receptor Agonists.   Aside from the naturally occurring compounds, dopamine
and norepinephrine, the drugs that are known to stimulate central DA and
NE receptors when injected systemically are apomorphine, which stimulates DA
receptors, and clonidine, which stimulates NE receptors. Since L-dopa is converted to dopamine and norepinephrine following injection, it can also stimulate
NE and DA receptors.

Synthesis Inhibitors.   Alpha-methyltyrosine (AMT) is an inhibitor of the enzyme
tyrosine hydrozylase, the rate-limiting enzyme in CA synthesis. Ro 4-4602 and
NSD 1055 also inhibit the synthesis of CAs by inhibiting the enzyme aromatic-L-
amino acid decarboxylase. Dopamine-β-hydroxylase (DBH), which only exists in
noradrenergic cells to convert dopamine to norepinephrine, is inhibited by FLa-63
and disulfiram.

Degradation Inhibitors.   The MAO inhibitors, nialamide, iproniazid, and pargyline alter the degradation of CAs by interfering with the enzyme responsible
for their destruction. CAs are also inactivated by COMT. COMT is inhibited by
pyrogallol.

Reuptake Blockers.   Amphetamine and benztropine block DA reuptake, whereas
amphetamine also blocks NE reuptake. Cocaine, nortriptyline and desmethyl-

TABLE 5-1. Prototypic drugs affecting processes within the noradrenergic and dopaminergic neuron

Process	Compound affecting DA system	Compound affecting NE system
Receptor stimulation	dopamine apomorphine	norepinephrine clonidine
Synthesis inhibition tyrosine hydroxylase	α-methyltyrosine	α-methyltyrosine
aromatic-L-amino acid decarboxylase	Ro-4-4602 NSD 1055	Ro-4-4602 NSD 1055
dopamine-beta- hydroxylase		disulfiram FLa-63
Degradative inhibition monoamine oxidase	nialamide pargyline iproniazid	nialamide pargyline iproniazid
catechol-O-methyl-transferase	pyrogallol	pyrogallol
Reuptake blockade	amphetamine benztropine	amphetamine cocaine nortriptyline desmethylimipramine imipramine
Receptor blockade	chlorpromazine haloperidol pimozide	chlorpromazine phenoxybenzamine phentolamine propranolol
Storage	reserpine tetrabenazine	reserpine tetrabenazine
Neurotoxin	6-hydroxydopamine	6-hydroxydopamine

imipramine (sometimes called desipramine) selectively block NE reuptake. Imipramine also blocks norepinephrine reuptake, but is less selective because it also blocks the reuptake of serotonin.

Receptor Blockers. Several drugs block DA receptors, including haloperidol, pimozide and chlorpromazine (and possibly other phenothiazines). Not all of these drugs block dopamine receptors selectively. Chlorpromazine also blocks NE as well as other receptors. In addition, the specificity of haloperidol has not been established. Phenoxybenzamine, phentolamine and propranolol are among the compounds that block central NE receptors.

Drugs That Interfere With Storage. Reserpine depletes both norepinephrine and dopamine (Holzbauer and Vogt, 1956; Carlsson *et al.*, 1957) and serotonin (Brodie and Shore, 1957) from brain and other tissues. Reserpine is thought to deplete catecholamines and serotonin by interfering with their storage (see Chapters 3 and 4). Tetrabenazine also interferes with the storage of CAs, although its duration of action is much shorter than that of reserpine.

Neurotoxin. 6-Hydroxydopamine (6-HDA) injected directly into the brain in the ventricular system produces a long-lasting depletion of brain DA and NE by destroying catecholaminergic neurons. Apparently, 6-HDA is taken up by catecholaminergic nerve terminals, and causes destruction of the terminals which is followed by retrograde degeneration.

Intraventricular injection of 6-hydroxydopamine has been studied primarily in the rat; typically between 100 and 250 μg of 6-HDA is administered. Depending upon the dose of 6-HDA, the number of injections and other drugs injected prior to administration of 6-HDA, a number of behavioral effects have been observed, including some long range behavioral deficits (Longo, 1973; Kostrzewa and Jacobowitz, 1974).

After 6-HDA administration, norepinephrine shows greater depletion from brain than dopamine. However, either dopamine or norepinephrine can be selectively depleted by 6-HDA, depending upon the pattern of administration and other relevant pharmacological pretreatments. Two or three small doses of 6-HDA selectively deplete norepinephrine from brain, whereas pretreatment with an MAO inhibitor, such as pargyline, causes depletion of both dopamine and norepinephrine. Desmethylimipramine (also called DMI or desipramine) selectively prevents uptake of 6-hydroxydopamine into norepinephrine terminals, thereby preventing destruction of NE cells and subsequent depletion of NE. Since DMI pretreatment does *not* prevent uptake in dopamine cells, dopamine is selectively depleted. Serotonergic cells are only minimally affected by the intraventricular administration of 6-hydroxydopamine (10–15% decrease in 5-HT), and peripheral catecholaminergic nerve terminals are not affected at all by intracisternal or intraventricular injection of 6-hydroxydopamine. The relatively selective depletion of catecholamines caused by 6-hydroxydopamine is a useful tool for investigating the function of catecholaminergic cells in physiological and behavioral processes.

It should be pointed out that the intraventricular injection of 6-hydroxydopamine produces irreversible changes in catecholamine neurons in the central nervous system. This permanent effect contrasts with the effects of other amine-depleting agents such as reserpine and AMT, in that the effects of these drugs are temporary, albeit some last longer than others. In this respect, the effect of 6-hydroxydopamine is more similar to the effect of a discrete CNS lesion than to temporary drug-induced depletion of CAs. However, unlike a lesion which affects neurons located in a particular anatomical locus (see Cooper *et al.*, 1974), 6-HDA affects all catecholaminergic neurons when given in sufficient doses.

THE ROLE OF CATECHOLAMINES IN BEHAVIOR

General Approach

In order to infer a causal relationship between brain amines and behavior, one must observe more than a concomitant alteration of the two. Additional experimental evidence is necessary to show that the two events are dependent upon one another. This evidence often consists of reversing the behavioral effect observed by manipulating one or more of the amines thought to be responsible for the effect. For example, if reserpine administration produces a change in some behavior, the biochemical mechanisms underlying that effect might be investigated by replacing one or more of the amines depleted by reserpine and observing concomitant alterations in the behavior.

Since no single approach is adequate to investigate the function of endogenous chemicals in the mediation of behavior, a variety of approaches are generally used. It will be the purpose of this chapter to investigate the various approaches that have been used to examine relationships between CAs and behavior. The student should realize that the investigation of CAs and behavior (like the investigation of 5-HT and behavior) is an extremely active field of research. Generalizations made upon the basis of data available today, may be compromised or fall on the basis of newer data.

In order to investigate the role of catecholamines in behavior, three approaches are generally used. These include: (1) reduction of CA levels; (2) elevation of CA levels; and (3) agonism/antagonism of CA receptor sites in the CNS. Frequently two or even three of these approaches are combined.

Reduction of CA Levels. Catecholamines can be reduced in the following way:

1. Reserpine and tetrabenazine deplete NE, DA and 5-HT by interfering with storage in granules.
2. Several drugs interfere with CA synthesis (see Table 5-1), but AMT has been more frequently used than any other agents.
3. 6-HDA depletes catecholamines by destroying catecholaminergic nerve cells; this destruction, while relatively selective, appears to extend to other types of cells as well (e.g., there is a small loss in 5-HT).
4. Stereotaxically placed electrolytic lesions in the brain reduce CAs in specific regions.

Elevation of CA Levels. Catecholamines can be elevated or replaced through administration of their metabolic precursor, L-dopa, which, unlike DA or NE, crosses the blood-brain barrier.   Replacement can also be achieved by the in-traventricular or intracerebral infusion of NE and DA.   Each technique has limitations.   L-dopa is decarboxylated in nerve cells that do not ordinarily con-tain DA or NE, and therefore the distribution of the CAs after L-dopa adminis-tration is not completely normal.   Catecholamines placed directly into brain regions or ventricles may be taken up or act upon nerve cells that under physio-logical conditions do not contain or respond to catecholamines.

Agonists/Antagonists.   CA function can be altered by the use of specific agonists and antagonists.   For example, apomorphine (see Table 5-1) is thought to be a dopaminergic agonist and clonidine a noradrenergic agonist.   While there is evi-dence to support this idea, the degree to which these drugs affect other systems in brain is not known.   Table 5-1 lists several drugs thought to have some spe-cificity as dopaminergic and noradrenergic blockers (see section on receptor blockade).

Motor Behavior

The importance of motor function in the expression and assessment of behavior is often overlooked relative to sensory, motivational and conditioning processes. However, it is obvious that impairment of motor function can be responsible for alterations in both simple and complex behavioral patterns.   Inability of an animal to perform a motor task may be quite as disruptive as is loss of discrimina-tive functions, alteration in food and water consumption or factors interfering with conditioning.   Motor behavior may become repetitive, grossly exaggerated or diminished, and thereby interfere with the performance of another behavior through the expression of competing motor responses.   In this section we will examine the role of dopamine and norepinephrine, as well as certain drugs that act on these amines, on various aspects of motor behavior. We will also examine the role of DA in a clinical syndrome that is manifested by abnormal motor be-havior, viz., Parkinson's disease.

Spontaneous Locomotor Activity.   Spontaneous locomotor activity is defined as grossly observable movements of an animal in a certain pattern. The stimuli that elicit or maintain the activity are not readily identifiable. (See Chapter 1 for a discussion of procedures used to measure spontaneous locomotor activity.)

Dopamine appears to play a primary role in the regulation of spontaneous locomotor activity.   The role of norepinephrine is less clear, but some evidence suggests that it can modulate dopaminergic effects on locomotor activity. Several lines of evidence support this conclusion.   First of all, dopamine is localized in a network of neurons with motor function (i.e., nigrostriatal system). Lesions of the nigrostriatal system produce substantial degeneration of dopaminergic neurons and also cause motor dysfunctions which include a decrease in spon-

taneous locomotion or akinesia. Second, drugs and chemicals that affect catecholamine concentrations produce changes in locomotor activity. Drugs which
affect catecholamine concentrations are often divided into two groups. In one
group, the drugs (e.g., a single dose of reserpine or AMT) produce a short term
depletion of catecholamines which persists 4 to 96 hours, depending on the particular drug and dose. In the other group, the drugs (e.g., repeated administration of reserpine or 6-HDA) produce a long-lasting depletion. 6-HDA depletion
is thought to be irreversible (see p. 125, this chapter).

1. *Short-Term Depletion in Catecholamines.* When catecholamines are depleted by a single dose of reserpine, locomotor activity decreases and postural
tone is changed. Replacement of the depleted catecholamines through L-dopa
administration reverses these effects (Blaschko and Chruściel, 1960; Carlsson

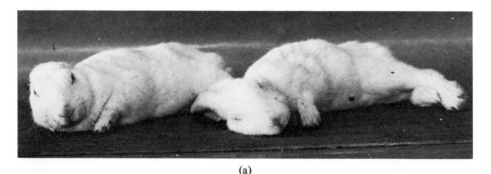

(a)

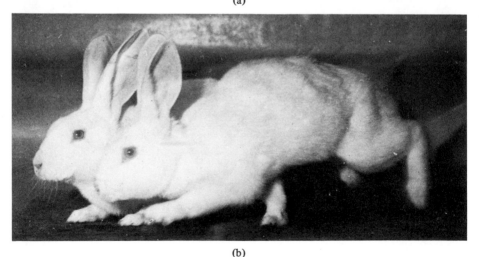

(b)

Fig. 5-5. (a) Rabbits treated with 5 mg/kg (iv) reserpine. Note resting posture, ptosis and
ear position. (b) Same rabbits 15 minutes after 200 mg/kg *dl*-dopa. Note that the effects of
reserpine are no longer visible. (From Carlsson, 1960.)

et al., 1957) (see Fig. 5-5). Catecholamine depletion by injections of AMT also reduces spontaneous locomotor activity (Rech *et al.*, 1966).

While L-dopa can reverse reserpine's effects on spontaneous locomotor activity, it also affects locomotor activity when given alone. Administration of L-dopa alone in a dose range between 100 and 1000 mg/kg has been reported by some investigators to increase spontaneous locomotor activity in mice and rats (Smith and Dews, 1962; Everett and Wiegand, 1962). The increased locomotor activity was accompanied by marked sympathetic signs, including piloerection, salivation, pupillary dilation, blanching of the peripheral vasculature, urination and hyperpnea. In some instances, lower doses of L-dopa suppressed locomotor activity. Increases in spontaneous locomotor activity following L-dopa correlated with increases in dopamine levels. NE levels did not increase noticeably as a result of L-dopa administration. Therefore, it has been assumed that DA and not NE is the important transmitter in motor activity. This assumption can only be made with caution, however, since NE may be formed from the DA, but show no increase in concentration due to a high rate of turnover (see Chapter 2, pp. 44–48).

These data suggest that L-dopa can both inhibit (low doses) and stimulate (high doses) locomotor activity. It has been suggested (Butcher and Engel, 1969) that L-dopa inhibits locomotor activity as a result of its peripheral autonomic effects and stimulates locomotor behavior as a result of its central effects. Butcher and Engel support their conclusion with three observations. First, when the conversion of L-dopa to DA is blocked in the peripheral ANS by administration of a small dose of a decarboxylase inhibitor, Ro 4-4602, a small dose of L-dopa which normally suppresses locomotor activity produces an increase in locomotor activity. Second, when the same small dose of L-dopa is given in conjunction with an injection of dopamine (which elevates peripheral DA concentration), locomotor activity decreases (Fig. 5-6). Third, dopamine alone produces the same autonomic signs that are present after L-dopa alone, but are absent with L-dopa plus the peripheral decarboxylase inhibitor. These data support Butcher and Engle's conclusion that locomotor behavior is decreased as a result of dopamine's peripheral effects and increased as a result of increased DA in the CNS. While this interpretation is consistent with the data presented, other interpretations are possible. For example, when the peripheral decarboxylation of L-dopa is blocked, a larger amount of L-dopa would reach brain parenchyma (neurons) cells, and therefore more dopamine would be formed in brain. The fact that DA decreased motor activity when given alone mitigates against this interpretation, but in the absence of dose-response data on both the effects of DA and L-dopa in the presence of peripheral decarboxylase inhibition, it is difficult to exclude the alternative interpretation.

Several studies have attempted to differentiate the role of NE and DA in the mediation of motor behavior. Andén *et al.* (1973) treated mice with reserpine

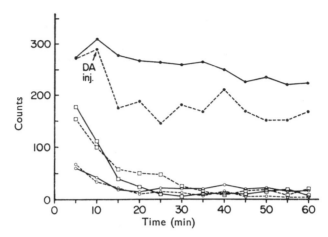

Fig. 5-6. Spontaneous locomotor activity as a function of time following several drug regimens. Locomotor activity was measured in a box equipped to count movement. The doses and time of injection before the start of session are as follows: Ro 4-4602, 50 mg/kg, 75 min; L-dopa, 150 mg/kg, 45 min; dopamine (DA), 150 mg/kg, 5 min. In the Ro 4-4602-dopa-dopamine regimen, the time of dopamine administration is indicated at the arrow. Each point represents the mean of 10 values. Ro 4-4602 + L-dopa ●——●. Ro 4-4602 + L-dopa + dopamine ●— —●. Control □—□. Ro 4-4602 □— —□. L-dopa ○—○. Dopamine ○— —○. (From Butcher and Engel, 1969.)

and observed a concomitant decrease in locomotor activity. When apomorphine (a DA agonist) was administered, motor activity was temporarily restored. Clonidine (a NE agonist) did not restore motor activity; however, simultaneous administration of clonidine and apomorphine caused a greater increase in locomotor behavior than that following apomorphine alone. These results indicate that DA mediates locomotor activity, but that NE can enhance or modulate DA function. It should be noted that this interpretation rests on the tenuous assumption that apomorphine acts only on DA receptors and clonidine only on NE receptors (see Benkert *et al.*, 1973a, b; Guldberg and Marsden, 1972).

On the other hand, some studies suggest that NE levels in brain are not important in maintaining motor behavior. Ahlenius (1974c) found that AMT administration produced a decrease in locomotor activity which could be restored by a low dose of L-dopa (10 mg/kg). When the formation of NE was blocked by the dopamine-beta-hydroxylase inhibitor, FLa-63, motor activity was still restored.

Other attempts to differentiate the role of DA and NE in the mediation of motor behavior have used agents that block either DA or NE receptors. For example, Przegalinski and Kleinrok (1972) found that both DA and NE were important in locomotor activity by using a combination of DA and NE agonists and antagonists. First of all, they administered L-dopa and observed the usual increases in motor activity. When DA receptors were blocked by haloperidol or chlorpromazine, the L-dopa-induced stimulation of locomotor activity was blocked. When the reuptake of NE was blocked by nortriptyline, L-dopa-induced locomotor stimulation increased. (Recall that when NE reuptake is blocked, the concentration of NE accumulating at the receptors is increased.)

The importance of DA and NE in locomotor behavior was also demonstrated by Geyer *et al.* (1972). Dopamine or norepinephrine was perfused into the ventricles of an unrestrained rat, and a dose-dependent increase in motor activity was observed. Since the increase was greater following NE administration, the authors suggested that NE played a greater role in the mediation of motor behavior than DA. They also suggested that DA increased motor activity either by being converted to NE in the appropriate neurons or by displacing NE. These data are difficult to reconcile with other data which suggest that DA plays a primary role in the mediation of locomotor activity, although there are some data to suggest that NE plays a secondary, modulating role in locomotor activity.

2. *Long-Term Depletion of Catecholamines.* While short-term depletion of CAs decreases locomotor activity, long-term depletion of catecholamines (i.e., 7 days or longer) only decreases locomotor activity initially. After a week to 10 days, animals appear normal. Long-term depletion of CAs can be produced in two ways, either by daily injections of small doses of reserpine or by intraventricular administration of 6-HDA.

Daily administration of very small doses of reserpine to either rabbits or mice (Häggendal and Lindqvist, 1963, 1964) caused slow amine depletion and the appearance of autonomic (hypothermia, ptosis, mydriasis, diarrhea) and gross behavioral (sedation) signs. These signs reached maximum effect after 10 days of treatment, and were well correlated with maximum amine depletion. With continued daily administration of the same small dose of reserpine, the animals returned to normal within four hours after each reserpine injection. When the animals were sedated, brain amine levels were 5% of normal. During recovery, brain amines rose to 15% of normal. Therefore, function was restored following only a 10% rise in brain catecholamines.

These results might be explained in terms of amine storage. Recall from Chapter 3 that amines are either bound within granules, free inside the cell (where presumably they are inactivated by MAO) or active at the synaptic cleft. It has been suggested that there may be two pools of stored amines, i.e., a pool that is readily releasable and another which is firmly bound. The readily releasable pool is derived from newly synthesized amines, and presumably the granular pool is derived from amines that are not immediately released. There is some evidence to suggest that the newly synthesized pool is the more important on a functional basis (Häggendal and Lindqvist, 1963, 1964). Therefore, while reserpine interferes with the storage of amines, the small increase in amines seen after recovery from reserpine might have been sufficient to restore function even though the level of stored amines was low.

On the other hand, the notion of a rather small, newly synthesized pool of critical functional importance in behavior does not fit well with evidence from studies in which AMT has been given to produce a short-term depletion of catecholamines. If AMT decreases catecholamine synthesis by inhibiting tyrosine hydroxylase, the newly synthesized pool of amines should be affected by AMT first. Moreover, if the newly synthesized pool is more important functionally, one might expect the effects of AMT to occur before the depletion of a large proportion of CAs; however, changes in spontaneous motor activity following AMT administration occur only if the CA content of the brain is decreased to a level of about 30% of normal. This dilemma could be resolved if the size of the so-called newly synthesized and functional pool were known, but presently it poses difficulties in interpreting AMT effects on locomotor behavior as well as on other behaviors.

Nevertheless, other studies have shown changes in spontaneous motor behavior as a result of prolonged CA depletion following 6-hydroxydopamine (6-HDA) administration. Recall that when 6-hydroxydopamine is injected into the cerebrospinal fluid by means of either an intracisternal injection or an intraventricular injection, it is taken up into catecholaminergic cells, where it acts as a neurotoxin and destroys the CA cells (see p. 125, this chapter). Brain catecholamine levels slowly decrease as the CA cells degenerate, although sometimes there is a transient increase in CAs in some areas of the brain several hours after 6-HDA administration (Bell *et al.*, 1970). Injection of 6-HDA into the ventricles produces short-term suppression of spontaneous locomotor activity that lasts from one to eight days (Uretsky and Schoenfeld, 1971; Burkard *et al.*, 1969; Evetts *et al.*, 1970; Fibiger *et al.*, 1972). Several days following administration of 6-HDA (which depletes brain NE by 80% and DA by 75%), animals are normal in terms of general appearance and motor activity. They groom, eat, drink and move about like untreated control rats. Therefore, treatment with 6-HDA that is sufficient to produce a permanent 75–80% decrease in brain catecholamine levels only has temporary effects on spontaneous locomotor activity. The fact that these effects are transient suggests that the role of CAs in the mediation of behavior might not be as important as previous work with reserpine, AMT, L-dopa and other drugs affecting the catecholaminergic system would indicate.

While 6-HDA alone does not produce long-term changes in locomotor activity, several studies have shown that the effects of various drugs on locomotor activity can be altered by treatment with 6-HDA. The effects of L-dopa and apomorphine on locomotor activity are potentiated by pretreatment with 6-HDA, and the effects of amphetamine on locomotor activity are blocked with 6-HDA. For example, Uretsky and Schoenfeld (1971) demonstrated that 6-HDA treatment enhanced stimulation of locomotor activity by L-dopa (Fig. 5-7). Two groups of rats were examined; one group was pretreated with 6-HDA prior to receiving L-dopa and a peripheral decarboxylase inhibitor; the other group was not pre-

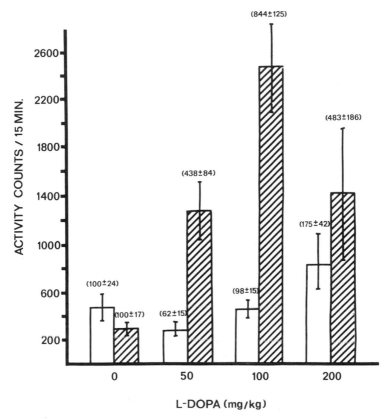

Fig. 5-7. Effect of L-dopa on the motor activity of 6-hydroxydopamine (6-HDA) and vehicle-treated rats. The striped bars indicate activity of 6-HDA-treated rats; the clear bars refer to vehicle-treated rats. The numbers in parentheses represent motor activity expressed as a percentage of the activity of vehicle-treated and 6-HDA rats not injected with dopa. Each value is the mean ± S.E.M. of at least four rats. (From Uretsky and Schoenfeld, 1971.)

treated with 6-HDA, but it was given L-dopa and a peripheral decarboxylase inhibitor. 6-HDA was given in a dose which reduced CA levels by 75–80%. L-dopa increased DA formed in brain in a dose-dependent manner in both groups of rats; however, neither group showned an increase in NE levels as a result of the L-dopa injection. The effects of apomorphine (a DA receptor agonist) on locomotor activity were also increased following 6-HDA administration, supporting the notion that DA receptors are important in the expression of locomotor activity.

Uretsky and Schoenfeld (1971) have proposed possible mechanisms at the synaptic level which may explain their results. They suggest that the potentiation of the effect of L-dopa on locomotor activity by 6-HDA is due to destruction of CA terminals which normally take up and thereby inactivate the CA transmitter. Without this mechanism of inactivation, the effects of the transmitter are enhanced. Uretsky and Schoenfeld also suggest that 6-HDA administration may increase the sensitivity of the catecholamine receptors. These two explanations have been used to explain increases in drug efficacy after nerve cell destruction (called *supersensitivity* or *denervation supersensitivity*). The mechanism by which supersensitivity occurs is not well understood, but it has been reported in a variety of situations.

Breese *et al.* (1973a) also found enhanced stimulation of locomotor activity with L-dopa following 6-HDA administration. They found that motor activity was enhanced in 6-HDA rats following L-dopa, but enhancement only occurred in those rats with selective depletion of DA. In rats that were selectively depleted of NE there was no enhancement of motor activity by L-dopa. According to the model proposed by Uretsky and Schoenfeld (1971), these results suggest that DA receptors become supersensitive when DA is selectively depleted, and the supersensitivity results in enhanced locomotor activity after L-dopa administration, strengthening the suggestion that DA is of primary functional importance in the maintenance of locomotor activity. These results are difficult to interpret, however, since in animals selectively depleted of NE, brain NE levels were still 40% of control. We have already seen that with both NE and DA, 5–10% of the normal values may be sufficient to maintain function.

The role of DA in the maintenance of normal locomotor activity is also supported by experiments in which 6-HDA is injected into the substantia nigra (see Butcher *et al.*, 1973). This treatment causes almost complete depletion of striatal DA levels (greater than 99%), and some depletion of forebrain NE. Rats with 6-HDA lesions of the substantia nigra show loss of motor activity and are supersensitive to the locomotor stimulating effects of apomorphine and L-dopa (Ungerstedt, 1971a; Iversen and Creese, 1975). A role for NE cannot be entirely eliminated by these experiments, however, since 6-HDA produces a decrease in both DA and NE. The interpretation rests on the specificity of apomorphine on DA receptors.

In summary, we have reviewed evidence that depletion of brain catecholamines by any one of a number of methods can produce at least a temporary reduction in spontaneous motor activity. Much of the data points to a primary role for DA in the maintenance of normal locomotion, although the role of NE cannot be discounted. A few experiments suggest that NE is important in the maintenance of motor activity, but in general most of the data supports a primary role for DA with NE playing a secondary role in modifying locomotor activity. Moreover, we have seen that no single experiment by itself can conclusively demonstrate a point; a combination of several experiments asking the same or similar questions is necessary before general inferences can be drawn.

Parkinson's Syndrome. Parkinson's disease is characterized by muscular rigidity, difficulty in initiating movements (akinesia) and tremors. The patient with Parkinson's disease often exhibits an immobility of facial muscles which extends to the neck and causes difficulty in coughing and swallowing. Hornykiewicz (1966) has speculated that the tremor and rigidity are due to an over-activity in certain motor brain areas caused by the degeneration of systems which normally exert inhibitory control on motor behavior. Much evidence has accrued over the past years to suggest that degeneration in the extrapyramidal system is the cause of the disease. The extrapyramidal system is believed to be involved in the regulation of normal muscle tone and movement. The most frequent neuropathological change seen during autopsy of patients with Parkinson's disease is degeneration in the substantia nigra, particularly the pars compacta. It has been found that the cell bodies originating in the substantia nigra and projecting to other striatal nuclei contain dopamine. Furthermore, patients with Parkinson's disease excrete less dopamine and its metabolites in urine; and on autopsy the Parkinson's patient is found to have less dopamine in the nigrostriatal system.

There are several lines of evidence which suggest that the symptomatology of Parkinsonism is due to the lack of dopamine (at least in part) in the nigrostriatal system. L-dopa, the metabolic precursor of dopamine, antagonizes some of the motor deficits, particularly the akinesia and rigidity, and to a lesser extent the tremors of Parkinsonism. Since the enzyme for the decarboxylation of L-dopa is ubiquitous, high doses of L-dopa (4–8 grams per day) must be administered to obtain sufficient levels of dopamine in brain. Moreover, both chlorpromazine (which is thought to block dopaminergic and noradrenergic receptor sites) and reserpine can induce Parkinsonian-like effects. These effects can be antagonized by L-dopa.

Although the above data are consistent with the hypothesis that lack of dopamine plays a role in the functional deficits of Parkinson's disease, other compounds such as acetylcholine may be of importance as well. The nigrostriatal system has a cholinergic component, and drugs which have anticholinergic effects in the CNS are also effective in mitigating against some of the symptoms of Parkinsonism. Indeed, anticholinergic agents were in use before L-dopa in the treatment of Parkinson's disease. Furthermore, while L-dopa is probably the most valuable compound for treatment of Parkinsonism symptoms (Costall and Naylor, 1975), its use is complicated by severe side effects including gastrointestinal, cardiovascular and genitourinary problems and motor dyskinesis (Barbeau *et al.*, 1971). The search for dopaminergic agonists not having these side effects is one of the main directions of current research in this area (McDowell and Sweet, 1975; Rondot *et al.*, 1975). (See also Narotzky *et al.*, 1973; Klawans, 1973a, b; Klawans *et al.*, 1970; Cotzias *et al.*, 1970.)

Aggressive Behavior

In Chapter 4 we discussed the relationship between 5-HT depletion and the occurrence of aggressive behavior. It was suggested that the 5-HT system might play a role in the inhibition of certain types of "aggressive" behavior. Experimentation also suggests that the CA system may be involved in the elaboration of fighting behavior.

Spontaneous Fighting. Several investigators have reported increases in spontaneous fighting in mice and rats following administration of L-dopa alone or of L-dopa in combination with MAO or dopamine-beta-hydroxylase inhibitors (Everett and Wiegand, 1962; Scheel-Krüger and Randrup, 1967, 1968; Senault, 1970). Based on these experiments it would seem as if stimulation of DA receptors in brain is involved in spontaneous fighting.

Moreover, severe fighting in rats housed eight per cage occurs when 6-HDA treatment is followed by administration of L-dopa in the presence of a peripheral decarboxylase inhibitor. Neither (1) 6-HDA alone nor (2) L-dopa alone with a peripheral decarboxylase inhibitor elicited fighting behavior. When the dopamine-beta-hydroxylase inhibitor, FLa 63, was given to 6-HDA-treated rats along with L-dopa and a peripheral decarboxylase inhibitor, fighting also occurred. Therefore, while formation of NE does not seem to be important in the expression of L-dopa-induced fighting behavior, both DA depletion and destruction of DA presynaptic neurons increase the occurrence of spontaneous fighting seen after L-dopa administration.

Shock-Induced Fighting. In a shock-induced fighting procedure, two rats are placed in one chamber, and relatively intense foot shock (2 ma) is administered. The number of attacks per 50 shocks is often used as the measure of aggression. Shock-induced fighting increases following intracisternal administration of 6-HDA (Thoa *et al.*, 1972a, b), suggesting CA involvement in shock-induced fighting. Replacement of CAs with L-dopa or stimulation of DA receptors by apomorphine antagonizes the increased fighting. When synthesis of DA and NE is blocked by AMT or when NE synthesis is blocked by FLa-63, shock-induced fighting does not increase.

It has been suggested that CAs mediate aggressive behavior by inhibiting it (as was suggested for 5-HT in Chapter 4). If this is true, increases in aggressive behavior should follow a decrease in brain catecholamine content. We have seen that shock-induced fighting does increase when CAs are reduced by 6-HDA but not when CAs are reduced by AMT or FLa-63. The reason for this discrepancy might be related to the terminal degeneration that occurs following 6-HDA. It has been suggested that terminal degeneration following 6-HDA increases the sensitivity of receptors to DA, as evidenced by increased sensitivity (supersensitivity) to L-dopa in rats pretreated with 6-HDA.

It should also be noted that aggression is a complicated behavior, which has many forms including territorial, predatory and defensive aspects. Changes in one measure of aggression may not correlate with changes in another measure. Clearly, further research is necessary to reconcile apparent conflicts (see Eichelman and Thoa, 1973; Redmond *et al.*, 1971; Reis, 1974).

Food Intake

Destruction of the ventromedial hypothalamus (VMH) in rats and other animals leads to a hyperphagia and an increase in body weight, while destruction of the lateral hypothalamic area (LHA) leads to hypophagia, with a decrease in body weight and death in a certain proportion of lesioned animals. In addition, electrical and chemical stimulation in the LHA, particularly the perifornical area (PA), elicit feeding in sated animals. From this evidence it has been proposed that the ventromedial hypothalamus functions in satiety, and the lateral hypothalamic area and the perifornical area function in feeding. Food intake, therefore, is thought to be, in part, a function of the relative activity of these three loci in the hypothalamus. While there are many unresolved questions regarding the regulation of food intake, for the purposes of this chapter, we will assume certain functional and anatomical characteristics of this system.

Before proceeding to an investigation of the chemical systems which might mediate feeding behavior we will briefly examine some of the important variables in the regulation of food intake and its control by hypothalamic sites. For example, while it has been found that destructive lesions of the ventromedial hypothalamus cause hyperphagia and obesity, this occurs mainly in female rats. Moreover, while hyperphagia occurs following VMH lesions when rats are offered fresh food or milk sweetened with saccharin, hypophagia is reported when rats are offered unpalatable food. Therefore, the palatability of the diet can influence the hyper- or hypophagic response. In addition, the extent of food deprivation, ambient temperature, the size of the individual subject, as well as the frequency of meals, can influence whether hyperphagia or hypophagia occurs. It should also be pointed out that drinking and eating bear a close relationship. The amount of eating behavior observed in a given situation will depend in part on the amount of water deprivation of the organism (see Myers and Martin, 1973; Myers, 1974).

In general, two techniques have been used to examine biochemical involvement in feeding behavior. In one technique, NE is directly injected into the various hypothalamic regions. Data obtained from work with this technique suggest that NE plays an important role in the regulation of feeding. The other technique commonly used to investigate biochemical involvement in feeding behavior involves the prolonged depletion of catecholamines by 6-HDA. In general, work in this area suggests that DA plays an important role in feeding.

Intracranial Chemical Stimulation and Feeding. In 1960, Grossman demonstrated that direct application of crystalline norepinephrine in the lateral hypothalamic area (LHA) elicited feeding in sated rats. Crystalline norepinephrine was applied through a permanently indwelling cannula in the lateral hypothalamus. This finding has been questioned on the following grounds: (1) the concentration of NE at the tip of the cannula was far above physiological concentrations and therefore created rather extensive lesions at the tip of the cannula (see Routtenberg, 1972; Singer and Montgomery, 1973, for a review of methodology in intracranial stimulation); (2) the dose of NE and the extent of diffusion of NE into other areas of the brain could not be ascertained. However, subsequent research with refined injection techniques in which NE was administered in solution and in nanogram quantities has confirmed Grossman's original finding that NE elicits feeding behavior when applied in the hypothalamus (Booth, 1968; Slangen and Miller, 1969).

Subsequently, the anatomical localization and the nature of the receptor site have been examined, and the connection between regulation of feeding by the lateral hypothalamic area, the perifornical area and the ventromedial hypothalamus has been explored. In general, the results show that the PA, and to a lesser extent the LHA, is rich in noradrenergic receptors that control feeding behavior. Application of alpha noradrenergic agonists to this area elicits feeding, while beta noradrenergic agonists decrease feeding. The generality of these findings is tempered, however, by other factors important in the control of feeding, such as the palatability of the food, the phase of the diurnal cycle and the sex of the animal.

Booth (1967, 1968) proposed that an alpha noradrenergic system elicited feeding. His proposal was based on the following findings: Booth injected NE in solution close to the stria medullaris and its confluence with lateral cortico-olfacto-habenular tracts at the rostral tip of the lateral hypothalamus, i.e., the perifornical area (PA). Food consumption was measured at intervals over a two-hour period. A reliable eating response was obtained from sated rats following administration of 2.5 μg of norepinephrine. In general, the amount of food consumed increased as the quantity of norepinephrine injected was increased. *l-*Epinephrine (an alpha agonist) also elicited eating, while other noradrenergic agonists whose primary effects are on beta receptors did not. Moreover, injection of NE into the LHA did not elicit feeding behavior in sated rats. When the alpha blockers phenoxybenzamine or phentolamine were injected directly into the PA, effects of norepinephrine were blocked. Beta blockers had no effect, suggesting that the feeding response is elicited by the alpha receptors (Table 5-2).

TABLE 5-2. Effects of direct application of noradrenergic agonists and antagonists to hypothalamic areas in the rat

Area	Chemicals	Response	Reference
LHA[1]	NE (α agonist)	increased feeding	Grossman (1960)
LHA	NE	increased Metracal consumption	Wagner and DeGroot (1963)
LHA	NE	no effect on feeding	Booth (1967, 1968)
LHA	isoproterenol (β agonist)	decreased feeding	Leibowitz (1970)
PA[2]	NE and E (α agonists)	increased feeding	Booth (1967, 1968); Slangen and Miller (1969); Leibowitz (1970)
PA	NE	decreased milk consumption	Margules (1970a, b)
PA	isoproterenol (β agonist)	decreased feeding	Leibowitz (1970)
PA	phentolamine (α blocker) followed by NE	blocked NE-induced feeding	Booth (1968); Slangen and Miller (1969)
PA	phentolamine	blocked deprivation-induced feeding	Leibowitz (1970)
PA	phentolamine	increases milk consumption, but if milk treated with quinine, milk consumption is decreased	Margules (1970a)
PA	propanolol followed by NE	no change in NE-induced feeding	Booth (1968); Slangen and Miller (1969)
PA	propanolol (β blocker) followed by isoproterenol	blocks isoproterenol-induced decrease in feeding	Leibowitz (1970)
VMH[3]	E	drinking of Metracal	Wagner and DeGroot (1963)
VMH	NE, E	increased feeding	Leibowitz (1970)
VMH	isoproterenol	no effect	Leibowitz (1970)

[1]LHA: Lateral hypothalamic area.
[2]PA: Perifornical area.
[3]VMH: Ventromedial hypothalamus.

Moreover, increases in feeding behavior produced by NE were potentiated by desmethylimipramine (DMI) which blocks reuptake of NE (Booth, 1968; Slangen and Miller, 1969). When DMI was injected by itself into the lateral hypothalamus, food consumption was increased in rats that were food-deprived, but consumption did not increase in sated rats (Montgomery et al., 1971). Montgomery suggested that NE was released from the lateral hypothalamus in deprived rats and therefore DMI potentiated the effects of the released NE by preventing its reuptake. If NE is not released in nondeprived rats, then DMI can have no effect (see Miller et al., 1964).

Leibowitz (1972) extended Booth's proposal that an alpha noradrenergic system elicits feeding to include a beta system which inhibits feeding. This proposal is based on an examination of food intake in rats following injections of a norepinephrine solution and of other agonists and antagonists into the periforical area or the ventromedial hypothalamus. An injection of norepinephrine (primarily an alpha agonist) into the PA enhanced food intake in both sated and food-deprived rats in a dose-related manner. The enhanced feeding was blocked by phentolamine (an alpha blocker). On the other hand, injection of isoproterenol (a beta agonist) at the same site decreased food intake in food-deprived rats. This effect was blocked by propanolol (a beta blocker). When the site of injection was in the ventromedial hypothalamus, food intake was enhanced following alpha agonists and attenuated with an alpha blocker. Injection of beta agonists into the medial hypothalamus did not alter food intake (Table 5-2).

Leibowitz suggested from these findings that noradrenergic neurons terminating on alpha receptors in the ventromedial hypothalamus inhibit a satiety system and, as a result of this inhibition, cause feeding. Similarly, she suggested that noradrenergic cells terminating on beta receptors in the PA inhibit the feeding system and as a result suppress feeding. (See also Broekkamp and Van Rossum, 1972.) In summary, according to Leibowitz's scheme, there is an alpha system that inhibits satiety and "turns on" or releases feeding and a beta system that inhibits food intake and thereby "turns off" or suppresses feeding (see Table 5-2).

While both Leibowitz and Booth found that solutions of NE introduced directly into the PA increased food intake, Margules (1970a, b) found that crystalline NE introduced into the PA decreased milk consumption (Table 5-2). Milk consumption was increased, however, when NE was administered in the presence of an alpha blocker. The alpha blocker did not increase milk consumption when the milk was treated with quinine to make it unpalatable, suggesting that palatability is an important factor in food intake. Margules also reported that a beta agonist, isoproterenol, decreased intake with unpalatable food, but caused no change with palatable food. When a beta blocker was introduced into the system, intake increased for both palatable and unpalatable food. On the basis of these data, Margules proposed that the beta system is a satiety system which is responsive to external cues (e.g., food taste) rather than internal cues such as an empty stomach or low blood sugar (Rabin, 1972; Grossman, 1972).

The fact that norepinephrine produces an increase in feeding in some situations (Leibowitz, 1970) and a decrease in others (Margules, 1970a, b) can be explained by examining the environmental conditions under which NE was administered. Margules and his colleagues (1972) showed that the effect of NE on the lateral hypothalamus depended on whether NE was administered during the light or dark phase of the diurnal cycle. During the dark phase of the diurnal cycle, crystalline NE inhibited the milk-drinking response; but during the light phase of the diurnal cycle, treatment with the same dose of NE facilitated feeding behavior. Leibowitz administered NE in the light phase of the cycle, while

Margules usually administered it in the dark phase. Armstrong and Singer (1974) also found that feeding was dependent on the diurnal cycle; however, in contrast to all other results, they did not find that NE enhanced food intake when injected into the perifornical area. In interpreting these divergent results, it is important to note that these studies differ in a number of ways, including differences in the form of NE (crystalline or solution), the dose, the type of food consumed (rat chow or milk), the precise anatomical site of injection and/or state of deprivation.

Nevertheless, the work of Grossman, Leibowitz, Booth and Margules implicates norepinephrine in feeding and satiety in the lateral and ventromedial nuclei of the hypothalamus (see Table 5-2). The fact that NE is normally found in neurons at these anatomical sites suggests that endogenous NE may play a role in normal feeding behavior. On the other hand, Friedman *et al.* (1973) have suggested that both hypothalamic NE and DA function in feeding behavior (see also Coscina *et al.*, 1973). Friedman *et al.* found that NE injected into the lateral hypothalamus elicited eating in nondeprived but not in deprived rats, while DA enhanced feeding in deprived rats. This finding suggests that NE may disinhibit feeding in nondeprived rats, while DA has an excitatory influence in deprived rats. The reasons for this apparent discrepancy are not clear, but several possibilities exist. Recall that DA plays an important role in motor function. Myers (1974) and Rolls *et al.* (1974) have suggested that decreases in feeding may be secondary to changes in motor function since food consumption involves complex motor functions.

Prolonged Catecholamine Depletion and Feeding. In general, 6-HDA produces a transient but severe aphagia in rats. When the rats are force-fed so that food intake is maintained during the most severe periods of aphagia, feeding partially returns approximately seven days after the 6-HDA injection; however, body weights of 6-HDA rats are often lower than for controls. Evidence will be reviewed that the feeding deficits are a function of the prolonged depletion of dopamine by 6-HDA.

Ungerstedt (1971a, 1973) has shown that bilateral lesions produced by an injection of 6-HDA in the nigrostriatal system produce both a decrease in DA and severe aphagia and adipsia. In addition, rats lesioned in either the lateral hypothalamus or the substantia nigra, all exhibited the typical lateral hypothalamic syndrome of severe aphagia and adipsia of such proportions that death occurred if the rats were not tube-fed for at least five or six days. After five to six days of tube feeding, rats were put on a special diet of preferred foods. Spontaneous feeding and drinking resumed in about three to five weeks.

Ungerstedt also found that lesions which produced severe aphagia and adipsia destroyed the dopamine-containing nigrostriatal tract. Aphagia and adipsia were not produced by selective lesions of the noradrenergic system or of the dopaminergic system supplying axons to the nucleus accumbens or the olfactory tubercle. Ungerstedt (1973) suggested that degeneration of DA nerve terminals leading to the striatum was responsible for the aphagia and adipsia, which has been called the "lateral hypothalamic syndrome."

Zigmond and Stricker (1972) have also demonstrated that dopamine plays an important role in the maintenance of normal feeding behavior. They investigated the effects of 6-HDA or electrolytic lesions on feeding. 6-HDA produced a moderate aphagia and failure to maintain body weight that was similar to the effects of a lesion in the lateral hypothalamus. The lateral hypothalamic lesions produced depletion of telencephalic NE and striatal DA. When 6-HDA was injected, NE was depleted by 95% and DA was depleted by 60%. When pargyline (MAO inhibitor) was administered prior to 6-HDA, the aphagia was more severe and the depletion of NE and DA was over 95%. Rats slowly recovered from the severe aphagia produced by 6-HDA and pargyline, but the brain CA levels did not increase. With severe depletion of striatal DA, special feeding regimens (e.g., a diet of highly palatable food) had to be instituted to obtain a gradual recovery of feeding. While most rats did recover normal feeding behavior, they did not respond normally to glucose deprivation. Moreover, food intake was decreased by AMT alone. When AMT was given following 6-HDA, food intake was further decreased. On the basis of this evidence, Zigmond and Stricker concluded that partial recovery of feeding behavior following 6-HDA treatment is due to compensatory processes within the damaged system. For example, it was suggested that DA neurons not destroyed by 6-HDA increase their synthetic capacity and turnover, thereby producing partial recovery of function.

Further evidence for the role of DA in aphagia has been provided by studies producing selective depletion of either DA or NE (Smith *et al.*, 1973). Dopamine or norepinephrine can be selectively deplected by injecting 6-HDA in combination with other drugs (see p. 125). It has been shown that when DA is decreased and NE remains normal, sucrose consumption is decreased in rats. On the other hand, when NE is decreased and DA remains normal, sucrose consumption is normal (also see Breese *et al.*, 1973b).

This evidence suggests that DA plays a primary role in feeding behavior. It is important to note, however, that while selective depletion of DA following a combination of 6-HDA and certain other drugs (e.g., DMI) leads to a decrease in feeding behavior, this does not eliminate the importance of NE. 6-HDA may interfere with the utilization of NE at the receptors by direct receptor blockade or by decreasing NE turnover. Moreover, some small functional pool in the lateral hypothalamus could be selectively depleted by this treatment but go unmeasured in terms of whole brain levels.

In summary, work with direct chemical application of NE to the lateral hypothalamus, suggests a primary role for NE in feeding behavior. Evidence from studies in which 6-HDA is used to deplete catecholamines suggests that DA also plays a primary role in feeding behavior. It should be noted, however, that direct application of NE does not ensure that NE only stimulates the lateral hypothalamus. Norepinephrine may diffuse to proximal areas containing DA fibers and produce its effects by stimulating the nigrostriatal system. In addition, it is important to recognize that high concentrations of NE were directly applied to the LH and that much of the injected compound may have been metabolized. It is not possible to determine just how much of the injected NE actually reached the receptor sites (see section in Chapter 2 on routes of drug administration). Moreover, work with NE has focused on only two hypothalamic sites believed to be involved in the regulation of food intake. While lesion, stimulation and drug studies make this account highly attractive, it seems unlikely that feeding regulation would be confined to only two areas. The crucial innervation of, and interconnections in, the feeding regulation system have not been worked out. More detailed investigation of the anatomical, chemical and behavioral variables involved is necessary to promote understanding of feeding regulation. (See Grossman, 1972, for a review of extrahypothalamic systems involved in food intake.) The strength and significance of the work we have just described lies in the fact that it provides both some consistent data and a methodological approach to this problem.

Schedule-Controlled Behavior

In the preceding pages we have presented evidence that dopamine and norepinephrine play a role in motor behavior, aggressive behavior and food intake. Knowledge in these areas is not precise or definitive, but it seems fair to conclude that the evidence to date does indicate that catecholamines play a role in these three types of behavior. Dopamine is involved in the expression of normal motor activity, while norepinephrine in the hypothalamus and dopamine in the striatum seem to be involved with regulation of food intake. Both catecholamines play a role in aggressive behavior. The question therefore arises as to what other forms of behavior depend on normal function of the brain catecholamines.

In this section, data will be presented which suggest that both DA and NE in the CNS play an important role in the mediation of behavior that is maintained by negative and positive reinforcement. In particular it will be shown that DA plays a primary role in the maintenance of avoidance behavior and both DA and NE play a role in the maintenance of behavior maintained by positive reinforcement. Both data which fit these generalizations as well as some exceptions will be discussed.

Negative Reinforcement. Reserpine, like many other drugs used in the treatment of pyschosis (antipsychotics) interferes with the maintenance of previously acquired avoidance responses (see Chapter 9). Furthermore, reserpine interferes with the avoidance component of this behavior in a dose range that does not affect the escape component. That is, the response to the stimulus that signals shock is decreased, while the response to the shock remains relatively intact. The reserpine-induced suppression of avoidance responding can be partially and temporarily antagonized by administration of L-dihydroxyphenylalanine (L-dopa), the precursor of dopamine and norepinephrine. In the following paragraphs we will describe: (1) the generality of this effect across species; (2) the relative function of L-dopa, dopamine and norepinephrine in avoidance; (3) the importance of spontaneous motor activity in the reserpine effect; and (4) the function of peripheral and central catecholamines in the maintenance of avoidance. The results of this work are summarized in Table 5-3.

Seiden and Carlsson (1963) trained mice to perform an avoidance response in a shuttle box. A buzzer signaled the shock (see Chapter I for details of the paradigm). Several responses were examined: (1) avoidance responses—when the animal crossed from one side of the shuttle box to the other in the presence of the buzzer; (2) escape responses—when the animal crossed in the presence of the buzzer and shock; (3) response failures—when the animal failed to cross after a specified period of time during both buzzer and shock; and (4) spontaneous crosses—when the animal crossed from one side to the other in the absence of the buzzer or the buzzer-shock complex. After repeated pairing of the buzzer and shock, avoidance responses occurred to a criterion of 90% within 60 to 100 trials.

TABLE 5-3. Avoidance behavior: drug, behavioral, neurochemical effects

Drug	Neurochemical effect	Avoidance response
Reserpine	depletes 5-HT, DA, NE	suppressed
Reserpine + L-dopa	large increase in DA; small increase in NE	partially restores avoidance suppressed by reserpine
Reserpine + 5-HTP	increase in 5-HT; no change in DA or NE	suppressed
Reserpine + D-dopa	depletes 5-HT, DA, NE	suppressed
Reserpine + Ro 4-4602 (large dose) + L-dopa	blocks L-dopa increases in DA and NE; no change in 5-HT	blocks L-dopa restoration of avoidance suppressed by reserpine
Reserpine + disulfiram + L-dopa	increase in DA; no formation of NE; no change in 5-HT	partially blocks L-dopa restoration of avoidance suppressed by reserpine
Reserpine + Ro 4-4602 (small dose) + L-dopa	increase in DA in brain parenchyma	potentiates L-dopa restoration of avoidance suppressed by reserpine
AMT	decrease DA, NE	suppressed
AMT + L-dopa	replace DA, NE	restored

When mice were treated with reserpine (2.5 mg/kg) 20 hours prior to testing, the previously established avoidance response was completely suppressed, while escape responses were only suppressed by about 50%. L-dopa injection resulted in a partial and temporary restoration of the avoidance response, and complete restoration of the escape response (Fig. 5-8). The restoration of avoidance occurred between 15 and 35 minutes after the L-dopa injection; by 80 minutes after L-dopa, avoidance responding was suppressed again; the mice appeared sedated and showed typical reserpine-induced parasympathetic and motor signs. D-dopa did not restore avoidance. (D-dopa unlike L-dopa is not metabolized to dopamine.) 5-Hydroxytryptophan (5-HTP) was not effective in restoring the avoidance response, suggesting that serotonin is not involved in the maintenance of this response. Moreover, mice did not reacquire the avoidance response under

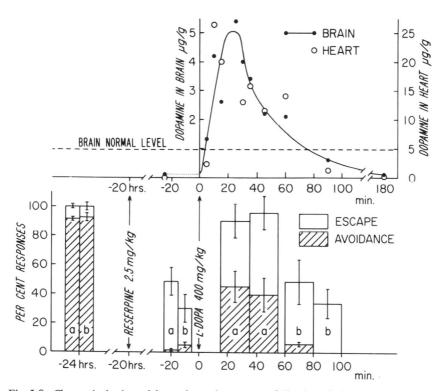

Fig. 5-8. Change in brain and heart dopamine content following administration of L-dopa (above) and corresponding changes in the avoidance and escape responses (below). Experiments (a) and (b) are separate experiments. The controls for each of these experiments appear at 24 hr and at 25 min before L-dopa administration. Each control session has a duration of 20 min. Vertical lines = standard error of the mean. Experiment (a): $N = 7$. Experiment (b): $N = 6$. (From Seiden and Carlsson, 1964).

reserpine. The possibility of reacquisition of the response under the influence of reserpine was of concern since testing occurred for a number of trials in the presence of shock and buzzer.

Control mice were treated in a similar fashion with the same doses of reserpine and L-dopa, and the brains and hearts of these mice were assayed for their DA and NE content. Reserpine, as expected, caused a marked reduction of both DA and NE. L-Dopa administration produced a marked increase in DA but no increase in NE; furthermore, the time course of the DA elevation in brain (but not heart) roughly corresponded to the period during which the avoidance response was restored (Seiden and Carlsson, 1964). Further experiments along these same lines showed that L-dopa could antagonize reserpine-induced suppression of avoidance in rats and cats as well as in certain other strains of mice (Seiden and Carlsson, 1963; Seiden and Hanson, 1964).

Furthermore, the time during which L-dopa had its maximal effect on locomotor activity did not correspond with the time during which L-dopa acted on avoidance responding. One strain of mice showed maximal effects on spontaneous crossing behavior several minutes after avoidance responding was suppressed. The dissociation over time of spontaneous locomotor responses from avoidance responses strongly suggests that the effects of reserpine and L-dopa cannot be accounted for simply in terms of effects on locomotor activity. Moreover, the time period during which the reserpine-induced suppression of avoidance was antagonized corresponds to the period during which DA was synthesized.

While this suggests that DA is necessary for the maintenance of avoidance, it is possible that L-dopa alone was responsible for the observed effects. To examine the role of L-dopa alone in avoidance responding, the following experiment was run: the same avoidance-reserpine-L-dopa experimental paradigm was used except that a decarboxylase inhibitor (Ro 4-4602; 400 mg/kg) was administered before the L-dopa injection (see Table 5-4). By administering 400 mg/kg of Ro 4-4602, 42 minutes prior to testing, the decarboxylation of L-dopa in brain was completely inhibited, but the endogenous levels of brain DA were unchanged. Reserpine-suppressed avoidance responding was not antagonized by L-dopa in the presence of the decarboxylase inhibitor, indicating that L-dopa alone is not responsible for restoring avoidance. When the decarboxylase inhibitor was given alone, it did not interfere with the maintenance of avoidance. If the decarboxylase inhibitor itself interfered with avoidance, it could not be concluded that the decarboxylation of L-dopa into dopamine was critical in restoring avoidance responding suppressed by reserpine (Seiden and Peterson, 1968b).

Despite the fact that an elevation in brain NE was not observed following L-dopa administration, it is possible that NE also plays a role in avoidance behavior. Small amounts of NE might have been formed following L-dopa administration but not stored, and therefore rapidly utilized and metabolized. The function of NE in L-dopa reversal of avoidance suppression can be examined

TABLE 5-4. Avoidance behavior: effects of L-dopa and dopa decarboxylase inhibition[1]

Group	N	Pre-reserpine	20-hr post-reserpine (or vehicle)	12-min post-dopa (or saline)
		Avoidance %	Avoidance %	Avoidance %
Reserpine—I	8	96.2 ± 1.6	0.0 ± 0.0	35.6 ± 7.9
Reserpine and Ro 4-4602—II	7	94.3 ± 2.0	0.0 ± 0.0	0.7 ± 0.7
Ro 4-4602—III	4	96.2 ± 2.4	88.8 ± 3.8	86.2 ± 5.9

Group I: Reserpine (2.5 mg/kg), 0.9% NaCl (10 ml/kg, administered 30 min before L-dopa) and L-dopa (400 mg/kg).
Group II: Reserpine (2.5 mg/kg), Ro 4-4602 (400 mg/kg, administered 30 min before L-dopa) and L-dopa (400 mg/kg).
Group III: Reserpine vehicle (10 ml/kg), Ro 4-4602 (400 mg/kg, administered 30 min before saline) and 0.9% NaCl (40 ml/kg).
Groups I and II differ significantly at the 12-min post-dopa period ($P < .005$).
Results are given ± S.E.
[1]Seiden and Peterson (1968b).

with disulfiram, a dopamine-beta-hydroxylase inhibitor which blocks the conversion of DA to NE. When NE conversion was blocked with disulfiram following L-dopa administration, the reserpine-induced suppression of avoidance responding was only *partially attenuated* (50%).

Biochemical evidence also suggests that both DA and NE play a role in the maintenance of avoidance. While early evidence (Seiden and Carlsson, 1964) indicated that NE was not formed in brain following L-dopa administration in mice pretreated with reserpine (see p. 146), subsequent evidence (Seiden and Peterson, 1968a) indicated that L-dopa produced a small, but significant increase in NE in brain as well as the large increase in DA previously reported. The increase in NE was in the nanogram range (10^{-9} gram), whereas the increase in DA was in microgram range (10^{-6} gram) and exceeded normal brain DA concentrations by several times (Seiden and Peterson, 1968a). The very small increase in NE was blocked when the conversion of DA to NE was blocked by disulfiram. It was concluded, therefore, that both DA and NE play a role in the maintenance of avoidance.

Further evidence for the role of NE in avoidance stems from the following study: Mice were treated with a monoamine oxidase (MAO) inhibitor following pretreatment with reserpine. When L-dopa was subsequently administered, the reserpine-suppressed avoidance response was potentiated by a factor of ten. That is, in the presence of an MAO inhibitor, between 15 and 30 mg/kg of L-dopa was sufficient to restore the avoidance response by 50%; without MAO inhibition between 200 and 400 mg/kg of L-dopa was required to produce an equivalent reversal of the reserpine-suppressed avoidance response. Furthermore, without MAO inhibition, L-dopa increased DA values to greater than five times normal, while NE only increased to 15% of normal; with MAO inhibition and lower doses of L-dopa, L-dopa increased DA to about normal and NE to about 50% of normal. This provides evidence consistent with the conclusion that both DA and NE are involved in the maintenance of avoidance.

There has existed considerable interest and controversy over the extent to which the maintenance of autonomic tone is responsible for the maintenance or acquisition of avoidance behavior. Wenzel and Jeffrey (1967) found that normal development of the sympathetic nervous system in mice was necessary for the acquisition or performance of an avoidance response as well as other behaviors. In this context it is important to remember that both central and peripheral catecholamines are depleted by reserpine and restored by L-dopa administration. Therefore the question arises as to whether the effect of these compounds on avoidance is mediated by the peripheral autonomic or central nervous system (see Pappas and Sobrian, 1972).

It has been shown that restoration of reserpine-suppressed avoidance responding depends on central and *not* peripheral catecholamine formation. In order to separate the effects of central and peripheral CA formation, small doses of Ro 4-4602 that inhibit peripheral decarboxylase without inhibiting central decarboxylase can be used (Bartholini *et al.*, 1969). In mice pretreated with reserpine, and then treated with Ro 4-4602 and L-dopa, no dopamine is formed in the heart, whereas dopamine is formed in the brain. Moreover, the time course of DA formation in brain resulting from a single L-dopa injection is prolonged (Fig. 5-9) in the presence of Ro 4-4602. Groups of mice were trained to perform an avoidance response in the manner already described. After reserpine administration, they were treated with different doses of L-dopa and Ro 4-4602 and tested at varying time intervals after the L-dopa and Ro 4-4602 injection. It was found that the L-dopa antagonism of reserpine suppression was potentiated when peripheral decarboxylation was inhibited by Ro 4-4602 (Fig. 5-10). The peripheral autonomic signs normally observed after L-dopa, such as piloerection, exophthalmos and salivation, were not present when peripheral decarboxylation was inhibited; to the contrary, parasympathetic signs normally seen after reserpine (ptosis, smooth fur, etc.) were observed (Seiden and Martin, 1969).

This experiment suggests that normal peripheral sympathetic nervous system tone is not necessary for maintenance of avoidance, but that central catecholaminergic function is necessary. The importance of CNS catecholaminergic function in avoidance is also supported by the fact that when Ro 4-4602 is given in doses large enough to inhibit decarboxylase centrally, L-dopa does not reverse reserpine-induced avoidance suppression. The potentiation of L-dopa reversal when peripheral decarboxylase is blocked (Fig. 5-10) is accounted for by the

Brain Dopamine

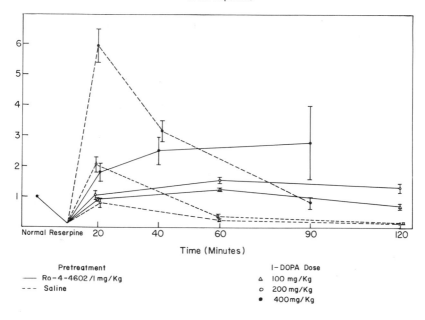

Time (Minutes)

Pretreatment	I-DOPA Dose
—— Ro-4-4602/I mg/Kg	△ 100 mg/Kg
--- Saline	○ 200 mg/Kg
	● 400mg/Kg

Heart Dopamine

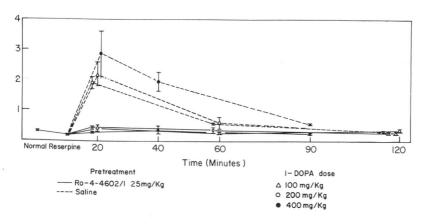

Time (Minutes)

Pretreatment	I-DOPA dose
—— Ro-4-4602/I 25mg/Kg	△ 100 mg/Kg
--- Saline	○ 200 mg/Kg
	● 400 mg/Kg

Fig. 5-9. Dopamine formed in heart and brain following administration of L-dopa in the presence and absence of decarboxylase inhibition. The mice were treated with reserpine (2.5 mg/kg) 20 hr prior to treatment with Ro 4-4602 (25 mg/kg) or saline; 30 min after Ro 4-4602 administration they were injected with varying doses of L-dopa and sacrificed at varying times for amine analysis. Abscissa is the time (min) after dopa injection. Ordinate is μg/g of brain DA. (From Seiden and Martin, 1971.)

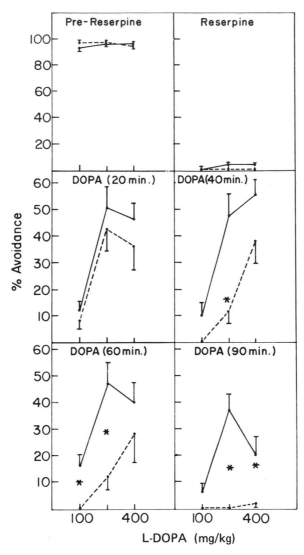

Fig. 5-10. Effect of Ro 4-4602 on the L-dopa reversal of reserpine-induced suppression of the avoidance response. Abscissa is plotted on a log dose scale. Numbers in parentheses indicate the time after L-dopa. Mice treated with reserpine, Ro 4-4602 and dopa; N = 5, 13 and 13 for the 100, 200 and 400 mg/kg doses of L-dopa respectively. Mice treated with reserpine, saline and L-dopa; N = 5, 6 and 5 for 100, 200 and 400 mg/kg doses. P less than 0.05 by t-test. —————Mice treated with reserpine, Ro 4-4602 and L-dopa--------- Mice treated with reserpine, saline and L-dopa. (From Seiden and Martin, 1971.)

fact that a larger amount of L-dopa reaches brain parenchyma (neurons) cells when the decarboxylation of L-dopa is blocked peripherally. Studies have shown that much of the dopamine formed "in the brain" following L-dopa is trapped inside brain capillary walls. In the presence of a peripheral decarboxylase inhibitor, decarboxylation within the capillary walls is also inhibited, and therefore L-dopa can pass from the blood through the capillaries into the brain before it is decarboxylated (Seiden and Martin, 1971).

Other investigators (Wada *et al.*, 1963; Moore, 1966; Rech *et al.*, 1966; Moore and Rech, 1967; Ahlenius and Engel, 1971) have confirmed and extended the finding that catecholamine depletion can suppress avoidance responding, which can in turn be reversed by L-dopa. Drugs such as tetrabenazine and AMT reduce levels of catecholamines in brain, and also interfere with maintenance of avoidance responding. Furthermore, L-dopa can antagonize the behavioral effects of these amine-depleting drugs. For example, Tanaka *et al.* (1972), depleted brain CA levels by multiple injections of AMT and demonstrated a concomitant decrease in responding on a continuous avoidance schedule and an increase in the number of shocks the rats received. Administration of L-dopa antagonized the AMT-induced suppression of lever pressing, but the number of shocks received was only reduced slightly. This is in contrast with the shuttle box situation (see above) where the number of shocks received is decreased when L-dopa is administered after reserpine or AMT.

Using a shuttle box avoidance procedure, Ahlenius (1974a,b) compared a difficult avoidance task (discrete trial successive discriminated avoidance) with a simple avoidance task not involving successive discrimination. The shuttle box avoidance procedure without the successive discrimination is described earlier in this chapter and in Chapter 1. The successive discrimination avoidance procedure uses the same type of shuttle box with the same preshock stimuli except that there are two passages between the compartments of the shuttle box. Above each passage is a lamp; when the lamps are lit, the rat has to pass through the right passage to avoid shock, when they are dark, the rat has to pass through the left passage. The rats are shocked following an incorrect choice.

Ahlenius found that responding in both avoidance tasks was suppressed by either tetrabenazine or AMT. The suppression produced by tetrabenazine in the successive discrimination task could not be reversed by administration of L-dopa. On the other hand, suppression produced by tetrabenazine or AMT on the simple avoidance task could be reversed by L-dopa (see Table 5-5). Ahlenius *et al.* (1971) related this difference in L-dopa antagonism to the different mechanisms by which AMT and tetrabenazine deplete CAs. Recall that AMT inhibits synthesis of CAs and tetrabenazine interferes with their granular storage. When L-dopa is given after AMT, the storage granules can be refilled with DA and NE; but when L-dopa is given after tetrabenazine, the granules are not refilled. In the

TABLE 5-5. Interaction of L-dopa with AMT and tetrabenazine on two avoidance procedures

Drug	Simple avoidance	Successive discriminated avoidance
AMT	suppresses	suppresses
AMT + L-dopa	antagonizes suppression	antagonizes suppression
Tetrabenazine	suppresses	suppresses
Tetrabenazine + L-dopa	antagonizes suppression	still suppressed

case of AMT, the amines replaced by L-dopa are stored in granules and released by nerve stimulation, whereas in the case of tetrabenazine, the amines replaced by L-dopa are probably leaking from the presynaptic neuron independently of nerve stimulation. Ahlenius (1974c) has speculated that postsynaptic stimulation of receptors independent of nerve stimulation may be sufficient to maintain "simpler types" of behavior, but as behavior becomes more complex (as with discriminated avoidance), a more controlled neuronal release of CAs is necessary for the maintenance of behavior.

Prolonged Depletion of Catecholamines and Negative Reinforcement. Smith *et al.* (1973) demonstrated that normal development of CAs could be prevented by injecting 6-HDA into neonatal rats. When tested at 60 days of age for acquisition of shuttle box avoidance responding, rats with low brain DA but normal NE did not acquire the avoidance response. Suppression of avoidance responding was well correlated with 6-HDA-produced depletion of DA. These effects did not occur when DA levels were normal. Moreover, when NE was selectively depleted and dopamine was normal, avoidance acquisition rate was enhanced over control rates. Rats selectively depleted of NE also showed enhanced locomotor activity; it is possible, therefore, that the increase in activity may account for the facilitation of avoidance acquisition. 6-HDA also produced a permanent suppression of responding in one-way shuttle box avoidance procedures (Breese *et al.*, 1973a; Cooper and Bresse, 1974). Shuttle box performance did not recover following 6-HDA, nor did brain amine levels return to normal.

The finding that DA depletion by 6-HDA treatment can interfere with maintenance and acquisition of avoidance responding is consistent with work reported above in which dopamine has been implicated as an important mediator of this behavior (Seiden and Carlsson, 1963, 1964). However, we have seen that NE also plays a role in avoidance behavior (Seiden and Peterson, 1968a). Since 6-HDA depletes NE by only about 60%, a substantial amount of NE is present in brain. Therefore, it is likely that remaining NE is still functionally important.

Positive Reinforcement. A series of studies will be discussed which show that the catecholamines play an important role in behavior maintained by positive reinforcement. Schoenfeld and Seiden (1969) trained rats to press a lever for a small amount of water. One group of rats was trained to respond on fixed ratio schedules (FR 1, 5 and 10). Training was carried out in the following sequence: FR 1, FR 5, FR 10. Another group was trained on fixed interval schedules (FI 30, 60 and 120 sec) in the following sequence: FI 30, FI 60, FI 120 sec. FR and FI schedules engendered characteristic rates and patterns of responding which depended on the parameter chosen for study. When alpha-methyltyrosine (AMT) was administered in doses that depleted brain catecholamines to about 20% of normal, a decrease in response rate was observed. Decreases in responding on the FR schedules depended on the FR requirement. Responding decreased by 34% on the FR 1 schedule, by 59% on the FR 5 schedule and by 78% on the FR 10 schedule (Fig. 5-11). In contrast, on all three FI schedules, responding decreased by 40%. When L-dopa was administered to rats maintained on the FR 10 schedule, the decreases in response rate produced by AMT were attenuated. This finding suggests that the depression in response rate was related to the reduction of catecholamines in brain. Concentrations of DA and NE in brain were measured after rats maintained on the FR 10 schedule of water presentation were treated with AMT plus various doses of L-dopa. Rate of responding was correlated with DA and NE concentrations (Schoenfeld and Seiden, 1969).

Alpha-methyltyrosine produced different effects on the time course of FR and FI performance. On the FR 10 schedule, lever pressing was decreased by 30% in the initial part of the session: within 20 minutes after the start of the session, responding had stopped. On the other hand, FI responding remained at 60% of control throughout the session (Fig. 5-12). These findings suggest that response rate may be a crucial element in determining the effect of AMT, and further suggest that the ongoing behavior may interact with the metabolism of

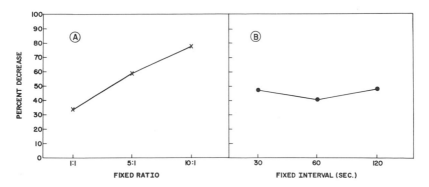

Fig. 5-11. Percent decrease in responding on three different fixed ratio schedules (FR 1, FR 5, FR 10) and three different fixed interval schedules (FI 30, FI 60, FI 120 sec) following AMT (two doses, 75 mg/kg). (From Schoenfeld and Seiden, 1969.)

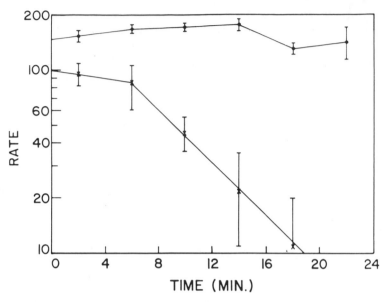

Fig. 5-12. Effect of AMT (two doses of 75 mg/kg) on rate of lever pressing during FR 10 performance (8.0 hr after first dose). Each value represents mean rate per min over consecutive 4-min periods of five animals. ●, 30-min control session; X, 30-min test session. (From Schoenfeld and Seiden, 1969.)

the catecholamines. The changes in metabolism produced by behavioral factors will be discussed in the next section of this chapter.

Other investigators have also shown that the catecholamines play a role in behavior maintained by positive reinforcement (Ahlenius *et al.*, 1971). AMT and tetrabenazine suppressed responding maintained on an FR 40 schedule of food presentation in rats. L-dopa antagonized the AMT-induced suppression but did not antagonize tetrabenazine-induced suppression, although L-dopa administration replenished CAs depleted from brain by both tetrabenazine or AMT. Ahlenius *et al.* (1971) related this difference in L-dopa antagonism to the different mechanisms by which tetrabenazine and AMT deplete CAs (see p. 151). Ahlenius *et al.* proposed that catecholamines replaced by L-dopa following depletion by AMT can be released by nerve stimulation, whereas catecholamines replaced by L-dopa following depletion by tetrabenazine are not stored and therefore leak from the presynaptic neuron independently of nerve stimulation. There are, however, other differences between AMT and tetrabenazine that may be important in this effect. First, alpha-methyltyrosine depletes NE to a greater extent than does tetrabenazine; second, replacement of NE is much greater with L-dopa following AMT pretreatment than following tetrabenazine pretreatment. Third, tetrabenazine depletes 5-HT from brain while AMT does not. It is possible that a combination of these differential effects could account for the different responses to L-dopa.

In summary, agents that reversibly deplete catecholamines from brain generally suppress behavior maintained by positive reinforcement. This effect depends upon the schedule of reinforcement controlling behavior, as well as the drug dose.

Prolonged Depletion of Catecholamines and Positive Reinforcement. In the following paragraphs, we will examine the effects of intraventricular or intracisternal injection of 6-HDA on behavior maintained by positive reinforcement. The results of these studies are puzzling when compared to the effects of pharmacological agents that temporarily deplete CAs from brain. The evidence generally indicates that AMT, reserpine and tetrabenazine decrease behavior maintained by either positive or negative reinforcement. We have seen that 6-HDA also decreases behavior maintained by negative reinforcement, and in this respect is similar to AMT, reserpine and tetrabenazine. The influence of 6-HDA on behavior maintained by positive reinforcement, however, differs in some ways from the effects of other amine depletors. 6-HDA often results in a temporary decrease in behavior a day or two after administration, followed by a return to control levels. This return of behavior to control levels occurs in spite of the fact that brain CA levels remain low because of permanent destruction of a large population of catecholaminergic neurons.

Schoenfeld and Zigmond (1970) examined the effects of 6-HDA on behavior maintained by positive reinforcement. Rats were trained to respond on an FR schedule for water and were treated with two doses of 6-HDA (250 μg/dose). Rats treated with 6-HDA showed transient suppression of lever pressing which lasted only three or four days (Fig. 5–13a), while brain CA levels remained permanently decreased (Schoenfeld and Zigmond, 1973). A dose of AMT that did not affect control rats completely suppressed responding in 6-HDA-treated rats (Fig. 5–13b). The increased sensitivity to the effects of AMT in 6-HDA-treated rats indicates that catecholaminergic function was not normal in 6-HDA rats. Cooper et al. (1972) obtained similar results with an FR 1 schedule of food presentation. While 6-HDA-treated rats showed no change in schedule-controlled behavior after brain NE and DA levels were depleted, low doses of reserpine or AMT that had no effect on behavior when given alone (see Cooper et al., 1973) suppressed behavior. The question therefore arises as to how behavior could be maintained with the low levels of catecholamines remaining. Schoenfeld and Zigmond suggested that behavior was maintained by the CA neurons that survived 6-HDA treatment, possibly through a mechanism of supersensitivity (see p. 134).

Further studies by Schoenfeld and Uretsky (1972) using a VI 90-sec schedule of water presentation with a 9-min time-out period in the middle of the session,

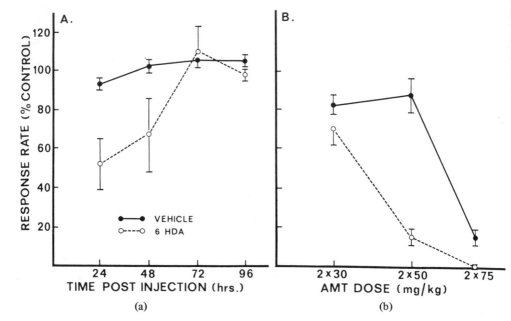

Fig. 5-13. (a) Effect of 6-HDA on FR 20 performance. Two hundred fifty micrograms of 6-HDA or vehicle was injected into alternate lateral ventricles (48 hr apart) under ether anesthesia. Twenty-four hours after the second injection, testing was continued. Each point represents the mean (± S.E.M.) response output as a percentage of each group's mean response output for three days prior to injection ($N = 6$). (b) Effect of α-methyltyrosine (AMT) on FR-20 performance of 6-HDA and vehicle-treated rats. D,L-α-methyltyrosine or saline was administered 6 and 3 hr prior to the session. Each point represents the mean (± S.E.M.) response output as a percentage of the previous day's response output ($N = 6$). (From Schoenfeld and Zigmond, 1973.)

demonstrated that rats treated with 6-HDA showed a permanent fourfold increase in response rate (Fig. 5-14), which developed over a number of weeks. Similarly increases in responding maintained on an FR 30 schedule of food presentation were reported by Peterson and Sparber (1973).

The increases in responding seen after 6-HDA treatment are difficult to reconcile with previous reports that the depletion of catecholamines leads to a decrease or no change in schedule-controlled behavior depending upon the schedule of reinforcement and extent of CA depletion. While different schedules of reinforcement may be more dependent on the integrity of catecholamine pools than others, there are no reports where CA depletion by any means other than 6-HDA leads to an increase in schedule-controlled behavior. Furthermore, the fact that treatment with 6-HDA causes a decrease in food and water intake (see section on feeding) is difficult to reconcile with the fact that rats treated with 6-HDA respond more for food or water than control rats. The explanation for these

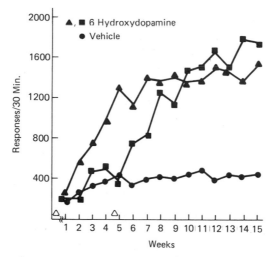

Fig. 5-14. Effect of 6-hydroxydopamine (6-HDA) on the response output of rats on a variable interval (VI) schedule of reinforcement. 6-HDA (▲——▲, $N = 8$) or vehicle (●——●, $N = 10$), was administered three weeks before training (first arrow). After four weeks of training (second arrow), three rats from the vehicle-treated group received 2×250 μg 6-HDA (■——■). Each point represents the mean number of responses of each group during a 30-min session. For clarity, only the data obtained from Wednesday of each week are plotted. (From Schoenfeld and Uretsky, 1972).

diverse findings is not apparent. Possibly there are other neurochemical systems affected by 6-HDA that may account for some of the observed effects. Supersensitivity to the locomotor stimulant effects of L-dopa has been observed after 6-HDA treatment (Schoenfeld and Uretsky, 1972), and it is possible that increases in responding result from this type of supersensitivity. If some small fraction of dopamine or norepinephrine remains following destruction of CA-containing fibers with 6-HDA, these remaining amines may be crucial to the maintenance of responding. The remaining amines along with receptors that are supersentitive to the amines may account for the increased behavior.

CHANGES IN CATECHOLAMINE METABOLISM PRODUCED BY BEHAVIORAL AND ENVIRONMENTAL FACTORS

In the preceding pages, evidence has been presented that a number of drugs, such as reserpine, AMT and 6-HDA affect catecholamine concentration in brain and thereby affect various behaviors. These studies provide strong evidence that dopamine and norepinephrine play an important role in the maintenance and development of normal behavior. Some behaviors are more sensitive to catecholamine alteration than others, however; while this may reflect a differential role for catecholamines in various behaviors, some data cannot be readily accounted for on this basis. For example, there is little reason to expect that large-valued fixed-ratio schedules are more dependent on CAs than lower-valued ratio schedules. Nevertheless, higher ratio schedules seem more sensitive to catecholamine-depleting effects of AMT than lower ratio schedules (see p. 153). A reasonable explanation of this finding is that the rate and pattern of ongoing behavior functionally alter the disposition and metabolism of the catecholamines. If catecholamines as transmitters in the central nervous system play a role in behavior, then a variety of factors such as sensory stimulation, stress and different behaviors would be expected to alter catecholamine release in the CNS.

Experimental evidence indicates that rather small subcellular amine pools maintain CNS function (see Schumann and Kroneberg, 1970). Alterations in a small functional pool of amines may be difficult to detect. Furthermore, the homeostatic mechanisms regulating the synthesis of amines can alter amine synthesis so that during periods of high amine utilization the rate of synthesis is increased, and correspondingly during periods of low utilization, synthesis is slowed down. Moreover, measurement of amine concentration may not be a true indicator of amine activity. Therefore, the rate of synthesis, release and catabolism should be measured in addition to changes in concentration. Changes in synthesis, release and catabolism are measured as alterations in turnover. The use of the term turnover must be qualified in this context, since we are dealing with a complicated system which involves not only synthesis and degradation (as in a more straightforward biochemical system), but also storage, release and re-

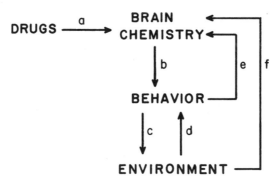

Fig. 5-15. Modification of behavior through the internal and external milieu. These might include: (a) alteration in brain chemistry by a drug as well as (b) the modification of behavior by alterations in brain chemistry (e.g., Seiden and Carlsson, 1964). Behavior also acts on the environment to produce a consequence (c) (see Chapter 1), and the environment itself may influence behavior (d) by providing the conditions necessary for the occurrence of behavior (e.g., Skinner, 1938; Reynolds, 1961; Terrace, 1963). Further (e) behavior may alter brain chemistry (e.g., Schoenfeld and Seiden, 1969; Lewy and Seiden, 1972). In addition (f), the environment may alter behavior by modifying brain chemistry (e.g., Rosenzweig *et al.*, 1962; Moore, 1963).

uptake of amines. Generally, in the experiments discussed below it is not possible to determine which factor or factors are altered; but for the present we will consider alterations in any of these processes as indicative of a change in metabolism or turnover. In the following pages, we will describe environmental and behavioral variables which cause alterations in either the concentration or turnover of the CAs. We will propose a neurochemical model by which differential drug effects on behavior may be understood (see Fig. 5-15).

Environmental Stress

While several investigators have demonstrated that various environmental factors such as intense electrical shock, forced motor activity or forced swimming for prolonged periods of up to several hours result in a decrease in the concentration of norepinephrine in brain and other tissues, other investigators have not found changes in NE content as a result of these or other forms of stress. Since the parameters of the various experimental situations used to examine this question differ so much, it is difficult to reconcile these discrepancies. Nevertheless, it is worthwhile to review some of these data since they are the basis for the notion that environmental factors influence the metabolism of putative CNS transmitters.

Bliss *et al.* (1966) investigated the effects of intense electrical shock on the levels and turnover rate of NE, DA and 5-HT in rats. In one experiment, they found that foot shock decreased brain NE concentration by about 30% one hour after administration. In other experiments, they found that decreases in NE levels were a function of shock intensity and duration. NE levels decreased by approximately the same amounts in the different neuroanatomical regions of the brain examined, including cerebral cortex, subcortex, brain stem, hypothalamus and cerebellum. AMT potentiated the decrease in NE, suggesting that NE was more rapidly released and metabolized as a result of the foot shock. Other stresses such as audiogenic seizures and electroconvulsive shock also decreased NE, suggesting that intense afferent stimulation results in increased neuronal discharge causing increased release of NE. A decrease in NE levels indicates that the rate of NE synthesis is unable to keep pace with the rate of release and catabolism.

Since the concentration of an amine does not necessarily reflect its functional levels, many investigators have measured changes in turnover as a function of afferent stimulation. For example, although concentrations of dopamine do not change as a result of foot shock, the turnover rate of DA is increased. (See Chapter 2 for a discussion of how turnover is measured.) In addition, increases in turnover rate of NE have been demonstrated as a result of a low shock which did not change NE concentration (Thierry *et al.*, 1968). Moreover, while exercise and exposure to cold do not produce changes in NE levels, they do produce a considerable increase in turnover rate as measured by the incorporation of ^{14}C-tyrosine into ^{14}C-NE, suggesting that exercise or cold exposure promotes increased synthesis of NE. Since tyrosine hydroxylase is the rate-limiting step in NE synthesis, it is reasonable to assume that the activity of this enzyme might be stimulated during periods of increased demand; however, the mechanism by which this occurs is not understood (Gordon *et al.*, 1966).

While these data indicate that environmental stress can influence the concentrations and turnover rate of brain amines, interpretation is confounded by the fact that some of the stimuli (e.g., shock or cold) were so intense that the animal could have been near death. If it were pushed to its limit, one could get dramatic changes in turnover rate through the death of the animal, but no one could seriously argue that this represents a specific, behaviorally dependent neurochemical change.

Behavioral-Environmental Factors

Several behaviors and environmental conditions alter the metabolism of amines in brain. For example, Draskóczy and Lyman (1967) demonstrated differences in catecholamine turnover rates in various tissues of the ground squirrel that depended on whether the squirrel was in an active or hibernating state. The stores of catecholamines were labeled by injection with tritiated L-dopa and the squirrels were killed at various times up to 96 hours after injection. Hibernation and activity were induced by controlling environmental temperature; hibernation was monitored by a thermal probe placed in the nest. When hibernation occurs, the temperature of the nest drops precipitously by several degrees. It was found that brown adipose tissue had the highest turnover rate of NE in the active state; lower turnover rates were found in heart and brain; the lowest turnover was obtained in the adrenal medulla. During hibernation, turnover rate decreased by 90% in the brain, whereas turnover rate remained the same in other tissues. Moreover, turnover rate decreased before the animals had reached a full state of hibernation, suggesting a causal relationship between central noradrenergic neural function and the onset of hibernation.

Aggressive behavior, the social conditions under which it is expressed, as well as antecedent conditions that elicit aggression, also modify catecholamine metabolism. Welch and Welch (1968) found that isolation induced fighting in mice. Moreover, they found that AMT depleted NE and DA at a slower rate in isolated than in grouped mice (see Welch and Welch, 1969). It has also been shown that isolation decreases the rate of catecholamine metabolism in brain (Modigh, 1973). Brain CA metabolism increased, however, when isolated mice were subsequently grouped and therefore engaged in vigorous fighting. In addition, turnover rates in isolated mice were significantly lower than in control mice. When mice were grouped and engaged in fighting, the turnover rates increased beyond normal values. Isolated and grouped mice also showed changes in CA utilization rate which was measured by inhibiting tyrosine hydroxylase with an AMT analogue (Modigh, 1974). This work emphasizes the importance of antecedent conditions and current environmental conditions in the control of brain catecholamine metabolism.

There is also evidence that training and performance of schedule-controlled behavior may produce neurochemical changes. For example, changes in catecholamine metabolism have been shown to occur as a function of avoidance responding (Hurwitz *et al.*, 1971). Rats were trained to avoid shock by pressing a lever whenever a tone sounded. Dopamine concentrations in brain were found to be higher, and norepinephrine concentrations lower in disulfiram-treated rats performing the avoidance task, when compared to an untrained control group (see Fig. 5-16). This effect was shown to be a function of both training *and* performance variables. Four major groups were compared: (1) untrained or trained, but not run in the experimental chamber on the day of the experiment (untrained Group and Group A in Fig. 5-16); both of these subgroups received saline injections; (2) untrained or trained, placed in the experimental chamber on the day of the experiment, but without the experimental contingencies in effect (untrained Group and Group B in Fig. 5-16); both of these subgroups were injected with disulfiram one hour before being placed in the experimental

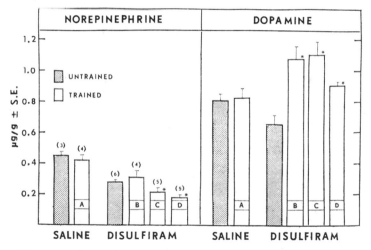

Fig. 5-16. Effect of saline or disulfiram (100 mg/kg) on brain catecholamines 3 hr after injection. Untrained and group *A* animals were not subjected to the experimental chambers before or after injection. Group *B* rats remained in the chambers 1 hr before and 3 hr after drug administration without performing, while *C* and *D* animals performed for 1 hr before and either remained inactive for 3 hr after treatment with the drug (*C*) or avoided during the 3rd hr (*D*). The numbers in parentheses refer to the total number of animals in each group. For those groups whose brain amine levels differed significantly from those of disulfiram-untrained animals, $P < 0.05$. (From Hurwitz *et al.*, 1971.)

chamber; (3) trained and performing before but not after disulfiram administration (Group C, Fig. 5-16); and (4) trained and performing both before and after disulfiram administration (Group D, Fig. 5-16). After engaging in one of these activities, rats were killed and their brains assayed for catecholamines. In the groups that were trained and performing (C and D), DA levels increased and NE levels decreased, compared to the untrained rats, while in the group trained but not performing (B), DA levels increased, but NE levels were unchanged. Therefore, DA levels increased following disulfiram in trained animals regardless of whether the rats performed the avoidance response or not; NE levels were further decreased by performance. It was concluded that *both* training *and* performance altered CA metabolism by increasing turnover. Since disulfiram inhibits dopamine-beta-hydroxylase, which converts DA to NE, an increase in DA and a decrease in NE can be accounted for by an increase in turnover rate. The importance of training in increasing turnover rates of NE is not entirely clear from this experiment however, since rats that were trained and did not perform after disulfiram did receive an hour of testing prior to disulfiram administration. It is possible that performance during this testing session had a carry over effect and that training *per se* did not increase turnover.

Changes in brain metabolism of NE also occur as a function of behavior maintained by positive reinforcement. Lewy and Seiden (1972) examined NE metabolism in three different behavioral situations. The following three groups of rats were used: (1) a group that was water-deprived and trained to press a lever for water on a variable-interval (VI) schedule; (2) a group that was similarly water-deprived but untrained; and (3) a group that was neither trained nor deprived. After the first group had about 15 days of VI training, all groups were injected with tritiated NE introduced into the brain via cannulas chronically implanted in one of the lateral ventricles. Immediately after the injection, the group trained on the VI schedule was run in an experimental session during which they responded on a VI schedule for water. The two control groups were returned to their home cages. Two hours later, animals were killed and endogenous NE, tritiated NE and its metabolites were measured in the brain-stem and hypothalamus. The specific activity (tritiated NE/endogenous NE) was lower in the trained-performing group than in either of the two control groups (Fig. 5-17), indicating that performance on a VI schedule increases the rate of NE metabolism. No differences were seen in endogenous NE concentration between the three groups. Differences in specific activity were due to the amount of ^{3}H-NE remaining in the brain-stem–hypothalamus after the two-hour period. Analysis of tritiated NE metabolites showed a larger percentage of O-methylated deaminated metabolites in the performing group than in either of the control groups. This finding is consistent with the notion that NE was released from nerve endings, and as a result of the release and subsequent metabolism, new NE was synthesized. Recall that the areas analyzed (i.e., brain-stem and hypoth-

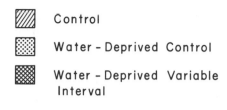

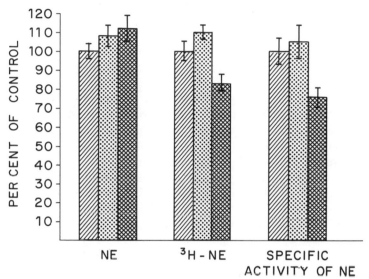

Fig. 5-17. The effect of operant behavior and water deprivation on the concentrations of NE and the specific activity of NE in the rat brain-stem–diencephalon. Values represent the mean of five animals ±S.E.M. Absolute values for the control group are 0.555 ± 0.022 μg of NE, 92.7 ± 5.3 mμc/g of ^{3}H–NE, and 168 ± 13 mμc/g specific activity of NE. (From Seiden *et al.*, 1973.)

alamus) contain both NE cell bodies and nerve endings where synthesis and release occur, respectively (see this chapter, p. 118). The fact that the water-deprived group did not differ from the nondeprived group suggests that the effect was not due to water deprivation, but rather that some aspect of the training or performance was responsible for the increased NE metabolism.

Further experiments revealed that the increased utilization of NE could not be attributed to motor activity or to training. One group of rats ran in a running wheel for several hours each day, while another group was handled similarly but given no running wheel experience. No difference in the metabolism of norepinephrine was seen between running wheel rats and control rats, nor was there any correlation in the running group between distance run and the turnover of NE. In another experiment, trained and performing rats were compared to rats that had been trained but were not performing the task on the experimental day. Differences in NE metabolism were observed between the performing group and a trained but nonperforming group. The difference between these groups was the same as between a performing group and a water-deprived group. This result suggests that neither motor activity nor training alone was sufficient to cause a change in NE metabolism in the brain-stem and hypothalamus. In rats trained to avoid a shock, however, alteration in NE metabolism is a function of *both* training and performance. These differences may be attributed to several factors, including: (1) the behavioral task; (2) the method used to measure NE metabolism; or (3) the neuroanatomical areas analyzed. The important point is that NE metabolism can be altered by ongoing behavior (see Sparber and Tilson, 1972; Stolk *et al.*, 1974).

Therefore, the status of the catecholaminergic system depends not only on the integrity of the synthetic, degradative and storage mechanisms in the CNS, but also upon behavior and the environment in which the behavior occurs. We have seen that intense afferent stimulation generally produces a decrease in brain concentration of NE. Isolation, aggression induced by isolation, hibernation, as well as behavior maintained by schedules of reinforcement, produce changes in the "turnover" of catecholamines in the central nervous system. Environmental and behavioral variables therefore are both affected by and affect the catecholamines. The fact that these factors influence catecholamine metabolism must be considered in examining interactions between drugs, behavior and neurochemistry.

SUMMARY

Catecholamines play a role in the maintenance and acquisition of several different behaviors, including motor behavior, aggressive behavior, feeding and behavior that is under schedule control. Dopamine appears to play a primary role in motor activity and in behavior under schedule control, with norepinephrine playing a modulating role. Both norepinephrine and dopamine appear to be involved in feeding. Generally, decreasing catecholamine levels in the central nervous system leads to an inhibition of behavioral function, and increasing catecholamine levels leads to an increase in function, except in the case of aggressive behavior. Drugs also affect catecholamine metabolism, and the behavioral effects of these drugs can sometimes be related to their effects on catecholamines. In addition, environmental factors as well as behavior influence catecholamine levels and metabolism. Therefore, behavioral, environmental and pharmacological variables all influence catecholamine metabolism.

While this work has shown that relationships between endogenous brain chemistry and behavior do exist, these data do not provide detailed functional relationships on which to base predictions. For example, chemical analyses are usually based on whole brain measures. Since neither amines nor behavior uniformly involve all areas of the brain, detailed neuroanatomical analysis is indicated for furture work. An anatomical-behavioral analysis is complicated by the fact that there is little reason to assume that one or only a few discrete brain areas might be involved in any behavior.

REFERENCES

Ahlenius, S. 1974a. Effects of L-Dopa on conditioned avoidance responding after behavioural suppression by alpha-methyltyrosine or reserpine in mice. *Neuropharmacology* 13: 729–739.

Ahlenius, S. 1974b. Effects of low and high doses of L-Dopa on the tetrabenazine or alpha-methyltyrosine-induced suppression of behaviour in a successive discrimination task. *Psychopharmacologia* 39: 199–212.

Ahlenius, S. 1974c. Reversal by L-Dopa of the suppression of locomotor activity induced by inhibition of tyrosine hydroxylase and DA-beta hydroxylase in mice. *Brain Res.* 69: 57–65.

Ahlenius, S. and J. Engel. 1971. Behavioral and biochemical effects of L-DOPA after inhibition of dopamine-β-hydroxylase in reserpine pretreated rats. *Naunyn-Schmiedebergs Arch. Exper. Path. Pharmakol.* 270: 349–360.

Ahlenius, S., N. E. Andén and J. Engel. 1971. Importance of catecholamine release by nerve impulses for free operant behavior. *Physiol. Behav.* 7: 931–934.

Andén, N. E., U. Strömbom and T. H. Svensson. 1973. Dopamine and noradrenaline receptor stimulation: Reversal of reserpine-induced suppression of motor activity. *Psychopharmacologia* 29: 289–298.

Armstrong, S. and G. Singer. 1974. Effects of intrahypothalamic administration of norepinephrine on the feeding response of the rat under conditions of light and darkness. *Pharmacol. Biochem. Behav.* 2: 811–815.

Barbeau, A., H. Mars and L. Gillo-Joffroy. 1971. Adverse clinical side effects of leva dopa therapy. *In* F. H. McDowell and C. H. Markham (eds.), *Recent Advances in Parkinson's Disease*. Davis, Philadelphia, pp. 204–237.

Bartholini, G., J. E. Blum and A. Pletscher. 1969. Dopa-induced locomotor stimulation after inhibition of extracerebral decarboxylase. *J. Pharm. Pharmacol.* 21: 297–301.

Bell, L. J., L. L. Iversen and N. J. Uretsky. 1970. Time course of the effects of 6-hydroxydopamine on catecholamine containing neurons in rat hypothalamus and striatum. *Brit. J. Pharmacol.* 40: 790–799.

Benkert, O., H. Gluba and N. Matussek. 1973a. Dopamine, noradrenaline and 5-hydroxytryptamine in relation to motor activity, fighting and mounting behaviour. I. L-DOPA and DL-threo-dihydroxyphenylserine in combination with Ro 4-4602, pargyline and reserpine. *Neuropharmacology* 12: 177–186.

Benkert, O., A. Renz and N. Matussek. 1973b. Dopamine, noradrenaline and 5-hydroxytryptamine in relation to motor activity, fighting and mounting behaviour. II. L-DOPA and DL-threo-dihydroxyphenylserine in combination with Ro 4-4602 and parachlorophenylalanine. *Neuropharmacology* 12: 187–193.

Blaschko, H. and T. L. Chruściel. 1960. The decarboxylation of amino acids related to tyrosine and their awakening action in reserpine-treated mice. *J. Physiol.* 151: 272–284.

Bliss, E. L., V. B. Wilson and J. Zwanziger. 1966. Changes in brain norepinephrine in self-stimulating and "aversive" animals. *J. Psychiat. Res.* 4: 59–63.

Booth, D. A. 1967. Localization of the adrenergic feeding system in the rat diencephalon. *Science* 158: 515–517.

Booth, D. A. 1968. Mechanism of action of norepinephrine in eliciting an eating response on injection into the rat hypothalamus. *J. Pharmacol. Exp. Ther.* 160: 336–348.

Breese, G. R., B. R. Cooper and R. D. Smith. 1973a. Biochemical and behavioural alterations following 6-hydroxydopamine administration into brain. *In* E. Usdin and S. H. Snyder (eds.), *Frontiers in Catecholamine Research*. Proc. of 3rd Int. Catecholamine Symposium. Pergamon Press, New York, pp. 701–706.

Breese, G. R., R. D. Smith, B. R. Cooper and L. D. Grant. 1973b. Alterations in consummatory behavior following intracisternal injection of 6-hydroxydopamine. *Pharmacol. Biochem. Behav.* 1: 319–328.

Brodie, B. B. and P. A. Shore. 1957. A concept for a role of serotonin and norepinephrine as chemical mediators in the brain. *Ann. N.Y. Acad. Sci.* 66: 631–642.

Broekkamp, C. and J. M. Van Rossum. 1972. Clonidine induced intrahypothalamic stimulation of eating in rats. *Psychopharmacologia* 25: 162–168.

Burkard, W. P., M. Jalfre and J. Blum. 1969. Effect of 6-hydroxydopamine on behaviour and cerebral amine content in rats. *Experientia* 25: 1295–1296.

Butcher, L. L. and J. Engel. 1969. Peripheral factors in the mediation of the effects of L-Dopa on locomotor activity. *J. Pharm. Pharmacol.* 21: 614–616.

Butcher, L. L., G. K. Hodge, G. K. Byran and S. M. Eastgate. 1973. Effects of precise motor responding of bilateral 6-hydroxydopamine infusion into the substantia nigra. *In* E. Usdin and S. H. Snyder (eds.), *Frontiers in Catecholamine Research*. Pergamon Press, New York, pp. 763–766.

Carlsson, A. 1960. Zur Frage der Wirkungsweise einiger Psychopharmaka. *Psychiat. Neurol.* 140: 220–222.

Carlsson, A., M. Lindqvist and T. Magnusson. 1957. 3,4-dihydroxyphenylalanine and 5-hydroxytryptophan as reserpine antagonists. *Nature* 180: 1200.

Cooper, B. R. and G. R. Breese. 1974. Relationship of dopamine neural systems to the behavioral alterations produced by 6-hydroxydopamine administration into brain. *Adv. Biochem. Psychopharmacol.* 12: 353–368.

Cooper, B. R., G. R. Breese, J. L. Howard and L. D. Grant. 1972. Enhanced behavioral depressant effects of reserpine and alpha-methyltyrosine after 6-hydroxydopamine treatment. *Psychopharmacologia* 27: 99–110.

Cooper, B. R., L. D. Grant and G. R. Breese. 1973. Comparison of the behavioral depressant effects of biogenic amine depleting and neuroleptic agents following various 6-hydroxydopamine treatments. *Psychopharmacologia* 31: 95–109.

Cooper, J. R., F. E. Bloom and R. H. Roth. 1974. *The Biochemical Basis of Neuropharmacology*. Oxford University Press, London.

Coscina, D. V., C. Rosenblum-Blinick, D. D. Godse and H. C. Stancer. 1973. Consummatory behaviors of hypothalamic hyperphagic rats after central injection of 6-hydroxydopamine. *Pharmacol. Biochem. Behav.* 1: 629–642.

Costall, B. and R. J. Naylor. 1975. Actions of dopaminergic agonists on motor function. *In* D. Caine, T. M. Chase and A. Barbeau (eds.), *Advances in Neurology* 9: 285–297. Raven Press, New York.

Cotzias, G. C., P. S. Papavasiliou, C. Fehling, B. Kaufman and I. Mena. 1970. Similarities between neurologic effects of L-Dopa and of apomorphine. *New Engl. J. Med.* 282: 31–33.

Dahlström, A. and K. Fuxe. 1964. Evidence for the existence of monoamine-containing neurons in the central nervous system. I. Demonstration of monoamines in the cell bodies of brainstem neurons. *Acta Physiologica. Scand. Suppl.* 232: 1–55.

Draskóczy, P. R. and C. P. Lyman. 1967. Turnover of catecholamines in active and hibernating ground squirrels. *J. Pharmacol. Exp. Ther.* **155**: 101–111.

Eichelman, B. S., Jr. and N. B. Thoa. 1973. The aggressive monoamines. *Biol. Psychiat.* **6**: 143–164.

Everett, G. M. and R. D. Wiegand. 1962. Central amines and behavioral states: A critique and new data. *In* W. D. M. Patent (ed.), *Proc. First Int. Pharmacological Meeting, Stockholm, Sweden. Pharmacological Analysis of Central Nervous Action* 8: 85–92. Pergamon Press, New York.

Evetts, K. D., N. J. Uretsky, L. L. Iversen and S. D. Iversen. 1970. Effects of 6-hydroxydopamine on CNS catecholamines, spontaneous motor activity and amphetamine induced hyperactivity in rats. *Nature* **225**: 961–962.

Fibiger, H. C., B. Lonsbury, H. P. Cooper and L. D. Lytle. 1972. Early behavioural effects of intraventricular administration of 6-hydroxydopamine in rat. *Nature New Biol.* **236**: 209–211.

Friedman, E., N. Starr and S. Gershon. 1973. Catecholamine synthesis and the regulation of food intake in the rat. *Life Sci.* **12**: 317–326.

Geyer, M. A., D. S. Segal and A. J. Mandell. 1972. Effect of intraventricular infusion of dopamine and norepinephrine on motor activity. *Physiol. Behav.* **8**: 653–658.

Gordon, R., S. Spector, A. Sjoerdsma and S. Udenfriend. 1966. Increased synthesis of norepinephrine and epinephrine in the intact rat during exercise and exposure to cold. *J. Pharmacol. Exp. Ther.* **153**: 440–447.

Grossman, S. P. 1960. Eating or drinking elicited by direct adrenergic or cholinergic stimulation of hypothalamus. *Science* **132**: 301–302.

Grossman, S. P. 1972. Neurophysiologic aspects: Extrahypothalamic factors in the regulation of food intake. *Adv. Psychosom. Med.* **7**: 49–72.

Guldberg, H. C. and C. A. Marsden. 1972. Brain monoamines and the increase in motor activity in the rat after amphetamine. *Brit. J. Pharmacol.* **44**: 347P–348P.

Häggendal, J. and M. Lindqvist. 1963. Behaviour and monoamine levels during long-term administration of reserpine to rabbits. *Acta Physiol. Scand.* **57**: 431–436.

Häggendal, J. and M. Lindqvist. 1964. Disclosure of labile monoamine fractions in brain and their correlation to behaviour. *Acta Physiol. Scand.* **60**: 351–357.

Heller, A. and R. Y. Moore. 1968. Control of brain serotonin and norepinephrine by specific neural systems. *Adv. Pharmacol., Part A* **6**: 191–206.

Holzbauer, M. and M. Vogt. 1956. Depression by reserpine of the noradrenaline concentration of the hypothalamus of the cat. *J. Neurochem.* **1**: 8–11.

Hornykiewicz, O. 1966. Dopamine (3-hydroxytyramine) and brain function. *Pharmacol. Rev.* **18**: 925–964.

Hurwitz, D. A., S. M. Robinson and I. Barofsky. 1971. The influence of training and avoidance performance on disulfiram-induced changes in brain catecholamines. *Neuropharmacology* **10**: 447–452.

Iversen, L. L. 1967. *The Uptake and Storage of Noradrenaline in Sympathetic Nerves.* Cambridge University Press, Cambridge.

Iversen, S. D. and I. Creese. 1975. Behavioral correlates of dopaminergic supersensitivity. *In* D. Caine, T. N. Chase and A. Barbeau (eds.), *Advances in Neurology* 9: 81–92. Raven Press, New York.

Klawans, H. L., Jr. 1973a. *The Pharmacology of Extrapyramidal Movement Disorders.* Karger, Basel, pp. 42–43.

Klawans, H. L., Jr. 1973b. The pharmacology of tardive dyskinesias. *Am. J. Psychiat.* **130**: 82–86.

Klawans, H. L., Jr., M. M. Ilahi and D. Shenker. 1970. Theoretical implications of the use of L-Dopa in Parkinsonism. *Acta Neurol. Scand.* **46**: 409–441.

Kostrzewa, R. M. and D. M. Jacobowitz. 1974. Pharmacological actions of 6-hydroxydopamine. *Pharmacol. Rev.* **26**: 199–288.

Krnjevic, K. 1974. Chemical nature of synaptic transmission in vertebrates. *Physiol. Rev.* **54**: 418–540.

Leibowitz, S. F. 1970. Reciprocal hunger-regulating circuits involving alpha- and beta-adrenergic receptors located, respectively, in the ventromedial and lateral hypothalamus. *Proc. Nat. Acad. Sci. U.S.A.* **67**: 1063–1070.

Leibowitz, S. F. 1972. Central adrenergic receptors and the regulation of hunger and thirst neurotransmitters. *Res. Publ. Assoc. Res. Nerv. Ment. Dis.* **50**: 327–357.

Lewy, A. J. and L. S. Seiden. 1972. Operant behavior changes in norepinephrine metabolism in rat brain. *Science* **175**: 454–456.

Lindvall, O. and A. Björklund. 1974. The organization of the ascending catecholamine neuron systems in the rat brain as revealed by the glyoxylic acid fluoresence method. *Acta Physiol. Scand.* Suppl. **412**: 1–48.

Longo, V. G. 1973. Central effects of 6-hydroxydopamine. *Behav. Biol.* **9**: 397–420.

Margules, D. L. 1970a. Alpha-adrenergic receptors in hypothalamus for the suppression of feeding behavior by satiety. *J. Comp. Physiol. Psychol.* **73**: 1–12.

Margules, D. L. 1970b. Beta-adrenergic receptors in the hypothalamus for learned and unlearned taste aversions. *J. Comp. Physiol. Psychol.* **73**: 13–21.

Margules, D. L., M. J. Lewis, J. A. Dragovich and A. S. Margules. 1972. Hypothalamic norepinephrine: circadian rhythms and the control of feeding behavior. *Science* **178**: 640–643.

McDowell, F. H. and R. Sweet. 1975. Actions of dopaminergic agonist in Parkinsonism. *In* D. Caine, T. M. Chase and A. Barbeau (eds.), *Advances in Neurology* **9**: 367–372. Raven Press, New York.

Miller, N. E., K. S. Gottesman and N. Emery. 1964. Dose response to carbachol and norepinephrine in rat hypothalamus. *Am. J. Physiol.* **206**: 1384–1388.

Modigh, K. 1973. Effects of isolation and fighting in mice on the rate of synthesis of noradrenaline, dopamine, and 5-hydroxytryptamine in the brain. *Psychopharmacologia* **33**: 1–17.

Modigh, K. 1974. Effects of social stress on the turnover of brain catecholamines and 5-hydroxytryptamine in mice. *Acta Pharmacol. Toxicol.* **34**: 97–105.

Montgomery, R. B., G. Singer, A. T. Purcell, J. Narbeth and A. G. Bolt. 1971. The effects of intrahypothalamic injections of desmethylimipramine on food and water intake of the rat. *Psychopharmacologia* **19**: 81–86.

Moore, K. E. 1963. Toxicity and catecholamine releasing actions of *d*- and *l*-amphetamine in isolated and aggregated mice. *J. Pharmacol. Exp. Ther.* **142**: 6–12.

Moore, K. E. 1966. Effects of alpha-methyltyrosine on brain catecholamines and conditioned behavior in guinea pigs. *Life Sci.* **5**: 55–65.

Moore, K. E. and R. H. Rech. 1967. Antagonism by monoamine oxidase inhibitors of alpha-methyltyrosine-induced catecholamine depletion and behavioral depression. *J. Pharmacol. Exp. Ther.* **156**: 70–75.

Moore, R. Y., R. K. Bhatnagar and A. Heller. 1971. Anatomical and chemical studies of a nigro-neostriatal projection in the cat. *Brain Res.* **30**: 119–135.

Myers, R. D. 1974. *Handbook of Drug and Chemical Stimulation of the Brain.* Van Nostrand Reinhold Co., New York.

Myers, R. D. and G. E. Martin. 1973. 6-OHDA lesions of the hypothalamus: Interaction of aphagia, food palatability, set point for weight regulation and recovery of feeding. *Pharmacol. Biochem. Behav.* **1**: 329–345.

Narotzky, R., D. Griffith, S. Stahl, W. Bondareff and E. A. Zeller. 1973. Effect of long-term L-Dopa administration on brain biogenic amines and behavior in the rat. *Exp. Neurol.* **38**: 218–230.

Pappas, B. A. and S. K. Sobrian. 1972. Neonatal sympathectomy by 6-hydroxydopamine in the rat: no effects on behavior but changes in endogenous brain norephinephrine. *Life Sci.* **11**: 653–659.

Peterson, D. W. and S. B. Sparber. 1973. Increased fixed-ratio response rates following norepinephrine depletion by 6-hydroxydopamine (6-HDA). *Fed. Proc.* **32**: 753.

Przegalinski, E. and Z. Kleinrok. 1972. An analysis of DOPA-induced locomotor stimulation in mice with inhibited extracerebral decarboxylase. *Psychopharmacologia* **23**: 279–288.

Rabin, B. M. 1972. Ventromedial hypothalamic control of food intake in satiety: A reappraisal. *Brain Res.* **43**: 317–342.

Rech, R. H., H. K. Borys and K. E. Moore. 1966. Alterations in behavior and brain catecholamine levels in rats treated with alpha-methyltyrosine. *J. Pharmacol. Exp. Ther.* **153**: 412–419.

Redmond, D. E., Jr., J. W. Maas, A. Kling, C. W. Graham and H. Dekirmenjian. 1971. Social behavior of monkeys selectively depleted of monoamines. *Science* **174**: 428–431.

Reis, D. J. 1974. Central neurotransmitters in aggression. *Res. Publ. Assoc. Res. Nerv. Ment. Dis.* **52**: 119–148.

Reynolds, G. S. 1961. Behavioral contrast. *J. Exp. Anal. Behav.* **4**: 57–71.

Rolls, E. T., B. J. Rolls, P. H. Kelly, S. G. Shaw, R. J. Wood and R. Dale. 1974. The relative attenuation of self-stimulation, eating and drinking produced by dopamine-receptor blockade. *Psychopharmacologia* **38**: 219–230.

Rondot, P., N. Bathien and J. L. Ribadeau Dumas. 1975. Indications of piribedil in L-Dopa treated Parkinsonian patients: physiopathologic implications. *In* D. Caine, T. M. Chase and A. Barbeau (eds.), *Advances in Neurology* **9**: 373–381, Raven Press, New York.

Rosenzweig, M. R., D. Krech, E. L. Bennett and M. C. Diamond. 1962. Effects of environmental complexity and training on brain chemistry and anatomy: A replication and extension. *J. Comp. Physiol. Psychol.* **55**: 429–437.

Routtenberg, A. 1972. Intracranial chemical injection and behaviour: A critical review. *Behav. Biol.* **7**: 601–641.

Scheel-Krüger, J. and A. Randrup. 1967. Stereotype hyperactive behaviour produced by dopamine in the absence of noradrenaline. *Life Sci.* **6**: 1389–1398.

Scheel-Krüger, J. and A. Randrup. 1968. Aggressive behaviour provoked by pargyline in rats pretreated with diethyldithiocarbamate. *J. Pharm. Pharmacol.* **20**: 948–949.

Schoenfeld, R. I. and L. S. Seiden. 1969. Effect of alpha-methyltyrosine on operant behavior and brain catecholamine levels. *J. Pharmacol. Exp. Ther.* **167**: 319–327.

Schoenfeld, R. I. and M. J. Zigmond. 1970. Effect of 6-hydroxydopamine (HDA) on fixed ratio (FR) performance. *The Pharmacologist* **12**: 227.

Schoenfeld, R. I. and N. J. Uretsky. 1972. Operant behavior in catecholamine neurons: Prolonged increase in lever-pressing after 6-hydroxydopamine. *Eur. J. Pharmacol.* **20**: 357–362.

Schoenfeld, R. I. and M. J. Zigmond. 1973. Behavioral pharmacology of 6-hydroxydopamine. *In* E. Usdin and S. H. Snyder (eds.), *Frontiers in Catecholamine Research. Proc. of 3rd International Catecholamine Symposium.* Pergamon, Press, New York, pp. 695–700.

Schumann, H. J. and G. Kroneberg (eds.). 1970. *New Aspects of Storage and Release Mechanisms of Catecholamines.* Springer-Verlag, New York.

Seiden, L. S. and A. Carlsson. 1963. Temporary and partial antagonism by L-Dopa of reserpine induced suppression of a conditioned avoidance response. *Psychopharmacologia* **4**: 418–423.

Seiden, L. S. and A. Carlsson. 1964. Brain and heart catecholamine levels after L-Dopa administration in reserpine treated mice: Correlations with a conditioned avoidance response. *Psychopharmacologia* 5: 178–181.

Seiden, L. S. and L. C. F. Hanson. 1964. Reversal of the reserpine-induced suppression of the conditioned avoidance response in the cat by L-Dopa. *Psychopharmacologia* 6: 239–244.

Seiden, L. S. and T. Martin. 1969. Dopa reversal of reserpine-induced CAR suppression after preferential inhibition of peripheral Dopa-decarboxylase. *Proc. 77th Ann. Conv. APA*, 877–878.

Seiden, L. S. and T. W. Martin, Jr. 1971. Potentiation of effects of L-Dopa on conditioned avoidance behavior by inhibition of extracerebral Dopa decarboxylase. *Physiol. Behav.* 6: 453–458.

Seiden, L. S. and D. D. Peterson. 1968a. Blockade of L-Dopa reversal of the reserpine-induced conditioned avoidance response suppression by disulfiram. *J. Pharmacol. Exp. Ther.* 163: 84–90.

Seiden, L. S. and D. D. Peterson. 1968b. Reversal of the reserpine-induced suppression of the conditioned avoidance response by L-Dopa: Correlation of behavioral and biochemical differences in two strains of mice. *J. Pharmacol. Exp. Ther.* 159: 422–428.

Seiden, L. S., R. M. Brown and A. J. Lewy. 1973. Brain catecholamines and conditioned behavior: mutual interactions. *In* H. Sabelli (ed.), *Chemical Modulation of Brain Function*. Raven Press, New York, pp. 261–276.

Senault, B. 1970. Comportement d'agressivité intraspécifique induit par l'apomorphine chez le rat. *Psychopharmacologia* 18: 271–287.

Skinner, B. F. 1938. *The Behavior of Organisms: An Experimental Analysis*. Appleton-Century-Crofts, New York.

Singer, G. and R. B. Montgomery. 1973. Specificity of chemical stimulation of the rat brain and other related issues in the interpretation of chemical stimulation data. *Pharmacol. Biochem. Behav.* 1: 211–221.

Slangen, J. L. and N. E. Miller. 1969. Pharmacological tests for the function of hypothalamic norepinephrine in eating behavior. *Physiol. Behav.* 4: 543–552.

Smith, C. B. and P. B. Dews. 1962. Antagonism of locomotor suppressant effects of resepine in mice. *Psychopharmacologia* 3: 55–59.

Smith, R. D., B. R. Cooper and G. R. Breese. 1973. Growth and behavioral changes in developing rats treated intracisternally with 6-hydroxydopamine: Evidence for involvement of brain dopamine. *J. Pharmacol. Exp. Ther.* 185: 609–619.

Sparber, S. B. and H. A. Tilson. 1972. Schedule controlled and drug induced release of norepinephrine-7-^{3}H into the lateral ventricle of rats. *Neuropharmacology* 11: 453–464.

Stolk, J. M., R. L. Conner, S. Levine and J. D. Barchas. 1974. Brain norepinephrine metabolism and shock-induced fighting behavior in rats: Differential effects of shock in fighting on the neurochemical response to common footshock stimulus. *J. Pharmacol. Exp. Ther.* 190: 193–209.

Tanaka, C., Y. J. Yoh and S. Takaori. 1972. Relationship between brain monoamine levels and Sidman avoidance behavior in rats treated with tyrosine and tryptophan hydroxylase inhibitors. *Brain Res.* 45: 153–164.

Terrace, H. S. 1963. Discrimination learning with and without "errors." *J. Exp. Anal. Behav.* 6: 1–27.

Thierry, A., F. Javoy, J. Glowinski and S. S. Kety. 1968. Effects of stress on the metabolism of norepinephrine, dopamine and serotonin in the central nervous system of the rat. I. Modifications of norepinephrine turnover. *J. Pharmacol. Exp. Ther.* 163: 163–171.

Thoa, N. B., B. Eichelman and L. K. Y. Ng. 1972a. Shock-induced aggression: Effects of 6-hydroxydopamine and other pharmacological agents. *Brain Res.* 43: 467–475.

Thoa, N. B., B. Eichelman, J. S. Richardson and D. Jacobowitz. 1972b. 6-Hydroxydopa depletion of brain norepinephrine and the facilitation of aggressive behavior. *Science* **178**: 75–77.

Ungerstedt, U. 1971a. Adipsia and aphasia after 6-hydroxydopamine induced degeneration of the nigrastriatal dopamine system. *Acta Physiol. Scand. Suppl.* **367**: 95–122.

Ungerstedt, U. 1971b. Stereotaxic mapping of the monoamine pathways in the rat brain. *Acta Physiol. Scand. Suppl.* **367**: 1–48.

Ungerstedt, U. 1973. Selective lesions of central catecholamine pathways: application in functional studies. *In* S. Ehrenprei and I. J. Kopin (eds.), *Chemical Approaches to Brain Function. Neurosciences Research* **5**: 73–96. Academic Press, New York.

Uretsky, N. J. and R. I. Schoenfeld. 1971. Effect of L-Dopa on the locomotor activity of rats pretreated with 6-hydroxydopamine. *Nature New Biol.* **234**: 157–159.

Wada, J. A., J. Wrinch, D. Hill, P. L. McGeer and E. G. McGeer. 1963. Central aromatic amine levels and behavior. *Arch. Neurol.* **9**: 69–89.

Wagner, J. W. and J. DeGroot. 1963. Changes in feeding behavior and intracerebral injections in the rat. *Am. J. Physiol.* **204**: 483–487.

Welch, B. L. and A. S. Welch. 1968. Greater lowering of brain and adrenal catecholamines in group-housed than in individually-housed mice administered DL-α-methyltyrosine. *J. Pharm. Pharmacol.* **20**: 244–246.

Welch, B. L. and A. S. Welch. 1969. Aggression and the biogenic amine neurohumors. *In* S. Garattini and E. B. Sigg (eds.), *Aggressive Behavior.* Excerpta Medica Foundation, Amsterdam, pp. 179–189.

Wenzel, B. M. and D. W. Jeffrey. 1967. The effect of immunosympathectomy on the behavior of mice in aversive situations. *Physiol. Behav.* **2**: 193–201.

Zigmond, M. J. and E. M. Stricker. 1972. Deficits in feeding behavior after intraventricular injection of 6-hydroxydopamine in rats. *Science* **177**: 1211–1214.

6
Interactions Between Psychoactive Drugs, Catecholamines and Serotonin

The previous two chapters have dealt with the function of serotonin (5-HT), norepinephrine (NE) and dopamine (DA) in the mediation of behavior. The notion that behavior is functionally related to these endogenous chemicals in brain arises from data which demonstrate that certain drugs affect behavior as well as the metabolism and distribution of 5-HT, NE and DA. The effects of several drugs on behavior are also thought to be mediated by brain catecholamines and/or 5-HT. On the basis of the interactions between drugs, endogenous chemicals and behavior, hypotheses have been formed concerning abnormal metabolism of various endogenous chemicals in psychiatric illnesses (see Schildkraut, 1973; Weil-Malherbe and Szara, 1971; Ellinwood, 1974; Angrst and Gershon, 1974; Snyder, 1973). This chapter will explore relationships between commonly used drugs, behavior and various endogenous chemicals. It is important to recall that a correlation between drug-induced neurochemical changes and behavioral effects does not prove that the behavioral and neurochemical changes are functionally related. Several lines of evidence are required to establish a functional relationship between brain neurochemicals, drugs and behavior.

Five major classes of drugs will be considered in this chapter: (1) psychomotor stimulants; (2) antidepressants; (3) antianxiety drugs, also called minor tranquilizers; (4) antipsychotic drugs, also called major tranquilizers; and (5) the narcotic analgesics. Each class is generally defined in terms of its clinical use. The classification of drugs on a clinical basis does not necessarily imply a chemical classification. For example, among the antipsychotic drugs there are several chemical classes, including the phenothiazines and butyrophenones. In addition, there are drugs in the same chemical class that do not have similar behavioral actions. However, attempts at grouping drugs by either their pharmacological action or chemical structures are useful as a handle for remembering their effects and for trying to make sense about their mechanism of action. Nevertheless, any classification scheme should be looked upon as flexible.

Research in psychopharmacology over the past two decades has centered around catecholaminergic and serotonergic mechanisms. Therefore, in this chapter, we will investigate the interaction between drugs and the putative neurotransmitters, serotonin, norepinephrine and dopamine. While emphasis is on the mediation of drug effects via catecholaminergic and serotonergic mechanisms, it should be noted that other compounds including glycine, histamine, gamma-aminobutyric acid, phenylethylamine and certain polypeptides are potential putative transmitters in the CNS (see Krnjevic, 1974). The relationship of these chemicals to drug action has not been explored extensively, but their importance cannot be underestimated. Since this area is just beginning to emerge, data are usually insufficient to warrant discussion.

This chapter will take the following format:

> *First,* prototypic drugs from each clinical class will be described in terms of their general effects on behavior in humans. Their behavioral actions in animals will also be discussed, although a detailed discussion will be deferred to Chapters 9–12. *Second,* the neurochemical effects of these drugs will be discussed. *Third,* exemplary studies will be presented that relate the neurochemical effects of these drugs to their behavioral effects.

PSYCHOMOTOR STIMULANTS

Amphetamine and related drugs (e.g., pipradrol, methylphenidate, phenmetrazine, methamphetamine) have probably received the most attention in the investigation of drug-neurochemical-behavioral interactions. Therefore, we will discuss these drugs extensively so that the procedures for investigating drug-behavior-neurochemical interactions can be fully described.

General Effects

Amphetamine has been used clinically in the treatment of fatigue, obesity, narcolepsy and some forms of depression, and more recently in the treatment of hyperkinetic syndrome in children with presumed minimal brain dysfunction (Klein and Davis, 1969). Because of suggestions that the drug might lead to dependence and produce behavioral and other physical pathology with prolonged use at high doses, its use has been curtailed (Honigfeld and Howard, 1973; *AMA Drug Evaluations,* 1973). The tricyclic antidepressants and MAO inhibitors have largely replaced amphetamine in the treatment of depression. Nevertheless, since amphetamine has been used as the prototypic psychomotor stimulant in the investigation of the neuropharmacology of drug action, we will discuss it here.

The general effects of amphetamine include the following: First of all, amphetamine causes anorexia (loss of appetite, decrease in food intake). Tolerance occurs rapidly to this effect, and within two or three weeks of daily treatment the drug no longer depresses food intake. Amphetamine is also a strong central stimulant (sympathomimetic); it decreases sleeping, causes a loss of fatigue and stimulates the medullary respiratory center. Amphetamine and related drugs have been widely used by the general population for their antifatigue properties. On occasion, amphetamine has been reported to produce repetitive motor activity (stereotyped behavior), which is sometimes manifested in the assembling and disassembling of a complex piece of mechanical equipment. Amphetamine is also reported to improve attention, especially during prolonged sleep deprivation. In addition, subjective reports indicate that amphetamine causes euphoria and an increased ability to concentrate (Goodman and Gilman, 1970; Klein and Davis, 1969). Amphetamine has also been reported to have some analgesic properties.

Amphetamine produces similar effects in animals. Its most noticeable effect in animals is stimulation at low doses of various behaviors including behavior under schedule-control (see Chapter 9) and spontaneous locomotor activity. Larger doses lead to repetitive motor sequences and "stereotyped behavior" characterized by sniffing, head bobbing, licking and gnawing. In some primates, stereotyped behavior includes picking of the skin, sometimes to the point of self-mutilation.

Methylphenidate, methamphetamine, pipradrol and cocaine are other psychomotor stimulants whose effects are somewhat similar to those of amphetamine (Goodman and Gilman, 1970).

Neurochemical Effects

Early research on the neurochemical effects of amphetamines led to the suggestion that amphetamine might exert its effects by inhibiting monoamine oxidase. While this action cannot be discounted at present, there is substantial evidence that the pharmacological actions of amphetamine are mediated by the release of catecholamines from CNS neurons. In addition, amphetamine is thought to block the reuptake of NE and increase the concentration of CAs at the receptor (see Costa and Garattini, 1970). The action of amphetamine is thought to be due to the action of CAs on receptors. This action is referred to as indirect since amphetamine is not thought to act on CA receptors itself, but presumably releases CAs which in turn act on receptors. Moreover, it has been suggested that amphetamine-induced release of CAs is dependent on newly synthesized CAs since amphetamine-induced release of CAs is blocked by alpha-methylparatyrosine (AMT), which inhibits the synthesis of CAs, but is not blocked by reserpine. Since reserpine is thought to interfere with the storage of catecholamines (as well as with serotonin storage), brain amine levels would be low after reserpine; and therefore amphetamine would have to release CAs from a newly synthesized or "extragranular" pool resistant to the effects of reserpine. Histofluorescence studies (Fuxe and Ungerstedt, 1970) also suggest that amphetamine causes release of newly synthesized catecholamines that are loosely bound in an extragranular pool. While the bulk of evidence at present is consistent with the view that amphetamine acts indirectly through the catecholamines, NE and DA, there is some evidence that it may have a direct action on catecholaminergic or serotonergic receptor sites (Moore *et al.*, 1970).

The evidence for the catecholamine-releasing action of amphetamine has been elucidated and summarized by Carlsson (1970b). Carlsson administered amphetamine to mice and found increased amounts of methylated catecholamines, indicating that catecholamines were released following amphetamine administration. Animals were then pretreated with reserpine and given amphetamine. The catecholamine-releasing action of amphetamine became greater following reserpine pretreatment as evidenced by an increase in the amount of methylated amines.

Further evidence that amphetamine causes release of catecholamines from central neurons comes from experiments using cerebroventricular perfusion techniques in which two cannulae were used. An inflow cannula was placed into the anterior horn of the lateral ventricle and an outflow cannula was placed into the cerebroaqueduct. Artificial cerebrospinal fluid was perfused at a constant rate (about 0.4 ml/min) through the ventricle. Radiolabeled ^{3}H-DA or ^{3}H-NE or their metabolic precursor (^{3}H-tyrosine) was introduced into the inflow cannula. Substances released from neurons were sampled via the outflow cannula. (See VonVoigtlander and Moore, 1971, for an elaboration of this technique as well as Chapter 2 for a discussion of pulse labeling.)

Moore and his colleagues (1970) pulse-labeled the stores of NE in brain with ^{3}H-NE by perfusing the lateral ventricle with ^{3}H-NE. They then measured changes in the amount of ^{3}H-NE and its tritiated metabolites which were released after amphetamine administration. After the pulse labeling, a rapid decrease in ^{3}H-NE and its metabolites was apparent, with ^{3}H-NE reaching a low constant level within about two hours. When amphetamine was perfused, the amount of ^{3}H-NE and its metabolites increased; furthermore, normetanephrine (O-methylated norepinephrine) levels also increased, indicating that NE was released from presynaptic onto postsynaptic sites following amphetamine administration (see model of noradrenergic neuron, Chapters 3 and 5).

In later experiments, Chiueh and Moore (1974) injected ^{3}H-dopamine into the cat ventricular system and perfused the ventricles until radioactivity in the collected perfusate was stable. When *d*-amphetamine was introduced into the perfusate, the amount of ^{3}H-DA increased, indicating that dopamine was released following amphetamine administration.

It is important to note that when transmitter substances such as DA and NE are administered intraventricularly, they may be taken up and produce effects in cells not normally containing them.   Since tyrosine can only be converted to catecholamines in cells that normally contain CAs, tyrosine administration does not have this drawback.   Chiueh and Moore (1975a,b) perfused ^{3}H-tyrosine into the cat ventricular system and measured the amount of ^{3}H-DA re-

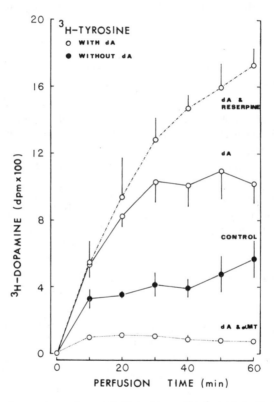

Fig. 6-1. Effects of reserpine and α-methyltyrosine on the d-amphetamine-induced release of endogenously synthesized dopamine.   CSF containing ^{3}H-tyrosine with or without d-amphetamine (dA, 1.1×10^{-8}M; 0.3 μg/ml base) was continuously infused into the ventricular system for 60 min, and 10-min samples of perfusate were analyzed for ^{3}H-dopamine.   Each point represents the mean and the vertical line represents 1 S.E.   Where no line is drawn, the S.E. was less than the radius of the symbol. $\bullet$—$\bullet$, CSF containing only ^{3}H-tyrosine (control N=3); $\circ$—$\circ$, CSF containing ^{3}H-tyrosine and d-amphetamine (N=4); $\circ$····$\circ$, CSF containing ^{3}H-tyrosine, d-amphetamine and 4×10^{-4}M α-methyltyrosine (N=3); $\circ$—·—·—$\circ$, CFS containing ^{3}H-tyrosine and d-amphetamine was perfused beginning two hours after the intravenous injection of 0.5 mg/kg reserpine (N=4).   (From Chiueh and Moore, 1975b.)

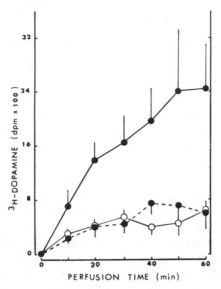

Fig. 6-2. Effect of methylphenidate on the efflux of endogenously synthesized ³H-dopa-mine in control and reserpine-pretreated cats. CSF containing ³H-tyrosine (○) or ³H-tyrosine and methylphenidate (●) was infused continuously into the ventricular system for 60 min, and 10-min samples of perfusate were analyzed for ³H dopamine. Each point represents the mean and the vertical line represents 1 S.E. ○—○, results of spontaneous efflux of ³H-dopamine obtained in three control cats; ●—●, results of methylphenidate-induced ³H-dopamine efflux obtained in four control cats; ●----●, results of methylphen-idate-induced ³H-dopamine efflux obtained in five cats injected intravenously with re-serpine (0.5 mg/kg) two hours prior to the start of the perfusion. (From Chiueh and Moore, 1975a.)

leased following intraventricular perfusion of d-amphetamine. Measurement was made in the presence of drugs that affect catecholamine storage and syn-thesis.   Reserpine pretreatment (iv) produced an increase in amphetamine-induced ³H-DA release over control levels.   On the other hand, AMT treatment attenuated the amount of tritiated DA released by amphetamine following intra-ventricular perfusion (Chiueh and Moore, 1975b; see Fig. 6-1). Methylphenidate also released ³H-DA (Chiueh and Moore, 1975a; Fig. 6-2), but this effect was blocked by reserpine.

Therefore, it appears that d-amphetamine-induced release of CAs (primarily DA) is dependent on newly synthesized CAs.   On the other hand, methylpheni-date-induced release is probably dependent on stored DA since release of DA by intraventricular administration of methylphenidate can be blocked by interfer-ing with storage.   The idea that d-amphetamine and methylphenidate may act at different intracellular sites is consistent with behavioral data presented below.

Drug, Behavioral, Neurochemical Interactions

In this section we will discuss evidence that the behavioral actions of amphetamine and related drugs are mediated by their catecholamine-releasing actions.

Stereotyped Behavior. Amphetamine and several other drugs classified as psychomotor stimulants elicit stereotyped patterns of behavior when given in relatively high doses. In rats, this pattern is characterized by repetitive licking and sniffing, periodically interrupted by gnawing on the cage floor or the rat's own forelegs (Randrup and Munkvad, 1968; Scheel-Krüger, 1971). The rat often assumes a characteristic crouched posture against the side of the cage. During periods of stereotyped behavior, the frequencies of other activities such as eating, drinking, grooming and forward locomotion are diminished greatly. Stereotyped patterns of behavior can be seen after amphetamine administration in several other species, although the topography of these patterns may differ. For example in cats, repeated head turning predominates, while in monkeys, high doses of amphetamine often produce stereotyped movement including fur picking, swipes at the air with the forelimbs or picking at one spot in the cage with a forehand. It should be emphasized that responses characterized by stereotyped behavior are not outside the animal's general repertoire, but are observed in caged animals under a variety of conditions, although they ordinarily occur at a much lower rate. They are classified as stereotyped when their rate increases and therefore the rate of other types of behavior decreases (e.g., eating and drinking).

Psychomotor stimulants which elicit stereotypic behavior fall into two groups (Randrup and Munkvad, 1970; Scheel-Krüger, 1972). In the first group the occurrence of stereotypic behavior can be blocked by AMT but cannot be blocked by reserpine. This group includes amphetamine, methamphetamine and phenmetrazine. In the second group, the occurrence of stereotypic behavior can be blocked by reserpine but not by AMT; this group includes pipradol and methylphenidate. The former group appears to release CAs from the newly synthesized pool while the latter group appears to release CAs from storage sites depleted by reserpine. Our discussion will center around the effect of amphetamine on stereotypic behavior, although some mention will be made of the effects of methlyphenidate.

Activation of dopamine receptors in the corpus striatum appears to be responsible for amphetamine-induced stereotyped behavior. This conclusion is based on a variety of experimental approaches including: (1) drug-drug interactions, (2) neurotoxin-drug interactions, and (3) lesion-drug interactions. In addition, evidence to support this notion has come from both biochemical and histofluorescent assays of transmitters.

1. *Drug-Drug Interactions.* It was noted above that AMT blocks amphetamine-induced stereotypy, while reserpine does not. From this finding it has

been suggested that amphetamine-induced stereotypy is dependent on the newly synthesized pool of catecholamines. L-Dopa can antagonize the AMT blockade of amphetamine-induced stereotypy, suggesting that DA plays an important role in stereotypic behavior. Administration of a dopamine-hydroxylase inhibitor (which blocks NE synthesis) does not antagonize the effect of L-dopa, suggesting that NE is not required for amphetamine-induced stereotyped behavior. The lack of a role for NE in stereotypic behavior is further supported by experimental data showing that neither alpha nor beta adrenergic blocking agents have an effect on stereotypy. On the other hand, either intraperitoneal administration of large doses of L-dopa or direct microinjection of DA into the caudate nucleus elicits stereotypy. The importance of DA in stereotyped behavior is also supported by evidence which indicates that DA acts at postsynaptic sites to produce stereotypic behavior.   The methylated metabolite of dopamine (methoxytyramine) has been shown to increase after an effective dose of amphetamine in both reserpine-pretreated and normal animals (Randrup and Munkvad, 1970).

2. *Neurotoxin-Drug Interactions.* Creese and Iversen (1973) used the neurotoxin 6-hydroxydopamine (6-HDA) in a series of experiments designed to examine the importance of the nigrostriatal dopaminergic system in the mediation of amphetamine-induced stereotypy in rats. Recall that 6-HDA destroys presynaptic CA terminals. Rats were treated with 6-hydroxydopamine intraventricularly at 5, 7 and 9 days of age, and testing was started at 90 days of age. Control rats were injected in the same manner but with the 6-HDA vehicle. It should be noted that although special feeding procedures were necessary after weaning, the 6-HDA rats were at normal body weights with a normal diet when tested. When control rats were given 5 mg/kg of *d*-amphetamine, stereotypic behavior occurred throughout the two-hour experimental session, whereas when 6-HDA-treated rats were given the same dose of *d*-amphetamine, stereotypy did not occur (Fig. 6-3). Similarly, a 10 mg/kg dose of *d*-amphetamine elicited stereotypy in controls, but very little, if any, stereotypy in 6-HDA-treated animals. On the other hand, apomorphine, a putative dopaminergic agonist, elicited stereotypic behavior in 6-HDA-treated rats which was two to five times greater than in control rats (Fig. 6-4). Biochemical data indicated that following 6-HDA treatment tyrosine hydroxylase activity was only 2% of normal in the striatum, and DA levels were so low they could not be measured. On the other hand, tyrosine hydroxylase activity and NE levels in the hypothalamus were 58% and 35% of normal, respectively. These data indicate that DA plays a major role in the expression of stereotypy. The increased stereotypy in 6-HDA-treated rats following apomorphine suggests that the DA receptors were intact and functional following 6-HDA. Indeed, they may have become supersensitive because of the destruction of presynaptic dopaminergic terminals (see Chapter 5, p. 134). The results also indicate that *d*-amphetamine-induced stereotypy depends upon intact presynaptic DA neurons and is mediated by DA release.

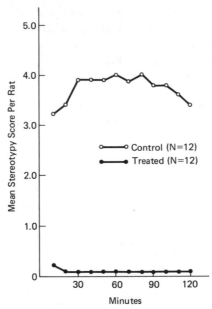

Fig. 6-3. Stereotypy response to 5 mg/kg d-amphetamine for adult 6-HDA, neonatally treated rats and controls ($N = 12$ and 12). The stereotypy response was rated blind by an independent observer according to the stereotypy rating scale developed from observations of the behavior of normal rats exposed to increasing doses of amphetamine. Mean stereotypy score per 10 min. (From Creese and Iversen, 1973.)

3. *Lesion-Drug Interactions.* Evidence from selective brain lesions also indicates that dopamine plays an important role in stereotyped behavior in adult rats. Creese and Iversen (1975) made substantia nigra lesions that caused a 99% decrease in striatal tyrosine hydroxylase activity and completely blocked amphetamine-induced stereotypy, whereas partial substantia nigra lesions that caused only an 80% decrease in tyrosine hydroxylase activity enhanced amphetamine-induced stereotypy. Lesions in the dorsal and ventral NE tracts caused no modification of drug-induced stereotypy. The fact that amphetamine-induced stereotypy was enhanced when striatal tyrosine hydroxylase was reduced by 80% and blocked when striatal tyrosine hydroxylase was reduced by 99% illustrates the importance of measuring the biochemical effects of a lesion. Had the experimenters only measured drug effects without measuring the biochemical effects, the results would have appeared inconsistent. Furthermore, the fact that the behavioral effects of amphetamine differed markedly depending on whether the lesion produced 80% or 99% depletion of tyrosine hydroxylase emphasizes the point made in Chapter 5 (p. 131) that small remaining pools of CAs may be of functional importance (see Fibiger *et al.*, 1973).

On the basis of discrete lesions in the DA system, Asher and Aghajanian

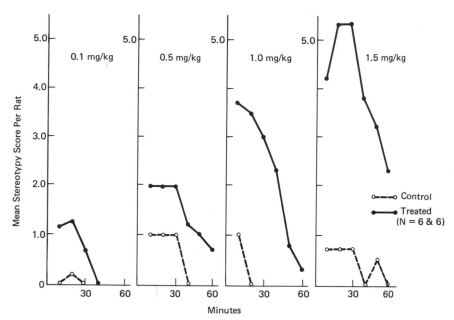

Fig. 6-4. Stereotypy response to 0.1, 0.5, 1.0 and 1.5 mg/kg apomorphine for adult 6-HDA, neonatally treated rats and controls (*N*=6 and 6). The graph represents the mean score on the stereotypy rating scale of each group of rats per 10 min, rated blind by an independent observer. (From Creese and Iversen, 1973.)

(1974) concluded that only lesions which reduced levels of DA in the caudate (i.e., nigrostriatal lesions) blocked stereotypy, and that limbic system DA is not necessary for amphetamine-induced stereotypy. On the other hand, other evidence questions whether the nigrostriatal dopaminergic system is necessary for stereotypy. Costall *et al.* (1972) lesioned the substantia nigra electrolytically and found no change in amphetamine-induced stereotypic behavior; moreover, the response to apomorphine was decreased. Since Costall *et al.* did not report dopamine levels, it is impossible to draw conclusions concerning the functional state of the DA system (Fibiger *et al.*, 1973; Creese and Iversen, 1975).

Taken together these results suggest that amphetamine-induced stereotypic behavior is mediated by striatal dopamine. It is only through a diversity of approaches to a common problem (drug-drug interactions, neurotoxin-drug interactions, lesion-drug interactions) that a convergent conclusion such as this can be reached (see Scheel-Krüger, 1972; Kulkarni and Dandiya, 1972; Cheng and Long, 1974; Costall and Naylor, 1974).

Stimulation of Locomotor Activity. It has been suggested that nigrostriatal dopaminergic fibers mediate locomotor activity, and that NE neurons play a secondary role. Rech and Stolk (1970) demonstrated an increase in locomotor

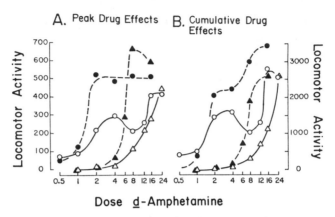

Fig. 6-5. Effects of α-methyl-tyrosine (AMT) and acute reserpine pretreatments on increased motor activity induced by *d*-amphetamine. Open symbols represent rats pretreated with saline alone, 24 hr before (o), or with saline plus 50 mg/kg AMT 135 min before (△). Solid symbols depict rats pretreated with 2 mg/kg reserpine alone, 24 hr before (•), or with reserpine 24 hr before plus the amino acid 135 min before (▲). (From Rech and Stolk, 1970.)

activity following amphetamine. As can be seen from Fig. 6-5, amphetamine increased locomotor activity in a dose-dependent manner. Reserpine did not block, but rather potentiated the effects of amphetamine, as indicated by a shift in the dose-response curve to the left (Fig. 6-5). α-Methyltyrosine blocked amphetamine-induced increases in locomotor activity in a dose-related fashion. In the presence of AMT, low doses of amphetamine did not increase locomotor activity, while high doses increased it (Fig. 6-5), indicating the importance of detailed dose-response investigations. Rech and Stolk reported similar effects in a continuous avoidance procedure. These results support the idea that newly synthesized catecholamines (probably DA) are important for amphetamine action; however, they also indicate that amphetamine may stimulate receptors directly at high doses (see Villarreal *et al.*, 1973).

Fibiger *et al.* (1973) used 6-HDA to examine the role of CAs in amphetamine-induced increases in locomotor activity. A vehicle control group was tested against three 6-HDA-treated groups that varied by degree of depletion of tyrosine hydroxylase in different brain regions. One group received 6-HDA in the substantia nigra, a second group received intraventricular 6-HDA and a third group received intraventricular 6-HDA following pretreatment with an MAO inhibitor. Tyrosine hydroxylase activity in various brain regions was taken as an index of CA depletion. In all groups, the effect of amphetamine on locomotor activity was attenuated. In the group in which tyrosine hydroxylase activity decreased extensively (6-HDA plus an MAO inhibitor), amphetamine had no effect at doses which increased the control rats' locomotor activity by a factor of four. The other groups showed an intermediate response to amphetamine and an intermediate decrease of tyrosine hydroxylase. It is important to compare the group of rats with nigral lesions with the group which received an MAO inhibitor. In both of these groups, tyrosine hydroxylase is decreased to 5-7% of normal in the striatum. In the group treated with 6-HDA and the MAO inhibitor, however, tyrosine hydroxylase activity decreased to a large extent in the midbrain and hypothalamus, areas rich in NE. Fibiger *et al.* concluded from these data that while the nigrostriatal pathway is primarily responsible for locomotor stimulation after amphetamine, NE plays a role as well. Recall that this is in keeping with the role of DA and NE in motor function discussed in Chapter 5.

Creese and Iversen (1973, 1975) also made selective CNS lesions using 6-HDA. In their experiments they depleted DA and NE by placing 6-HDA in the substantia nigra, or the ventral or dorsal NE bundles (see Chapter 5). Rats depleted of striatal DA showed a profound loss of amphetamine-induced locomotor activity, while NE depletion in the hypothalamus and cortex caused only slight modifications in amphetamine-induced locomotor activity (Fig. 6-6). They concluded that DA played a primary role and NE a modulating role in amphetamine-induced locomotion (see Tseng *et al.*, 1974; Tseng and Loh, 1974).

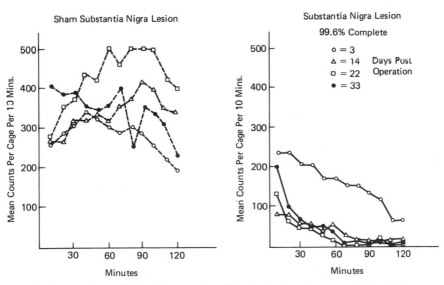

Fig. 6-6. Mean photocell beam interruptions/10 min for the sham-operated and the seven complete SN lesioned rats to 1.5 mg/kg *d*-amphetamine recorded on days 3, 14, 22 and 33 postoperation. The characteristic locomotor activity response to amphetamine was abolished in the SN lesioned rats. The response on day 3 in these animals records the presence of intense stereotypy. (From Creese and Iversen, 1975.)

The potential relationship between other drugs classified as psychomotor stimulants such as cocaine, methylphenidate, *l*-amphetamine and pipradrol and their action on locomotor activity vis à vis catecholaminergic mechanisms has not been worked out in the same detail as for *d*-amphetamine (see Scheel-Krüger, 1972; Ziegler *et al.*, 1972).

Self-Stimulation.   In 1954, Olds and Milner found that rats would press a lever when responding was followed by a weak electric pulse through an electrode implanted in the medial forebrain bundle (MFB) as well as in other brain regions. Recall for this discussion that the medial forebrain bundle is a prominent structure passing through the lateral hypothalamus which contains noradrenergic neurons which project to the cerebral cortex and limbic system (Chapter 5, p. 118). The importance of NE in the maintenance of self-stimulation is supported by several lines of evidence: (1) inhibition of dopamine-beta-hydroxylase (DBH) by disulfiram suppresses self-stimulation; (2) intraventricular infusion of *l*-norepinephrine (the *l*-isomer of norepinephrine is physiologically active but the *d*-isomer is inert) restores performance to normal; and (3) amphetamine facilitates self-stimulation in the medial forebrain bundle (MFB). Moreover, compounds that increase the available amount of NE potentiate the effect of amphetamine (e.g., tetrabenazine accompanied by an MAO inhibitor, alpha-methyl-metatyrosine, cocaine or imipramine).   Compounds that deplete CAs (e.g., reserpine, AMT and disulfiram) tend to antagonize the amphetamine-induced increase in self-stimulation.   If the rate-enhancing effect of amphetamine is blocked by the dopamine-beta-hydroxylase inhibitor disulfiram, an intraventricular injection of *l*-NE will restore self-stimulation while DA, 5-HT and *d*-NE will not (Fig. 6-7) (Wise and Stein, 1969; Wise and Stein, 1970).

In other experiments, Wise and Stein (1970) perfused the CNS with tritiated NE and measured the release of ^{3}H-NE from various areas of brain following stimulation (Fig. 6-8). It was found that stimulation of the MFB caused release of NE and O-methylated metabolites.   An increase in the formation of the O-methylated metabolites indicates that NE was released onto a postsynaptic site (see Chapter 3).   Moreover, since MFB stimulation caused an increase in the tritiated NE in the amygdala, but not in the hypothalamus, it was concluded that the amphetamine facilitation of medial forebrain bundle stimulation is due to release of norepinephrine in the forebrain.

Although Stein's work suggests an important role for NE in the maintenance of self-stimulation, other evidence suggests that both noradrenergic and dopaminergic systems are important.   For example, Liebman and Butcher (1973) placed electrodes either in the lateral hypothalamus or in the periaquaductal area of the mesencephalon; neither of these areas is a primary dopaminergic tract, although in the rat the lateral hypothalamus is close to dopamine fibers.   They then examined the effects of various drugs known to act on dopaminergic sys-

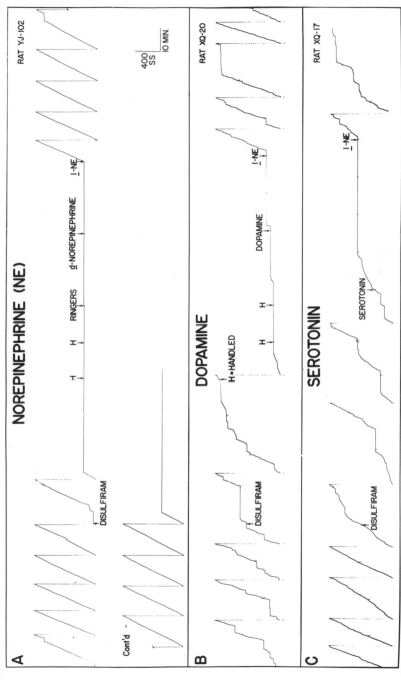

Fig. 6-7. Representative cumulative records showing suppression of responding maintained by self-stimulation by disulfiram (200 mg/kg) and reversal of behavioral suppression by intraventricular injection of l-norepinephrine (5 μg in A and B, 20 μg in C). Equivalent doses of d-norepinephrine, dopamine or serotonin did not restore self-stimulation. Note in A suppression of responding following disulfiram. Neither handling (H), ringers solution nor d-norepinephrine reversed this effect; however, injection of l-norepinephrine (l-NE) reversed the suppression. Note in B a similar suppression of responding following disulfiram which was not reversed by dopamine. Note in C that disulfiram-induced suppression of responding was not reversed by serotonin. (From Wise and Stein, 1969.)

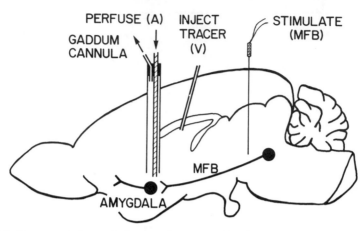

Fig. 6-8. Diagram of the perfusion experiment showing the relative locations of the stimulating electrode in the medial forebrain bundle (MFB), the perfusion cannula in the amygdala (A) and the needle for injection of radioisotopes into the lateral ventricle (V) on an outline of the rat brain. (From Wise and Stein, 1970.)

tems. The dopamingeric blocker, pimozide, as well as dopaminergic agonists (apomorphine or L-dopa) decreased the rate of self-stimulation. Disulfiram also reduced the rate of self-stimulation. In all cases, self-stimulation could be reinstated by doubling the amount of current delivered to the brain, suggesting that motor incapacity was not responsible for the drug effects. Phillips and Fibiger (1973) have also demonstrated that dopaminergic mechanisms are important in the maintenance of self-stimulation. They implanted electrodes in the substantia nigra, and self-stimulation was maintained at a high rate in this area. When either d- or l-amphetamine was given, the rate of self-stimulation was enhanced equally. On the other hand, when a stimulating electrode was placed in the lateral hypothalamus and d- or l-amphetamine was administered, the d-isomer was about ten times more potent than the l-isomer in maintaining self-stimulation. Snyder and his colleagues (Coyle and Snyder, 1969; Taylor and Snyder, 1970) have presented some data that might account for these differences. They found that the d-isomer is ten times more potent than the l-isomer in blocking reuptake of NE and that the two isomers have equal effects on DA reuptake.

Aggregation Toxicity. We have seen that amphetamine often produces increased motor activity in animals. Increases in motor activity following amphetamine are greater in mice aggregated in a small cage than in mice housed alone (Gunn and Gurd, 1940). Moreover, the lethal dose of amphetamine is decreased under aggregation conditions (this phenomenon is called aggregation toxicity). Increases in environmental temperature or noise also enhance the lethal effects of amphetamine under aggregation (Chance, 1946, 1947). Aggregation toxicity is of interest from both a pharmacological and a behavioral point of view since it demonstrates that environmental conditions are important determinants of drug action.

It has been suggested that the enhancement of amphetamine toxicity by aggregation is mediated by release of NE (Moore, 1963, 1964). Moore treated mice with the *d*- and *l*-isomers of amphetamine. With *d*-amphetamine, the LD50 was 20 mg/kg for aggregated mice and 100 mg/kg for isolated mice, whereas with the *l*-isomer, the LD50 was 90 mg/kg for aggregated mice and 130 mg/kg for isolated mice, indicating that the toxicity of *d*-amphetamine is increased more under aggregated conditions than is the toxicity of *l*-amphetamine. Both isomers caused depletion of NE in brain and heart in a dose-dependent manner in isolated mice, but only the *d*-isomer showed an increased depletion as a result of aggregation (Fig. 6-9). Furthermore, amphetamine-induced aggregation toxicity was reduced following reserpine and chlorpromazine. When drugs known to potentiate NE effects were given (e.g., monoamine oxidase inhibitors), the effects of aggregation were potentiated, supporting the notion that aggregation toxicity is mediated by NE release. These data suggest a role for NE in the response to aggregation and in *d*-amphetamine-induced aggregation toxicity. The basic findings of Moore have been confirmed by others (Lal and Chessick, 1964).

These findings have been disputed, however, by George and Wolf (1970), who found no difference in the NE levels of aggregated and isolated mice. When they analyzed the brains of surviving and nonsurviving mice following amphetamine administration, they found that surviving mice had lower NE levels than mice which died from amphetamine. No differences in NE were found between the two groups as a result of housing conditions. They propose that the differences observed in NE levels in Moore's studies were the result of pooling tissue samples of surviving and nonsurviving mice. While this may explain the differences in mice treated with *d*-amphetamine, it fails to account for the fact that Moore saw no differences in response to *l*-amphetamine as a result of aggregation. Moreover, it does not explain why various drugs that affect NE can antagonize or potentiate the amphetamine aggregation toxicity effect.

Catecholamine and Serotonin Interactions

In this section we will focus attention on data which suggest that although amphetamine exerts its behavioral action through the catecholaminergic system, the effects of amphetamine are also a result of functional alterations in the serotonergic system.

Parachlorophenylalanine (PCPA) depletes serotonin by inhibiting tryptophan hydroxylase. When PCPA was given in conjunction with *d*-amphetamine, the

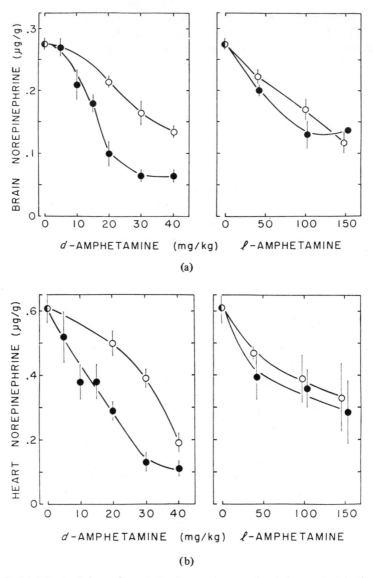

Fig. 6-9. (a) Effect of *d*- and *l*-amphetamine on the norepinephrine content in the brains of isolated (○) and aggregated (●) mice. Each point represents the mean of five to seven determinations, and the vertical line through the points represents the standard error of the mean. (b) Effect of *d*- and *l*-amphetamine on the norepinephrine content in the hearts of isolated (○) and aggregated (●) mice. Each point represents the mean of five to seven determinations, and the vertical line through the points represents the standard error of the mean. (From Moore, 1963.)

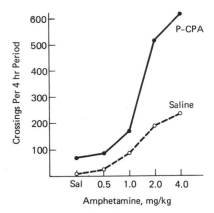

Fig. 6-10. Effect of amphetamine on mean levels of locomotor activity in rats pretreated with PCPA (300 mg/kg) or saline. (From Mabry and Campbell, 1973.)

locomotor stimulation normally produced by amphetamine was enhanced (Mabry and Campbell, 1973). The locomotor activity of rats increased as a function of the dose of *d*-amphetamine administered. When PCPA was given before amphetamine, the amphetamine effect was also enhanced (Fig. 6-10). PCPA had little effect on locomotor activity when given alone (Fig. 6-11). Furthermore, PCPA enhancement of amphetamine-induced motor activity could be antagonized by 5-HTP (the serotonin precursor, see Chapter 4), indicating that the PCPA-amphetamine interaction was related to 5-HT.

Green and Harvey (1974) also found that serotonin plays a role in determining

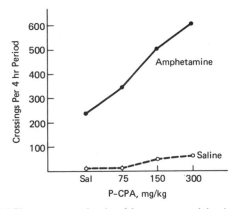

Fig. 6-11. Effect of PCPA on mean levels of locomotor activity in rats treated with amphetamine (4.0 mg/kg) or saline. (From Mabry and Campbell, 1973.)

the effects of amphetamine. They trained rats to respond on a VI 60-sec schedule of water presentation. Lesions were made in several brain areas, and the effects of amphetamine on response rate were determined. In rats with lesions that did not decrease 5-HT, amphetamine did not increase response rates at any dose. In rats with lesions that produced a large depletion of 5-HT, low doses of amphetamine caused a threefold increase in the rate of responding. At high doses of amphetamine, rate decreased in all rats. The changes seen could not be accounted for in terms of changes in baseline rate of responding, water consumption, body weight or changes in brain catecholamines. This experiment, like that of Mabry and Campbell (1973), suggests that a balance exists between the 5-HT and CA systems and that the action of amphetamine as well as other drugs may be best understood in terms of a balance between two systems (see Boston, 1971; Sparber and Tilson, 1972; Richardson *et al.*, 1974; Ellison and Bresler, 1974; Tilson and Sparber, 1972).

ANTIDEPRESSANTS: TRICYCLIC ANTIDEPRESSANTS

General Effects

The tricyclic antidepressants are used most often in the treatment of endogenous and reactive depression, although they are also effective in other types of depression. Since the tricyclics have fewer harmful side effects than other antidepressants, they are generally preferred over either the MAO inhibitors or electroconvulsive shock in the treatment of depression. The tricyclics exert their antidepressant effects slowly, and a period of four weeks is often required before a therapeutic effect can be determined. Imipramine is the prototypic drug in this series of compounds; amitriptyline, desmethylimipramine and chlorimipramine are also used clinically (see Klein and Davis, 1969; Carlsson, 1970a; Maitre *et al.*, 1974).

While imipramine is effective in the treatment of depression, it does not seem to have mood-elevating or other associated behavioral effects in normal subjects. On the contrary, in normal subjects imipramine causes dryness of mouth, feeling of fatigue, blurred vision and urinary retention. Some of these latter effects are typical of cholinergic blocking agents such as atropine.

Very little work has been done with the tricyclics in animals (see Chapter 9), probably because the compound must be administered for a prolonged period of time before effects are noticed. The behavioral studies that will be reviewed in this section have usually investigated imipramine or other tricyclics in combination with other drugs.

Neurochemical Effects

Imipramine, desmethylimipramine and other drugs such as cocaine and amphetamine interfere with reuptake mechanisms in noradrenergic nerve endings in both the peripheral autonomic and the central nervous system. Recall from Chapter 3 that reuptake of catecholamines into the presynaptic element is one of the major mechanisms of catecholamine inactivation. The criteria for determining when a compound interferes with the reuptake of amines are complicated (see Iversen, 1967, for a clear discussion of this point).

In the central nervous system, the tricyclic antidepressants only interfere with NE and 5-HT reuptake mechanisms; they do not interfere with the reuptake of DA (Carlsson *et al.*, 1969; Carlsson, 1970a; Maitre *et al.*, 1974). In addition, the various tricyclics have differential reuptake selectivities. Desmethylimipramine is much more effective in inhibiting reuptake of NE than either imipramine or chlorimipramine.   At low doses desmethylimipramine appears to inhibit NE reuptake selectively. The order of potency for inhibition of NE reuptake is desmethylimipramine > imipramine > chlorimipramine.   On the other hand, chlorimipramine inhibits 5-HT reuptake more effectively than imipramine or desmethylimipramine. The order of potency for inhibition of 5-HT reuptake is chlorimipramine > imipramine > desmethylimipramine. The fact that imipramine inhibits both NE and 5-HT reuptake is of interest with regard to possible NE and 5-HT interactions.

Drug, Behavioral, Neurochemical Correlates

Since there are only a very limited number of studies in which behavioral and neurochemical correlates of the tricyclic antidepressants have been examined, the evidence presented below must be regarded as preliminary. It is important because of the suggestions it makes about future work. One study in which neurochemical and behavioral correlations have been made involves the investigation of attack behavior in cats. Dubinsky *et al.* (1973) permanently implanted stimulating electrodes in the cat hypothalamus. Following stimulation of the hypothalamus with a threshold current, cats attack anesthetized rats placed in their chamber. Dubinsky *et al.* determined the minimum (threshold) current that elicited attack and recorded attack latency before and after administration of three tricyclic antidepressants, chlorimipramine, imipramine and desmethylimipramine. All three tricyclic antidepressants attenuated attack behavior at the minimum threshold current, but each differed in the dose at which attack was attenuated. The minimal dose at which chlorimipramine attenuated attack was 3.75 mg/kg; for imipramine it was 9.0 mg/kg. Desmethylimipramine had minimal effects in that half of the cats were not affected by the highest dose of desmethylimipramine (12 mg/kg). Recall that while these three tricyclics block 5-HT uptake, chlorimipramine inhibits reuptake more effectively than imipramine, and imipramine is more effective than desmethylimipramine. Therefore, the order of potency of these antidepressants in inhibiting 5-HT reuptake parallels their effectiveness in attenuating attack behavior. Chlorimipramine also elevated the threshold current necessary to elicit attack. This elevation was blocked by

PCPA. Furthermore, the effects of PCPA in blocking the effects of chlorimipramine could be reversed by a small dose of the serotonin precursor 5-HTP. Taken together, these results suggest that chlorimipramine suppresses attack behavior elicited by hypothalamic stimulation by interfering with 5-HT reuptake. These results are consistent with data presented in Chapter 4 which suggested that increased serotonin levels inhibit aggression.

ANTIDEPRESSANTS: MONOAMINE OXIDASE INHIBITORS

General Effects

The MAO inhibitor iproniazid was the first widely accepted pharmacological treatment for depression, but because of toxic effects caused by continued use, it was withdrawn from the market. Toxic effects include convulsions, orthostatic hypotension and adverse (sometimes fatal) reactions to other drugs and food (see Goodman and Gilman, 1970). Isocarboxazid, nialamide, phenelzine, tranylcypromine and pargyline are other MAO inhibitors that are used clinically. Very little is known about the effects of MAO inhibitors in normal (i.e., nondepressed) individuals. MAO inhibitors, like the tricyclics, exert their clinical effects slowly and often take several weeks to affect depression. Since the response to MAO inhibitors is variable (i.e., some patients are helped and some are not), it is difficult to manage these drugs on a clinical or research basis (Pare, 1972).

In spite of the problems associated with their use, the MAO inhibitors are both clinically and experimentally useful. Their effectiveness in the treatment of depression contributed to the formation of the amine hypothesis of depression, which states that in some cases depression is proportional to the amount of norepinephrine available at the synapse. If norepinephrine is low, depression occurs; when norepinephrine is increased as it is following administration of an MAO inhibitor, depression is decreased (Schildkraut, 1973).

Very little work has been done with the MAO inhibitors alone. They have, however, been used as research tools in the investigation of the function of dopamine, norepinephrine and serotonin in the CNS (see Chapters 4 and 5). They are usually given in combination with other drugs.

Neurochemical Effects

As their name implies, MAO inhibitors block the destruction of DA, NE and 5-HT by inhibiting the enzyme monoamine oxidase. This enzyme, which is primarily located in mitochondria in presynaptic nerve endings, controls the amount of "free" monoamine in cytoplasm. The MAO inhibitors form a complex with MAO; therefore inhibition is noncompetitive and irreversible. Recovery of MAO levels occurs when new enzyme is synthesized. The MAO inhibitors are not highly specific. They also inhibit other enzymes, indicated by the fact that metabolism of drugs other than the monoamines is slowed by MAO inhibition. Furthermore, some MAO inhibitors seem to prevent the release of NE (see Goodman and Gilman, 1970).

Currently, there has been a renewed interest in finding less toxic and more substrate-specific MAO inhibitors (Sandler et al., 1974; Martin and Biel, 1974). This interest stems from the recent discovery of multiple forms of MAO (Shih and Eiduson, 1974; Neff et al., 1974). Since work in this area is just emerging, the amount of behavioral data that exists is not sufficient to warrant a discussion of the detailed chemical data concerning the different forms of MAO.

Drug, Behavioral, Neurochemical Correlates

In general MAO inhibitors produce few effects on behavior when given alone. While some studies have reported increases in locomotor activity following MAO administration (Kulkarni and Dandiya, 1973; Gutwein et al., 1974; Corrodi, 1966), other studies report no change in locomotor activity (Green et al., 1975; Costall and Naylor, 1975; Scheel-Krüger and Jonas, 1973). Kulkarni and Dandiya (1973) found that when rats were given a single injection of either pargyline or nialamide, locomotor activity initially decreased; however, locomotor activity increased approximately threefold following daily treatment for up to 15 days. Gutwein et al. (1974) found that locomotor activity was increased by 50% thirty minutes after a single injection of pargyline to mice. At 24 hours after injection, locomotor activity was increased by 100%. Corrodi (1966) also reported that large doses of nialamide increased spontaneous locomotor activity and stereotyped head movement in mice within 2.5 to 3 hours after administration; these changes in behavior were correlated with increases in brain 5-HT and NE. Since neurochemical correlates of MAO administration have only been explored in a few of these studies, the results are difficult to interpret.

While very little behavioral work has been done with the MAO inhibitors alone, investigations have been carried out using MAO inhibitors in combination with other drugs (see Chapters 4 and 5). They have been used to investigate the mechanism of action of drugs which are thought to increase NE at the receptor site. Since it is not possible to measure NE at receptor sites, it is assumed that if a behavioral effect is mediated by increased NE concentration in the synaptic cleft, then this effect would be enhanced by a drug which increases the concentration of NE in the synaptic cleft. The MAO inhibitors increase NE at the synapse by interfering with the degradation of intraneuronal NE, while the tricyclics presumably increase NE by blocking reuptake.

In one study which examined the behavioral and neurochemical effects of MAO inhibition, rats were trained to avoid shock in a continuous avoidance procedure with an escape contingency (see Chapter 1). When alpha-methyl-metatyrosine (which is metabolized to metaraminol, which in turn displaces NE from its storage sites) was administered just prior to an experimental session, response rate increased; similarly, pretreatment with an MAO inhibitor caused a transient increase in responding. Moreover, responding also increased in rats given imipramine followed by tetrabenazine (a short-acting reserpine-like compound) (Scheckel and Boff, 1964a).

While the results of this work are consistent with the notion that a transient increase in rate is due to an increase in the concentration of NE available at the receptor, the interpretation of these results must be tempered by the fact that both tetrabenazine and imipramine have effects on 5-HT. Tetrabenazine interferes with 5-HT storage and thereby transiently releases 5-HT from nerve cells, and imipramine prevents 5-HT reuptake, thereby increasing 5-HT levels at receptors. Therefore, both 5-HT and NE may play a role in the behavioral effects described here (see Scheckel and Boff, 1964b; Kulkarni and Dandiya, 1972; Friedman and Gershon, 1972).

ANTIANXIETY DRUGS: BENZODIAZEPINES

Several drugs have been used in the treatment of anxiety, including ethanol, meprobamate, various barbiturates and the benzodiazepines. Only the benzodiazepines will be discussed here; however, it is interesting to compare the clinical efficacy of the benzodiazapines and the barbiturates.

General Effects

The benzodiazepines are the most frequently prescribed and the most effective antianxiety agents. They are now more commonly used than the barbiturates since they alleviate anxiety at doses which generally do not produce sedation or ataxia. The benzodiazepines are also used as preanesthetic agents and muscle relaxants. While they do have some sedative properties, these are not large and are rapidly tolerated (Klein and Davis, 1969; Goodman and Gilman, 1970). The benzodiazepines produce physical dependence with extensive use; however, physical dependence is much more severe with the barbiturates. Lethal overdosing with benzodiazepines is comparatively rare in contrast to the barbiturates (Goodman and Gilman, 1970).

There are several benzodiazepine compounds of clinical usefulness, including chlordiazepoxide, diazepam and oxazepam. While these drugs are not identical in their clinical activity, we will assume general similarities in order to describe their properties briefly.

In animals, the benzodiazepines are effective in reducing convulsions and aggression; they have been reported to tame monkeys that were difficult to handle without drugs. In addition, they have been shown to decrease avoidance responding at doses that do not interfere with escape responding. The benzodiazepines also increase behavior that has been suppressed by punishment (see Chapter 9).

Neurochemical Effects

Benzodiazepines have been shown to interact with several putative neurotransmitters, including catecholamines, serotonin, histamine and acetylcholine (Taylor and Laverty, 1973; Lidbrink et al., 1973; Bartholini et al., 1973; and Ladinsky et al., 1973). In the following pages, the effects of benzodiazepines on the CAs and 5-HT will be discussed; however, the possible role of other transmitters in the action of benzodiazepines on behavior should not be overlooked.

The benzodiazepines do not affect levels of DA, NE or 5-HT in brain; they do, however, retard the turnover of these monoamines. Taylor and Laverty (1973) studied the interaction of several benzodiazepines (chlordiazepoxide, diazepam and nitrazepam) with catecholamine turnover in various regions of the rat brain. Tritiated DA was introduced into the ventricles of three different groups of rats, each group pretreated with one of the three benzodiazepine derivatives. The rate of disappearance of tritiated NE formed from tritiated DA was examined in each group. Chlordiazepoxide, diazepam and nitrazepam retarded the rate of tritiated NE disappearance, indicating a decrease in the turnover rate of NE by 10–30%, depending on the brain region and particular benzodiazepine administered. Since the benzodiazepines do not affect either storage, reuptake or degradation, Taylor and Laverty postulated that the effect might result from decreased synthesis or release. On the basis of metabolic profiles of release, it appears that the benzodiazepines decrease catecholamine release. Decreases in NE turnover were noted in the thalamus-hypothalamus-midbrain, cerebral cortex and cerebellum; there was little effect in the pons-medulla. A large (50%) decrease in DA turnover was observed in the striatum. Similarly, Lidbrink et al. (1973) found that the benzodiazepines reduced the turnover of 5-HT as well as DA and NE.

Drug, Behavioral, Neurochemical Interactions

Taylor and Laverty (1973) have suggested that the benzodiazepines act by decreasing CA turnover. Since increases in turnover rate often lead to a reduction in whole-brain concentration of CAs, Taylor and Laverty examined a situation using prolonged footshock (see Chapter 5), which has also been reported to produce a reduction in the concentration of whole-brain NE. Taylor and Laverty found that the reductions in both endogenous and tritiated NE following footshock were antagonized by chlordiazepoxide, diazepam, and nitrazepam. The effect was largest in the thalamus-hypothalamus-midbrain, cortex and cerebellum.   The benzodiazepines also antagonized increases in DA turnover in the striatum.   Although it is tempting on the basis of these data to relate the pharmacological effects of the benzodiazepines to catecholamines, this evidence only suggests a relationship between the benzodiazepines and catecholamines.

One of the most noted effects of the benzodiazepines is that they increase behavior which has been suppressed by punishment (see Chapter 9). This effect has also been related to the action of the benzodiazepines on CA turnover in brain (Stein *et al.*, 1973; Wise *et al.*, 1972). Stein and Wise used the following punishment procedure to examine this relationship: responding was maintained

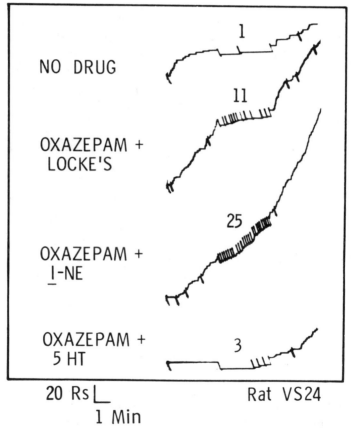

Fig. 6-12. Representative cumulative records in one rat showing a decrease in responding during periods in which every response was followed by shock (1). Responding increased following administration of oxazepam (11) and further increased following oxazepam plus *l*-norepinephrine (*l*-NE) (25).   Responding did not increase following oxazepam plus 5-HT (3). (From Stein *et al.*, 1973.)

on a VI 2-min schedule of sweetened milk presentation; during a tone every response was followed by milk and shock. (See Chapter 1 for details of this procedure.) Under control conditions (Fig. 6-12) responding during the tone was almost completely suppressed. The benzodiazepine, oxazepam, increased responding during the tone. An intraventricular administration of NE following oxazepam administration increased responding further. In contrast, oxazepam did not increase responding during the tone when given following intraventricular administration of 5-HT. Therefore, 5-HT appears to antagonize and NE appears to potentiate the effects of oxazepam on punished responding. In a separate experiment, it was shown that oxazepam, like other benzodiazepines, reduced NE and 5-HT turnover.

Biochemical and behavioral data also suggest that the benzodiazepines increase responding suppressed by punishment by reducing available 5-HT. This conclusion is consistent with the general notion that 5-HT plays a role in the inhibition of a variety of behaviors (see Chapter 4). Other investigators have also reported decreased suppression of punished behavior with 5-HT antagonists (Geller et al., 1974) or with PCPA (Geller and Blum, 1970).

These results are difficult to reconcile with evidence that the reduction of 5-HT produces hypersensitivity to shock (see Chapter 4; Tenen, 1968). If reduction in 5-HT produces hypersensitivity to shock, 5-HT might be expected to decrease further responding that has been suppressed by shock, rather than to increase responding as reported here. It should be noted, however, that these studies differ in a number of ways, including (1) the manner in which 5-HT was depleted (PCPA versus administration of a benzodiazepine), (2) the means by which 5-HT was replaced and (3) the behavioral measure (punished responding versus responding in a flinch-jump procedure). (See also Graeff and Schoenfeld, 1970.)

ANTIPSYCHOTIC DRUGS

General Effects

A variety of drugs are used in the treatment of psychosis. Generally, they fall into three classes: the phenothiazines, butyrophenones and thioxanthene derivatives. While these compounds differ in their chemical structure, they share many behavioral and neuropharmacological properties. Reserpine is also an antipsychotic drug, but it is more difficult to manage on a clinical basis and is not frequently used. Its importance as an experimental drug in elucidating catecholamine and serotonin function has been described in Chapters 4 and 5. For the purposes of this discussion, we will consider chlorpromazine, a prototypic phenothiazine derivative, and haloperidol, a butyrophenone derivative (see Goodman and Gilman, 1970; AMA Drug Evaluations, 1973).

The antipsychotic drugs (also called major tranquilizers) are used to modify the symptoms of chronic or acute psychotic states which are marked by some or all of the following symptoms: hallucinations, delusions, inappropriate affect, disorganized thought and behavior, as well as fear, panic and hostility. Patients diagnosed as schizophrenic exhibit psychotic behavior periodically but not continuously, and a diagnosis of schizophrenia is sometimes difficult to make. One of the problems in diagnosing the chronic condition is that acute psychotic states can be brought about by a variety of drugs, including LSD and *d*-amphetamine, and, occasionally, severe stress. While these so-called psychotomimetic drugs do not elicit exactly the same symptoms as the psychotic state associated with schizophrenia, there is enough similarity to make differential diagnosis difficult.

In the treatment of psychosis, the antipsychotics decrease combative, antisocial and withdrawn behavior, as well as ameliorate and prevent other psychotic symptoms. The drugs have a sedative effect when first administered, but sedation is rapidly tolerated while the antipsychotic effects.are not. The phenothiazines (e.g., chlorpromazine) have been the longest and most frequently used of the antipsychotics, and a great deal of research on their biochemical, pharmacological and behavioral effects has been done since their introduction two decades ago (for reviews see Goodman and Gilman, 1970; Klein and Davis, 1969; Matthysse, 1973). The most noted effect of these drugs in animals is on behavior maintained by negative reinforcement. In general, they decrease avoidance responding at doses that do not affect escape responding (see Chapters 1 and 9).

Neurochemical Effects

The antipsychotics have a broad spectrum of neurochemical effects, including effects on histamine, acetylcholine, 5-HT and CAs (Goodman and Gilman, 1970). All antipsychotics seem to influence the CAs, while effects on 5-HT or histamine are less universal.

In 1963 Carlsson and Lindqvist proposed that chlorpromazine and haloperidol block NE and DA receptors. The evidence for this proposal was based on the profile of CA metabolites following chlorpromazine administration and on inferences about the synthesis and subsequent release of CAs from presynaptic neurons. They found that administration of chlorpromazine or haloperidol to mice pretreated with an MAO inhibitor caused an increase in the level of DA and NE metabolites, i.e., 3-methoxytyramine (O-methylated DA) and normetanephrine (O-methylated NE). They suggested that the increase in O-methyl metabolites was caused by increased CA synthesis and release. This has been referred to as compensatory activation. Later investigators also found increased metabolites of DA after chlorpromazine or haloperidol administration when MAO was not blocked, again suggesting an increased rate of synthesis and release following chlorpromazine or haloperidol (Roos, 1965; DaPrada and Pletscher, 1966). Additional evidence that CA turnover is increased by chlorpromazine or haloperidol has been obtained by using radioisotopic techniques and tyrosine hydroxylase inhibitors (see Chapter 2). In view of these findings, it would appear that chlorpromazine and haloperidol increase CA turnover in brain.

Furthermore, characteristic motor responses elicited following administration of dopaminergic agonists or noradrenergic agonists were blocked by chlorpromazine or haloperidol (Andén et al., 1970; Gey and Pletscher, 1968; Fog et al., 1971; Corrodi et al., 1967a, b). The proposal that chlorpromazine and haloperidol block CA receptors is therefore supported by the following two lines of evidence: (1) chlorpromazine and haloperidol increase CA turnover, and (2) they antagonize the effects of CA agonists on a characteristic motor response.

Andén et al. (1970) suggested that, in general, antipsychotic agents block DA receptors but have variable effects on NE receptors. They used a variety of measures to examine receptor blockade, including measures of turnover, behavior and histofluorescence. The dose of an antipsychotic necessary to block DA receptors was usually lower than the dose necessary to block NE receptors. They concluded from this that the most potent and specific effect of the antipsychotic agents was to block DA receptors (see Matthysse, 1973).

Drug, Behavioral, Neurochemical Interactions

Haloperidol affects behavior maintained by schedules of positive reinforcement, and there is evidence that this effect is mediated by catecholamines. Rats were trained on an FR 40 schedule of food presentation and then injected with various doses of a tyrosine hydroxylase inhibitor, AMT-methylester, four hours before the test session. Doses as large as 50 mg/kg of AMT-methylester had no effect on rate of responding on the FR 40 schedule. In other experimental trials, rats were injected with various doses of haloperidol 15 minutes before the session; doses up to 0.05 mg/kg were found to have no effect on FR 40 responding. In subsequent experiments, both AMT-methylester and haloperidol were injected at four hours and at 15 minutes, respectively, before the session at doses that did not affect FR 40 responding when given alone. When the two drugs were given in this way, there was a marked disruption of responding. For example, 25 mg/kg of AMT-methylester and 0.01 mg/kg of haloperidol caused marked disruption of FR 40 responding. (Figure 6-13 shows data on one rat from this experiment.) Therefore, small doses of haloperidol that had no effect by themselves produced a marked decrease in responding when given in combination with AMT-methylester. These results indicate a potentiation between haloperidol and AMT and are consistent with the notion that haloperidol blocks CA receptors and leads to increased CA synthesis (Ahlenius and Engel, 1971).

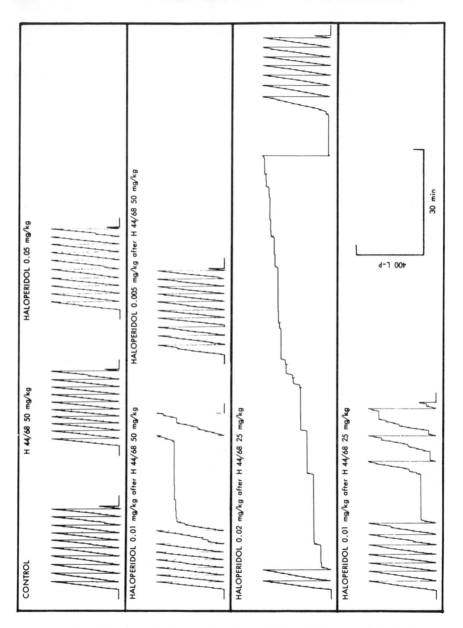

Fig. 6-13. Cumulative records showing the effect of haloperidol after tyrosine hydroxylase inhibition by H44/68 on operant behavior (fixed ratio 40). H44/68 was injected ip 4 h and haloperidol ip ·15 min before the start of the experimental session. The short downward deflections of the records indicate the delivery of food. L-P: lever presses. (From Ahlenius and Engel, 1971.)

Ahlenius and Engel (1971) suggested the following interpretation of these results: First of all, haloperidol is thought to produce a compensatory increase in synthesis and release of CAs in presynaptic neurons as a result of receptor blockade. When the dose of haloperidol is small, not all receptors are blocked, and therefore an increase in synthesis and release might compensate for partial receptor blockade. When tyrosine hydroxylase is inhibited, compensatory synthesis is partially blocked, and therefore the CAs available are not sufficient to act upon the remaining unblocked receptors.

Cooper *et al.* (1973) did not find any potentiation of the effects of haloperidol on FR 1 performance in rats treated with 6-HDA. This finding appears incompatible with the data of Ahlenius and Engel (1971); however, important differences between the two experiments may account for the apparent discrepancy. First of all, the schedules of reinforcement were different. We have already seen in Chapter 5 that this is an important variable. Its importance will be further discussed in Chapter 9. Furthermore, Cooper *et al.* (1973) used 6-HDA rather than a tyrosine hydroxylase inhibitor to deplete CAs. With partial depletion of DA and NE by 6-HDA in brain, the remaining cells may contain full or enhanced synthetic capacity and therefore may still respond to the compensatory synthesis induced by haloperidol (see Chapter 5—also see Gianutsos *et al.*, 1974; Fog *et al.*, 1971; Tarsy and Baldessarini, 1974). In summary, neurochemical and behavioral data derived from clinical and animal laboratory studies suggest that the antipsychotic drugs block DA or NE receptors in the central nervous system.

NARCOTIC ANALGESICS

General Effects

A number of drugs are classified as narcotic analgesics including: (1) opium alkaloids and purified derivatives of opium (morphine, hydromorphine and oxymorphine) and (2) synthetic compounds which resemble morphine in their pharmacological effects (meperidine, levorphanol, methadone and pimodine) (see *AMA Drug Evaluations*, 1973; Goodman and Gilman, 1970). Morphine is the prototypic narcotic analgesic. Clinically, the narcotic analgesics are used in the treatment of pain, dysentery and coughing.

Morphine's general effects include the following: First of all, morphine produces analgesia. Morphine-induced analgesia often occurs prior to or without sleep; drowsiness does occur, however. Morphine also relieves the distress associated with pain. Patients often report a sense of well-being and sometimes euphoria following morphine. On the other hand, in pain-free individuals, morphine can sometimes produce an unpleasant dysphoria, mild anxiety or fear and frequently nausea and vomiting, particularly when taken the first time.

Morphine also has euphoric effects after repeated use. The euphoric effects of morphine and related narcotic analgesics are thought to be responsible for their abuse in man. With repeated use, tolerance and physical dependence develop to morphine as evidenced by diminished potency of the drug and an increment in the dose necessary to produce the desired effect (e.g., euphoria). Physical dependence is marked by withdrawal signs when the drug is discontinued. These include gastrointestinal cramps, pilomotor activity resulting in "gooseflesh", insomnia, chills, increased blood pressure, nausea, vomiting, muscle pain and bone pain (Goodman and Gilman, 1970). The social, medical, legal and philosophical questions engendered by long-term nonmedical use of narcotics and other drugs is an extensive area of research (see Byrd, 1970; Hafen, 1973; Btesh, 1972; Blachly, 1970; Group for Advancement of Psychiatry, 1971; Fink *et al.*, 1973). Morphine also produces respiratory depression. Respiratory depression is often the cause of death following overdosage with morphine.

Morphine and related compounds exert analgesic effects in a variety of animals including rats, mice and primates (see Buxbaum *et al.*, 1973; Malis, 1973). In mice and rats, morphine generally elicits increased locomotor activity (see Eidelberg and Erspamer, 1975; Babbini and Davis, 1972; Rethy *et al.*, 1971), as well as various responses characterized as stereotypic behavior; whereas in primates, sedation usually occurs. Animals also become physically dependent and tolerant to morphine. The withdrawal syndrome in mice and rats consists of weight loss, diarrhea, tremors and shakes, stereotypic running and jumping (see Friedler *et al.*, 1972; Akera and Brody, 1968). In primates, it includes bradycardia, emesis and excessive salivation.

The narcotic antagonists should also be considered in a discussion of the narcotic analgesics. The narcotic antagonists are mainly used clinically to counteract excessive respiratory depression resulting from administration of morphine and related compounds. When given alone, some narcotic antagonists can cause respiratory depression and produce analgesia. Naloxone, nalorphine and levallophan are three fairly potent narcotic antagonists. Pentazocine is a weak narcotic antagonist which is used clinically as an analgesic. Narcotic antagonists can also precipitate the withdrawal syndrome in organisms physically dependent on morphine (Marshall, 1973), but they lack this effect in nondependent organisms (see Chapters 9 and 11).

Neurochemical Effects

In this section, the effects of morphine on catecholamines and/or serotonin are outlined. The reader should be aware, however, that other putative transmitters, hypothalamic-pituitary hormones, immune mechanisms and RNA and protein synthesis have been implicated in the acute and chronic effects of morphine and related compounds (see Clouet and Iwatsubo, 1975; Takemori, 1974; Dole, 1970; Chase and Murphy, 1973).

There is evidence that morphine when given to nontolerant animals: (1) depletes catecholamines, (2) increases CA turnover and (3) may affect 5-HT turnover, although the evidence for the effects of morphine on 5-HT turnover is not consistent. These effects have also been examined in tolerant animals, and in general it has been shown that tolerance to morphine reverses the effects seen following morphine administration in nontolerant animals, but again the effects on 5-HT turnover are difficult to interpret because of conflicting evidence.

In experimental animals, administration of morphine generally causes a reduction of NE and DA levels in brain during the first hour or two after administration. These effects depend on the dose given and the species examined. For example, in mice 20 mg/kg of morphine produced a 13% decrease in NE, while lower doses were without effect. On the other hand, in rats doses as high as 60 mg/kg of morphine were necessary to affect NE. Moreover, four hours after 60 mg/kg of morphine, rat brain NE levels were decreased, but 24 to 48 hours later, the NE levels were increased (see Way and Shen, 1971; Segal et al., 1972; Clouet and Iwatsubo, 1975). Morphine-induced depletion of CAs in mice (Rethy et al., 1971) can be blocked both by: (1) tolerance to morphine or (2) administration of a narcotic antagonist. Clouet et al. (1973) found that acute morphine administration in rats caused depletion of striatal DA as well as hypothalamic and cortical NE; but in tolerant rats DA levels were increased above normal, as were hypothalamic NE levels.

Morphine also affects CA turnover. It has been shown that acute administration of morphine increases the rate of incorporation of labeled tyrosine into labeled catecholamines in both mice and rats (Smith et al., 1970; Clouet and Ratner, 1970). Increases in turnover were found to be dose-dependent, and at the optimal dose (100 mg/kg) the increased incorporation was 200% (Smith and Sheldon, 1973). The increased synthesis was greatly attenuated when mice were made tolerant to morphine. Moreover, the increase in synthesis could be antagonized by administration of the narcotic antagonist naloxone. Furthermore, other narcotic analgesics such as levorphanol were found to increase CA turnover (Smith et al., 1972; Gunne et al., 1969; Clouet et al., 1973). Therefore, the evidence suggests that morphine both depletes CAs and increases CA turnover and that both effects can be reversed in animals tolerant to morphine or blocked by the administration of a narcotic antagonist.

In Chapter 4 we reviewed evidence (see Fig. 4-5, p. 98) that 5-HT turnover in mice was increased following morphine tolerance (Way et al., 1968; Shen et al., 1970). While this work has been confirmed by some investigators with morphine (Maruyama et al., 1971) and methadone (Bowers and Kleber, 1971), there are other reports that morphine does not increase 5-HT turnover as a result of tolerance (Marshall and Grahame-Smith, 1970; Cheney et al., 1971). For example, Yarbrough et al. (1973) did not report changes in 5-HT turnover in tolerant rats. Yarbrough and his colleagues administered various doses of morphine to rats which were not tolerant to morphine, and found that morphine initially increased the rate of 5-HT turnover in nontolerant rats. Following the first dose, the rats continued to receive morphine three times daily for six days, which produced tolerance. As the rats continued to receive morphine, 5-HT turnover returned to normal. Description of the effects of morphine on 5-HT are therefore complicated by this conflicting evidence.

Drug, Behavioral and Neurochemical Interactions

In rodents, as in man, morphine decreases reaction to painful stimuli and is therefore considered to be an analgesic. Morphine also stimulates locomotor activity in rodents, while in man it acts as a sedative. Many animal studies have focused on the relationship between the neurochemical effects of morphine and the locomotor stimulation and analgesia induced by single injections of morphine or by multiple injections that render animals tolerant and physically dependent on morphine. It is difficult to examine interactions between the behavioral and neurochemical effects of morphine, since the effects of morphine on 5-HT turnover are not agreed upon and therefore drug interaction studies involving behavior are difficult to interpret. Despite inconsistent results in respect to the action of morphine on 5-HT and limited evidence about the effects of morphine on other systems, recent experiments in this area will be discussed.

It has been suggested that 5-HT is involved in morphine analgesia. Tenen (1968) found that the 5-HT depletion by PCPA effectively antagonized morphine analgesia in a flinch-jump procedure using rats, but others (Harvey and Yunger, 1973) saw no change in morphine analgesia as a function of brain 5-HT levels. It has also been reported that reduction of 5-HT by PCPA interferes with the development of tolerance and physical dependence (Way *et al.*, 1968; Shen *et al.*, 1970). When tolerance occurred, the dose of morphine necessary to produce analgesia was higher than in nontolerant animals. Physical dependence was measured by characteristic jumping responses that occurred during naloxone-precipitated withdrawal. On the other hand, Cheney *et al.* (1971) found no effect on either tolerance to, or dependence upon, morphine as a result of depletion of 5-HT. Since the data are so divergent, no firm conclusions can be drawn about 5-HT and morphine-induced analgesia.

Catecholaminergic involvement in morphine analgesia is suggested by the finding that haloperidol potentiates morphine-induced analgesia but does not produce analgesia when given alone (Eidelberg and Erspamer, 1975). In addition, if haloperidol is injected daily along with morphine, the degree of tolerance to morphine is greater than when morphine is given alone. Insofar as haloperidol acts on dopaminergic sites, this is evidence for an interaction between DA and morphine (see Elchisak and Rosecrans, 1973; Friedler *et al.*, 1972; Ayhan and Randrup, 1973; Holtzman and Jewett, 1972).

There is evidence supporting the view that the narcotic analgesics produce an increase in locomotor activity in mice by causing increased synthesis and release of catecholamines from noradrenergic neurons. In the previous section, we discussed the fact that morphine and related compounds increased incorporation of labeled tyrosine into DA and NE. This effect is tolerated by repeated administration of morphine and can be antagonized with naloxone, a narcotic antagonist. Furthermore, repeated administration of morphine results in tolerance to its ability to stimulate locomotor activity. Tolerance and cross-tolerance develop to the locomotor-stimulating activity of the various narcotic analgesics, as well as to the effect of morphine in stimulating CA synthesis. Furthermore, the time courses of tolerance development to the behavioral and biochemical effects are roughly parallel. The fact that tolerance and cross-tolerance develop to both the behavioral and biochemical actions of morphine and can be blocked by naloxone suggests that the CAs play a role in morphine-induced behavior (Rethy et al., 1971; Smith et al., 1970, 1972; Smith and Sheldon, 1973). Reserpine and AMT markedly decrease the activity-increasing effect of morphine (Villarreal et al., 1973), confirming the involvement of CAs in morphine-stimulated locomotor behavior.

While evidence is not always consistent, data suggest that 5-HT and/or CAs play a role in morphine analgesia and in locomotor activity. There is evidence to support a role for 5-HT and perhaps to some extent the CAs in morphine-induced analgesia, but the inability to replicate directly some of these data casts doubt upon this interpretation. The evidence for an involvement of brain CAs in locomotor activity seems more consistent, but direct or indirect replication of these experiments has not been attempted. Moreover, investigations of other transmitters in the mediation of morphine's effects are needed. As Clouet and Iwatsubo (1975, p. 64) have concluded: "It is impossible to ascribe acute or chronic effects of opiate use to a single transmitter system in the CNS, although it is occasionally possible to define the neuronal pathway for a single effect of an opiate. The interaction between neurotransmitter systems must be considered when assessing the role played by a single transmitter."

SUMMARY

This chapter has examined the general behavioral and neurochemical effects of five major classes of drugs, and has explored experimental evidence which attempts to relate the effects of these drugs on catecholamine and/or serotonin to their effects on behavior. The combined use of pharmacological, biochemical and behavioral methods raises intriguing possibilities concerning neurochemical mechanisms that may account for the behavioral properties of these several different classes of drugs, but it is clear that delineation of the mechanisms depends upon further research.

REFERENCES

Ahlenius, S. and J. Engel. 1971. Behavioral effects of haloperidol after tyrosine hydroxylase inhibition. *Eur. J. Pharmacol.* **15**: 187–192.

Akera, T. and T. M. Brody. 1968. The addiction cycle to narcotics in the rat and its relation to catecholamines. *Biochem. Pharmacol.* **17**: 675–688.

AMA Drug Evaluations, 2nd edition. 1973. Publishing Sciences, Inc., Acton, Massachusetts.

Andén, N. E., S. G. Butcher, H. Corrodi, K. Fuxe and U. Ungerstedt. 1970. Receptor activity and turnover of dopamine and noradrenaline after neuroleptics. *Eur. J. Pharmacol.* **11**: 303–314.

Angrst, B. and S. Gershon. 1974. Dopamine and psychotic states: Preliminary remarks. *Advances in Biochemical Psychopharmacology* **12**: 211–219.

Asher, I. M. and G. K. Aghajanian. 1974. 6-hydroxydopamine lesions of olfactory tubercles and caudate nuclei: Effect on amphetamine-induced stereotyped behavior in rats. *Brain Res.* **82**: 1–12.

Ayhan, I. H. and A. Randrup. 1973. Behavioral and pharmacological studies on morphine-induced excitation of rats: Possible relation to brain catecholamines. *Psychopharmacologia* **29**: 317–328.

Babbini, M. and W. M. Davis. 1972. Time-dose relationships for locomotor activity of morphine after acute and repeated treatments. *Brit. J. Pharmacol.* **46**: 213–224.

Bartholini, G., H. Keller, L. Pieri and A. Pletscher. 1973. The effect of diazepam on the turnover of cerebral dopamine. *In* S. Garattini, E. Mussini and L. O. Randall (eds.), *The Benzodiazepines.* Raven Press, New York, pp. 235–240.

Blachly, P. H. (ed.). 1970. *Drug Abuse: Data and Debate.* C. C. Thomas, Springfield, Illinois.

Boston, J. E. 1971. Effect of *p*-chlorophenylalanine on avoidance conditioning and its interaction with amphetamine. *J. Ment. Deficiency Res.* **15**: 257–265.

Bowers, M. B. and H. D. Kleber. 1971. Methadone increases mouse brain 5-hydroxyindoleacetic acid. *Nature* **229**: 134–135.

Btesh, S. (ed.). 1972. *Drug Abuse: Non-medical Use of Dependence Producing Drugs.* Plenum Press, New York.

Buxbaum, D. M., G. G. Yarbrough and M. E. Carter. 1973. Biogenic amines and narcotic effects. I. Modification of morphine-induced analgesia and motor activity after alteration of cerebral amine levels. *J. Pharmacol. Exp. Ther.* **185**: 317–327.

Byrd, O. E. (ed.). 1970. *Medical Readings on Drug Abuse.* Addison-Wesley Publishing Co., Reading, Massachusettes.

Carlsson, A. 1970a. Effect of drugs on amine uptake mechanisms in brain. *In* H. J. Schumann and G. Kroneberg (eds.), *New Aspects of Storage and Release Mechanisms of Catecholamines.* Springer-Verlag, New York, pp. 223–233.

Carlsson, A. 1970b. Amphetamine and brain catecholamines. *In* E. Costa and S. Garattini (eds.), *Amphetamines and Related Compounds.* Proceedings of the Mario Negri Institute for Pharmacological Research. Raven Press, New York, pp. 289–300.

Carlsson, A. and M. Lindqvist. 1963. Effects of chlorpromazine or haloperidol on formation of 3-methoxytyramine and normetanephrine in mouse brain. *Acta Pharmacol. Toxicol.* **20**: 140–143.

Carlsson, A., H. Corrodi, K. Fuxe and T. Hökfelt. 1969. Effects of some antidepressant drugs on the depletion of intraneuronal brain catecholamine stores caused by 4, α-dimethyl-meta-tyramine. *Eur. J. Pharmacol.* **5**: 367–373.

Chance, M. R. A. 1946. Aggregation as a factor influencing the toxicity of sympathomimetic amines in mice. *J. Pharmacol. Exp. Ther.* **87**: 214–219.

Chance, M. R. A. 1947. Factors influencing the toxicity of sympathomimetic amines to solitary mice. *J. Pharmacol. Exp. Ther.* **89:** 289–296.

Chase, T. N. and D. Murphy. 1973. Serotonin and central nervous system function. *Ann. Rev. Pharmacol.* **13:** 181–197.

Cheney, D. L., A. Goldstein, S. Argeri and E. Costa. 1971. Narcotic tolerance and dependence: lack of relationship with serotonin turnover in brain. *Science* **171:** 1169–1170.

Cheng, H. C. and J. P. Long. 1974. Dopaminergic nature of apomorphine-induced pecking in pigeons. *Eur. J. Pharmacol.* **26:** 313–320.

Chiueh, C. C. and K. E. Moore. 1974. Effects of alpha-methyltyrosine on *d*-amphetamine-induced release of endogenously synthesized and exogenously administered catecholamines from the cat brain *in vivo*. *J. Pharmacol. Exp. Ther.* **190:** 100–108.

Chiueh, C. C. and K. E. Moore. 1975a. Blockade by reserpine of methylphenidate-induced release of brain dopamine. *J. Pharmacol. Exp. Ther.* **193:** 559–563.

Chiueh, C. C. and K. E. Moore. 1975b. *d*-Amphetamine-induced release of "newly synthesized" and "stored" dopamine from the caudate nucleus *in vivo*. *J. Pharmacol. Exp. Ther.* **192:** 642–653.

Clouet, D. H. and K. Iwatsubo. 1975. Mechanisms of tolerance to and dependence on narcotic analgesic drugs. *Ann. Rev. Pharmacol.* **15:** 49–71.

Clouet, D. H. and M. Ratner. 1970. Catecholamine biosynthesis in brains of rats treated with morphine. *Science* **168:** 854–856.

Clouet, D. H., J. C. Johnson, M. Ratner, N. Williams and G. J. Gold. 1973. The effects of morphine on rat brain catecholamines: turnover *in vivo* in uptake in isolated synaptosomes. *In* E. Usdin and S. H. Snyder (eds.), *Frontiers in Catecholamine Research*. Pergamon Press, New York, pp. 1039–1042.

Cooper, B. R., L. D. Grant and G. R. Breese. 1973. Comparison of the behavioral depressant effects of biogenic amine depleting and neuroleptic agents following various 6-hydroxydopamine treatments. *Psychopharmacologia* **31:** 95–109.

Corrodi, H. 1966. Blockade of the psychotic syndrome caused by nialamide in mice. *J. Pharm. Pharmacol.* **18:** 197–198.

Corrodi, H., K. Fuxe and T. Hökfelt. 1967a. The effect of neuroleptics on the activity of central catecholamine neurons. *Life Sci.* **6:** 767–774.

Corrodi, H., K. Fuxe and T. Hökfelt. 1967b. The effect of some psychoactive drugs on central monoamine neurons. *Eur. J. Pharmacol.* **1:** 363–368.

Costa, E. and S. Garattini. 1970. *Amphetamine and Related Compounds*. Raven Press, New York.

Costall, B. and R. J. Naylor. 1974. The involvement of dopaminergic systems with the stereotyped behavior patterns induced by methylphenidate. *J. Pharm. Pharmacol.* **26:** 30–33.

Costall, B. and R. J. Naylor. 1975. The behavioral effects of dopamine applied intracerebrally to areas of the mesolimbic system. *Eur. J. Pharmacol.* **32:** 87–92.

Costall, B., R. J. Naylor and J. E. Olley. 1972. The substantia nigra and stereotyped behavior. *Eur. J. Pharmacol.* **18:** 95–106.

Coyle, J. T. and S. H. Snyder. 1969. Catecholamine uptake by synaptosomes in homogenates of rat brain: Stereospecificity in different areas. *J. Pharmacol. Exp. Ther.* **170:** 221–231.

Creese, I. and S. D. Iversen. 1973. Blockage of amphetamine induced motor stimulation and stereotypy in the adult following neonatal treatment with 6-hydroxydopamine. *Brain Res.* **55:** 369–382.

Creese, I. and S. D. Iversen. 1975. The pharmacological and anatomical substrates of the amphetamine response in the rat. *Brain Res.* **83:** 419–436.

DaPrada, M. and A. Pletscher. 1966. Acceleration of the cerebral dopamine turnover by chlorpromazine. *Experientia* 22: 465–466.

Dole, V. P. 1970. Biochemistry of addiction. *Ann. Rev. Biochem.* 39: 821–840.

Dubinsky, B., J. K. Karpowicz and M. E. Goldberg. 1973. Effects of tricyclic antidepressants on attack elicited by hypothalamic stimulation: Relation to brain biogenic amines. *J. Pharmacol. Exp. Ther.* 187: 550–557.

Eidelberg, E. and R. Erspamer. 1975. Dopaminergic mechanisms of opiate actions in brain. *J. Pharmacol. Exp. Ther.* 192: 50–57.

Elchisak, M. A. and J. A. Rosecrans. 1973. Effect of central catecholamine depletions by 6-hydroxydopamine on morphine antinociception in rats. *Res. Comm. Chem. Pathol. Pharmacol.* 6: 349–352.

Ellinwood, E. H. 1974. Behavioral and EEG changes in the amphetamine model of psychosis. *Advances in Biochemical Psychopharmacology* 12: 281–297.

Ellison, G. D. and D. E. Bresler. 1974. Tests of emotional behavior in rats following depletion of norepinephrine, of serotonin, or of both. *Psychopharmacologia* 34: 275–288.

Fibiger, H. C., H. P. Fibiger and A. P. Zis. 1973. Attenuation of amphetamine-induced motor stimulation and stereotypy by 6-hydroxydopamine in the rat. *Brit. J. Pharmacol.* 47: 683–92.

Fink, M., A. M. Freedman, R. Resnick and A. Zaks. 1973. Clinical status of the narcotic antagonists in opiate dependence. *In* H. W. Kosterlitz, H. O. J. Collier and J. E. Villarreal (eds.), *Agonist and Antagonist Actions of Narcotic Analgesic Drugs*. University Park Press, Baltimore, pp. 266–276.

Fog, R., A. Randrup and H. Pakkenberg. 1971. Intrastriatal injection of quaternary butyrophenones and oxypertine: Neuroleptic effect in rats. *Psychopharmacologia* 19: 224–230.

Friedler, G., H. N. Bhargava, R. Quock and E. L. Way. 1972. The effect of 6-hydroxydopamine on morphine tolerance and physical dependence. *J. Pharmacol. Exp. Ther.* 183: 49–55.

Friedman, E. and S. Gershon. 1972. L-Dopa and imipramine: Biochemical and behavioral interaction. *Eur. J. Pharmacol.* 18: 183–188.

Fuxe, K. and U. Ungerstedt. 1970. Histochemical, biochemical and functional studies on central monoamine neurons after acute and chronic amphetamine administration. *In* E. Costa and S. Garattini (eds.), *Amphetamines and Related Compounds*. Proceedings of the Mario Negri Institute for Pharmacological Research. Raven Press, New York, pp. 257–288.

Geller, I., R. J. Hartmann, D. J. Croy and B. Haber. 1974. Attenuation of conflict behavior with cinanserin, a serotonin antagonist: Reversal of the effect with 5-hydroxytryptophan and alpha-methyltryptamine. *Res. Comm. Chem. Pathol. Pharmacol.* 7: 165–174.

Geller, I. and K. Blum. 1970. The effects of 5-HTP on parachlorophenylalanine (PCPA) attenuation of "conflict" behavior. *Eur. J. Pharmacol.* 9: 319–324.

George, D. J. and H. H. Wolf. 1970. Amphetamine toxicity and endogenous noradrenaline concentrations in isolated and aggregated mice. *J. Pharm. Pharmacol.* 22: 947–949.

Gey, K. F. and A. Pletscher. 1968. Acceleration of turnover of [14]-C catecholamines in rat brain by chlorpromazine. *Experienta* 24: 335–336.

Gianutsos, G., R. B. Drawbaugh, M. D. Hynes and H. Lal. 1974. Behavioral evidence for dopaminergic supersensitivity after chronic haloperidol. *Life Sci.* 14: 887–898.

Goodman, L. S. and A. Gilman. 1970. *The Pharmacological Basis of Therapeutics*. Macmillan Co., New York.

Graeff, F. G. and R. I. Schoenfeld. 1970. Tryptaminergic mechanisms in punished and unpunished behavior. *J. Pharmacol. Exp. Ther.* 173: 277–283.

Green, T. K. and J. A. Harvey. 1974. Enhancement of amphetamine action after interruption of ascending serotonergic pathways. *J. Pharmacol. Exp. Ther.* 190: 109–117.

Green, A. R., J. P. Hughes and A. F. C. Tordoff. 1975. The concentration of 5-methoxy-tryptamine in rat brain and its effects on behaviour following its peripheral injection. *Neuropharmacology* 14: 601–606.

Group for the Advancement of Psychiatry, Committee on Mental Health Services. 1971. *Drug Abuse: A Psychiatric View of a Modern Dilemma*. Scribner, New York.

Gunn, J. A. and M. R. Gurd. 1970. The action of some amines related to adrenaline. Cyclohexyalkylamines. *J. Physiol.* 97: 453–470.

Gunne, L. M., J. Johsson and K. Fuxe. 1969. Effects of morphine intoxication on brain catecholamine neurons. *Eur. J. Pharmacol.* 5: 338–342.

Gutwein, B. M., D. Quartermain and B. S. McEwen. 1974. Dissociation of cycloheximide's effects on activity from its effects on memory. *Pharmacol. Biochem. Behav.* 2: 753–756.

Hafen, B. O. (ed.). 1973. *Drug Abuse: Psychology, Sociology, Pharmacology*. Brigham Young University Press, Provo, Utah.

Harvey, J. A. and L. M. Yunger. 1973. Relationship between telencephalic content of serotonin and pain sensitivity. *In* J. Barchas and E. Usdin (eds.), *Serotonin and Behavior*. Academic Press, New York, pp. 179–189.

Holtzman, S. G. and R. E. Jewett. 1972. Some actions of pentazocine on behavior and brain monoamines in the rat. *J. Pharmacol. Exp. Ther.* 181: 346–356.

Honigfeld, G., and A. Howard. 1973. *Psychiatric Drugs, A Desk Reference*. Academic Press, New York.

Iversen, L. L. 1967. *The Uptake and Storage of Noradrenaline in Sympathetic Nerves*. Cambridge University Press, Cambridge.

Klein, D. F. and J. M. Davis. 1969. *Diagnosis and Drug Treatment of Psychiatric Disorders*. Williams and Wilkins, Baltimore.

Krnjevic, K. 1974. Chemical nature of synaptic transmission in vertebrates. *Physiol. Rev.* 54: 418–540.

Kulkarni, S. K. and P. C. Dandiya. 1972. On the mechanism of potentiation of amphetamine induced stereotype behavior by imipramine. *Psychopharmacologia* 27: 367–372.

Kulkarni, S. K. and P. C. Dandiya. 1973. Effects of antidepressant agents on open field behavior in rats. *Psychopharmacologia* 33: 333–338.

Ladinsky, H., S. Consolo, G. Peri and S. Garattini. 1973. Increase in mouse and rat brain acetylcholine levels by diazepam. *In* S. Garattini, E. Mussini and L. O. Randall (eds.), *The Benzodiazepines*. Raven Press, New York, pp. 241–242.

Lal, H. and R. D. Chessick. 1964. Biochemical mechanisms of amphetamine toxicity in isolated and aggregated mice. *Life Sci.* 3: 381–384.

Liebman, J. M. and L. L. Butcher. 1973. Effects on self-stimulation behavior of drugs influencing dopaminergic neurotransmission mechanisms. *Naunyn-Schmiedebergs Arch. Pharmacol.* 277: 305–318.

Lidbrink, P., H. Corrodi, K. Fuxe and L. Olson. 1973. The effects of benzodiazepines, meprobamate, and barbiturates on central monoamine neurons. *In* S. Garattini, E. Mussini and L. O. Randall (eds.), *The Benzodiazepines*. Raven Press, New York, pp. 203–224.

Mabry, P. D. and B. A. Campbell. 1973. Serotonergic inhibition of catecholamine-induced behavioral arousal. *Brain Res.* 49: 381–391.

Maitre, L., P. C. Waldmeier, P. A. Baumann and M. Staehelin. 1974. Effect of maprotiline, a new antidepressant drug, on serotonin uptake. *Advances in Biochemical Psychopharmacology* 10: 297–310.

Malis, J. L. 1973. Analgesic testing in primates. *In* H. W. Kosterlitz, H. O. J. Collier, J. E. Villarreal (eds.), *Agonist and Antagonist Actions of Narcotic Analgesic Drugs*. University Park Press, Baltimore, pp. 106–109.

Marshall, I. 1973. The morphine withdrawal syndrome and its modification by drugs.

In H. W. Kosterlitz, H. O. J. Collier and J. E. Villarreal (eds.), *Agonist and Antagonist Actions of Narcotic Analgesic Drugs.* University Park Press, Baltimore, pp. 192–197.

Marshall, I. and D. G. Grahame-Smith. 1970. Unchanged rate of brain serotonin synthesis during chronic morphine treatment and failure of parachlorophenylalanine to attenuate a withdrawal syndrome in mice. *Nature* 228: 1206–1208.

Martin, Y. C. and J. H. Biel. 1974. Some considerations in the design of substrate and tissue specific inhibitors of monoamine oxidase. *Advances in Biochemical Psychopharmacology* 12: 37–48.

Maruyama, Y., G. Hayashi, S. E. Smits and A. E. Takemori. 1971. Studies on the relationship between 5-hydroxytryptamine turnover in brain and tolerance and physical dependence in mice. *J. Pharmacol. Exp. Ther.* 178: 20–29.

Matthysse, S. 1973. Antipsychotic drug actions: a clue to the neuropathology of schizophrenia? *Fed. Proc.* 32: 200–205.

Moore, K. E. 1963. Toxicity and catecholamine releasing actions of *d*- and *l*-amphetamine in isolated and aggregated mice. *J. Pharmacol. Exp. Ther.* 142: 6–12.

Moore, K. E. 1964. The role of endogenous norepinephrine in the toxicity of *d*-amphetamine in aggregated mice. *J. Pharmacol. Exp. Ther.* 144: 45–51.

Moore, K. E., L. A. Carr and J. A. Dominic. 1970. Functional significance of amphetamine-induced release of brain catecholamines. *In* E. Costa and S. Garattini (eds.), *Amphetamines and Related Compounds.* Proceedings of the Mario Negri Institute for Pharmacological Research. Raven Press, New York, pp. 371–384.

Neff, N. H., H. Y. T. Yang and J. A. Fuentes. 1974. The use of selective monoamine oxidase inhibitor drugs to modify amine metabolism in brain. *Advances in Biochemical Psychopharamacology* 12: 49–58.

Olds, J. and P. Milner. 1954. Positive reinforcement produced by electrical stimulation of septal area and other regions of rat brain. *J. Comp. Physiol. Psychol.* 47: 419–427.

Pare, C. M. B. 1972. Clinical implications of monoamine oxidase inhibition. *Advances in Biochemical Psychopharmacology* 5: 441–444.

Phillips, A. G. and H. C. Fibiger. 1973. Dopaminergic and noradrenergic substrates of positive reinforcement: Differential effects of *d*- and *l*-amphetamine. *Science* 179: 575–577.

Randrup, A. and I. Munkvad. 1968. Behavioral stereotypies induced by pharmacological agents. *Pharmakopsychiatrie Neuro-Psychopharmakologie* 1: 18–26.

Randrup, A. and I. Munkvad. 1970. Biochemical, anatomical and psychological investigations of stereotyped behavior induced by amphetamines. *In* E. Costa and S. Garattini (eds.), *Amphetamines and Related Compounds.* Proceedings of the Mario Negri Institute for Pharmacological Research. Raven Press, New York, pp. 695–713.

Rech, R. H. and J. M. Stolk. 1970. Amphetamine drug interactions that relate brain catecholamines to behavior. *In* E. Costa and S. Garattini (eds.), *Amphetamines and Related Compounds.* Proceedings of the Mario Negri Institute for Pharmacological Research. Raven Press, New York, pp. 385–414.

Rethy, C. R., C. B. Smith and J. E. Villarreal. 1971. Effects of narcotic analgesics upon the locomotor activity and brain catecholamine content of the mouse. *J. Pharmacol. Exp. Ther.* 176: 472–479.

Richardson, J. S., N. Cowan, R. Hartman, and D. W. Jacobowitz. 1974. On the behavioral and neurochemical actions of 6-hydroxydopa and 5,6-dihydroxytryptamine in rats. *Res. Comm. Chem. Pathol. Pharmacol.* 8: 29–44.

Roos, B. E. 1965. Effects of certain tranquilisers on the level of homovanillic acid in the corpus striatum. *J. Pharm. Pharmacol.* 17: 820–821.

Sandler, M., S. B. Carter, B. L. Goodwin, C. R. J. Ruthven, B. M. H. Youdim, E. Hanington, M. F. Cuthbert and C. M. B. Pare. 1974. Multiple forms of monoamine oxidase: some *in vivo* correlations. *Advances in Biochemical Psychopharmacology* 12: 3–10.

Scheckel, C. L. and E. Boff. 1964a. Behavioral effects of interacting imipramine and other drugs with d-amphetamine, cocaine, and tetrabenzine. *Psychopharmacologia* 5: 198–208.

Scheckel, C. L. and E. Boff. 1964b. Behavioral stimulation in rats associated with a selective release of brain norepinephrine. *Arch. Int. Pharmacodyn. Ther.* 152: 479–490.

Scheel-Krüger, J. 1971. Comparative studies of various amphetamine analogs demonstrating different interactions with the metabolism of the catecholamines in brain. *Eur. J. Pharmacol.* 14: 47–59.

Scheel-Krüger, J. 1972. Some aspects of the mechanism of actions of various stimulant amphetamine analogues. *Psychiat. Neurol. Neurochir.* 75: 179–192.

Scheel-Krüger, J. and W. Jonas. 1973. Pharmacological studies on tetrabenazine-induced excited behavior of rats pretreated with amphetamine or nialamide. *Arch. Int. Pharmacodyn. Ther.* 206: 47–65.

Schildkraut, J. J. 1973. Neuropharmacology of the affective disorders. *Ann. Rev. Pharmacol.* 13: 427–454.

Segal, M., G. A. Deneau and M. H. Seevers. 1972. Levels and distribution of central nervous system amines in normal and morphine-dependent monkeys. *Neuropharmacology* 11: 211–222.

Shen, F. H., H. H. Loh and E. L. Way. 1970. Brain serotonin turnover in morphine tolerant and dependent mice. *J. Pharmacol. Exp. Ther.* 175: 427–434.

Shih, J. C. and S. Eiduson. 1974. Some interrelated properties of brain monoamine oxidase. *Advances in Biochemical Psychopharmacology* 12: 29–36.

Smith, C. B. and M. I. Sheldon. 1973. Effects of narcotic analgesic drugs on brain noradrenergic mechanisms. *In* H. W. Kosterlitz, H. O. J. Collier and J. E. Villarreal (eds.), *Agonist and Antagonist Actions of Narcotic Analgesic Drugs.* University Park Press, Baltimore, pp. 164–175.

Smith, C. B., M. I. Sheldon, J. H. Bednarczyk and J. E. Villarreal. 1972. Morphine-induced increases in the corporation of C^{14} tyrosine into C^{14} dopamine and C^{14} norepinephrine in the mouse brain: antagonism by naloxone and tolerance. *J. Pharmacol. Exp. Ther.* 180: 547–557.

Snyder, S. H. 1973. Amphetamine psychosis: "A model." Schizophrenia mediated by catecholamines. *Am. J. Psychiat.* 130: 61–67.

Sparber, S. B. and H. A. Tilson. 1972. The releasability of central norepinephrine and serotonin by peripherally administered d-amphetamine before and after tolerance. *Life Sci.* 11: 1059–1067.

Stein, L., C. D. Wise and B. D. Berger. 1973. Antianxiety action of benzodiazepines: Decrease in activity of serotonin neurons in the punishment system. *In:* S. Garattini, E. Mussini, L. O. Randall (eds.), *The Benzodiazepines.* Raven Press, New York, pp. 299–326.

Takemori, A. E. 1974. Biochemistry of drug dependence. *Ann Rev. Biochem.* 43: 15–33.

Tarsy, D. and R. J. Baldessarini. 1974. Behavioural supersensitivity to apomorphine following chronic treatment with drugs which interfere with the synaptic function of catecholamines. *Neuropharmacology* 13: 927–940.

Taylor, K. M. and R. Laverty. 1973. Interaction of chlordiazepoxide, diazepam, and nitrazepam with catecholamines and histamine in regions of the rat brain. *In* S. Garattini, E. Mussini and L. O. Randall (eds.), *The Benzodiazepines.* Raven Press, New York, pp. 191–202.

Taylor, K. M. and S. H. Snyder. 1970. Amphetamine: Differentiation by d- and l-isomers of behavior involving brain norepinephrine or dopamine. *Science* 168: 1487–1489.

Tenen, S. S. 1968. Antagonism of the analgesic effect of morphine and other drugs by p-chlorophenylalanine, a serotonin depletor. *Psychopharmacologia* 12: 278–285.

Tilson, H. A. and S. B. Sparber. 1972. Studies on the concurrent behavioral and neuro-chemical effects of psychoactive drugs using the push-pull cannula. *J. Pharmacol. Exp. Ther.* **181**: 387–398.

Tseng, L. F. and H. H. Loh. 1974. Significance of dopamine receptor activity in methoxy-amphetamine and *d*-amphetamine-induced locomotor activity. *J. Pharmacol. Exp. Ther.* **189**: 717–724.

Tseng, L. F., R. J. Hitzemann and H. H. Loh. 1974. Comparative effects of *dl-p*-methoxy-amphetamine and *d*-amphetamine on catecholamine release and reuptake *in vitro*. *J. Pharmacol. Exp. Ther.* **189**: 708–716.

Villarreal, J. E., M. Guzman and C. B. Smith. 1973. A comparison of the effects of *d*-amphetamine and morphine upon locomotor activity of mice treated with drugs which alter brain catecholamine content. *J. Pharmacol. Exp. Ther.* **187**: 1–7.

VonVoigtlander, P. F. and K. E. Moore. 1971. The release of H^3-dopamine from cat brain following electrical stimulation of the substantia nigra and caudate nucleus. *Neuropharmacology* **10**: 733–741.

Way, E. L. and F. H. Shen. 1971. Catecholamines and 5-hydroxytryptamine. *In* D. H. Clouet (ed.), *Narcotic Drugs: Biochemical Pharmacology*. Plenum Press, New York, pp. 229–253.

Way, E. L., H. H. Loh and F. H. Shen. 1968. Morphine tolerance, physical dependence and synthesis of brain 5-hydroxytryptamine. *Science* **162**: 1290–1292.

Weil-Malherbe, H. and S. I. Szara. 1971. *The Biochemistry of Functional and Experimental Psychosis*. Charles C Thomas, Springfield, Illinois.

Wise, C. D. and L. Stein. 1969. Facilitation of brain self-stimulation by central administration of norepinephrine. *Science* **163**: 299–301.

Wise, C. D. and L. Stein. 1970. Amphetamines: facilitation of behavior by augmented release of norepinephrine from the medial forebrain bundle. *In* E. Costa and S. Garattini (eds.), *Amphetamines and Related Compounds*. Proceedings of the Mario Negri Institute for Pharmacological Research. Raven Press, New York, pp. 463–485.

Wise, C. D., B. D. Berger and L. Stein. 1972. Benzodiazepines: Anxiety-reducing activity by reduction of serotonin turnover in the brain. *Science* **177**: 180–183.

Yarbrough, G. G., D. M. Buxbaum and E. Sanders-Bush. 1973. Biogenic amines and narcotic effects. II. Serotonin turnover in the rat after acute and chronic morphine administration. *J. Pharmacol. Exp. Ther.* **185**: 328–335.

Ziegler, H., P. DelBasso and V. G. Longo. 1972. Influence of 6-hydroxydopamine and of alpha-methyl-*p*-tyrosine on the effects of some centrally acting agents. *Physiol. Behav.* **8**: 391–396.

7
Acetylcholine and Behavior

Drugs that act on cholinergic mechanisms in the CNS have profound effects on several types of behavior. In the following chapter, the function of acetylcholine (ACh) in the maintenance of behavior will be discussed, as well as methods used to draw inferences about its function in behavior. The pharmacology and biochemistry of acetylcholine in the central nervous system will be reviewed briefly. For a more thorough understanding of the neuroanatomical, neurophysiological, biochemical and pharmacological aspects of ACh, the following reviews should be consulted: Hubbard, 1970; Katz, 1969; Koelle, 1969; Hrdina, 1974; Pepeu, 1973; Krnjevic, 1974; Fonnum, 1973.

Acetylcholine was the first naturally occurring biochemical to receive widespread attention and eventual acceptance as a neurotransmitter. Recall from Chapter 3 the discoveries by Dixon, Hunt and Traveau and Dale that strongly implicated acetylcholine as the chemical active in parasympathetic discharge. Subsequently, the classic experiments of Otto Loewi (1921) demonstrated that stimulation of a nerve caused the release of acetylcholine, which in turn stimulated the muscle innervated by that nerve. The role of acetylcholine as a chemical transmitter of nerve impulses at the parasympathetic neuromuscular junction, the nerve endings of striated muscle and ganglia in the autonomic nervous system is firmly established. The evidence for cholinergic transmission in the CNS is not quite so firm as for the peripheral nervous system.

BIOCHEMISTRY AND PHARMACOLOGY

Distribution in the CNS

The concentration of acetylcholine (ACh) in the central nervous system is of the same order of magnitude as that of catecholamines and serotonin in the CNS. As with the catecholamines and serotonin (see Chapters 4 and 5), its distribution in the CNS is confined to specific areas, implying that it may only function in those areas of the brain. The highest concentrations of ACh are found in the striatum (caudate plus putamen) and the lowest concentrations are found in the cerebellum. Intermediate concentrations of ACh are found in several areas of the brain, including the medulla, pons, midbrain, hypothalamus and cerebral cortex. While the cholinergic pathways have not been thoroughly mapped, existing evidence suggests that there are three major cholinergic systems (see Fig. 7-1)—(1) the dorsal tegmental pathway: cell bodies of this pathway are located in the cuneate nucleus of the medulla and axons project to the thalamus; (2) the ventral tegmental pathway: cell bodies of this pathway are located in the ventral tegmentum and substantia nigra and send projections to the subthalamus, hypothalamus and basal forebrain areas; (3) the septal pathway: cell bodies of this pathway are within the septal area and axons project to the hippocampus, cerebral cortex and mesencephalon. Of these pathways, the septal pathway has been the most extensively mapped (see Shute and Lewis, 1967; Hrdina, 1974; Harvey, 1973; Butcher and Butcher, 1974; Sethy *et al.*, 1973; Pepeu *et al.*, 1973).

At present, no technique exists for the localization of acetylcholine in nerve cells that is comparable to the histofluorescence method for localization of catecholamines and serotonin in nerve cells. Available evidence based on CNS lesions indicates that ACh is localized predominantly in nerve terminals (Cooper *et al.*, 1974). On a gross neuroanatomical basis, it is often tentatively assumed that distribution of acetylcholine follows the distribution of acetylcholinesterase (AChE), for which histochemical stain exists; however, there is not agreement concerning the accuracy with which the distribution of AChE reflects that of ACh. Further electrophysiological and neurochemical work, as well as direct application of ACh to various brain regions, is needed to determine the functional distribution of ACh as a transmitter within the CNS (see Hoskin, 1972).

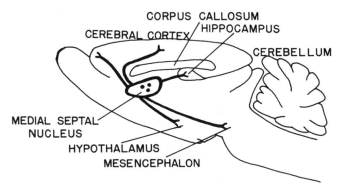

Fig. 7-1. Cholinergic projections from the medial septal nucleus. The dorsal and ventral tegmental pathways are not shown (see text). (From Harvey, 1973.)

Metabolism and Storage

Acetylcholine (ACh) is synthesized from acetate and choline according to the following simple reaction (see Chapter 3):

$$ATP^1 + Acetate + Choline \longrightarrow ACh + AMP^2 + Pyrophosphate$$

This reaction is catalyzed by the enzyme choline acetylase, and the acetate participating in the reaction must be in the active form of acetyl CoA. The source of the acetyl CoA is from metabolism of sugars, according to the following reactions:

$$ATP + Acetate \longrightarrow Adenyl\ acetate + Pyrophosphate$$

$$Adenyl\ acetate + CoA^3 \longrightarrow Acetyl\ CoA + AMP$$

Choline is probably the rate-limiting factor in the synthesis of acetylcholine, but the source of choline as a substrate is not clear. Choline is found in the diet, but it may also be synthesized from ethanolamine through a series of transmethylation reactions. Choline is probably reutilized after the breakdown of ACh by acetylcholinesterase (AChE). The catabolic step shown below is the primary way in which ACh is broken down:

$$ACh \longrightarrow Acetate + Choline$$
$$(AChE)$$

Choline acetylase[4] appears to be a cytoplasmic enzyme. In general, the distribution of choline acetylase follows the distribution of ACh and AChE. Acetylcholine appears to be stored in subcellular organelles called vesicles which are concentrated at the synapse. According to existing evidence, these storage vesicles (or granules) are synthesized in cell bodies and then transported down the axon to the nerve ending (see Cooper *et al.*, 1974; Hebb, 1972).

Acetylcholinesterase (AChE) is a membrane-bound enzyme associated with postjunctional neuromuscular sites, and post synaptic sites in the CNS, as well as glia. Acetylcholine is hydrolyzed in the presence of AChE. This is a rapid reaction and apparently the main mechanism for the inactivation of ACh. There is no evidence that reuptake of the transmitter ACh occurs, as is the case with noradrenergic neurons, but diffusion away from the active site may also play a small role in its inactivation. The properties of AChE have been extensively studied. It should be pointed out that there are a number of esterases that can hydrolyze both acetylcholine and other choline esters. Differentiation of these enzymes in an assay for the total level of cholinesterase is

[1] ATP: adenosine triphosphate.
[2] AMP: adenosine monophosphate.
[3] CoA: coenzyme A.
[4] Also called choline acetyltransferase.

an important variable in studies that measure the amount of AChE present as a result of a drug treatment, lesion or other experimental procedures. If proper controls are not employed, estimates of the level of the hydrolyzing enzyme in tissue are not accurate. Methods for differentiating the alloesterases (or pseudocholinesterase) from true acetylcholinesterase have been described (see Hoskin, 1972).

One of the major sources of difficulty in working on the cholinergic system has been the lack of a reliable and simple ACh assay method. Generally, the degree of contraction of a leech muscle or a frog rectus muscle in response to ACh is used to estimate ACh quantities (see Katz, 1969; Hoskin, 1972; Goldberg and McCaman, 1973). This method is extremely sensitive and can detect ACh concentrations in the nanogram range. In this assay, the isolated muscle is bathed in a nutrient medium and attached to a strain gauge so that contractility may be recorded. The system is standardized by addition of known concentrations of ACh (see Chapter 2 for more detail). Since contractile properties of muscle change with time, temperature and ACh concentration, constant restandardization is necessary. Recently, physical-chemical methods such as gas chromatography and mass spectrometry have been applied to the measurement of ACh in tissues; although these methods are reliable and sensitive, they have not been used widely to study ACh-behavior interactions (Stavinoha *et al.*, 1973).

Synaptic Transmission in the CNS

Acetylcholine meets several of the criteria necessary to establish it as a transmitter in the CNS. First, acetylcholine has been found in CNS areas rich in nerve endings like the hippocampus. Septal lesions that interfere with the cholinergic input to hippocampus are accompanied by a reduction of ACh in this area. Moreover, the enzymes necessary for the synthesis and degradation of acetylcholine are present in the CNS, and in many areas the activities of acetylcholinesterase and choline acetylase are well correlated. Second, release of ACh by stimulation has been demonstrated by several investigators in different areas of the CNS (see Krnjevic, 1974; Pepeu, 1973; Hrdina, 1974; Somogyi and Szerb, 1972).

It should also be pointed out that acetylcholine affects transmission in the CNS in three ways: (1) by excitation that appears to be nicotinic in nature since it can be blocked by nicotinic blockers; (2) by excitation that appears to be muscarinic since it can be blocked by muscarinic blockers; (3) by inhibition that appears to be muscarinic since it can be blocked by muscarinic blockers (see Krnjevic, 1974). A model of the cholinergic neuron in the peripheral nervous system is presented in Chapter 3, p. 79.

Drug Effects

Drugs that affect various aspects of the cholinergic system were reviewed in Chapter 3 (see pp. 81–84). A brief summary is presented here to focus on the drugs to be discussed in this chapter. Many of the drugs discussed in Chapter 3 are quaternary nitrogen compounds which only have peripheral action because they do not readily penetrate into brain except with extremely high doses. Drugs that have tertiary nitrogens affect both central and peripheral systems. In this chapter, drugs that are able to enter brain will be emphasized, since their behavioral effects have been most widely investigated. It should be noted, however, that drugs which have effects on the CNS also have peripheral effects. In fact, a behavioral effect might be due to a drug's effect on the peripheral nervous system or to a combination of its peripheral and central effects. The behavioral effects of some cholinergic or anticholinergic drugs are thought to be mediated mainly through the CNS (see Pradhan and Dutta, 1971; Aquilonius et al., 1972; Warburton, 1969), while others are thought to have a major peripheral component (Glow et al., 1966, 1967). The central nervous system mechanism of drug action is usually inferred from its peripheral mechanism of action. While this approach may be justified in some cases, in others it may not be appropriate. For excellent reviews regarding the methods by which data are obtained and limits on their interpretation, see Weiss and Heller (1969) and Russell (1969).

Cholinergic Agonists. Acetylcholine is the main cholinergic agonist. When acetylcholine is administered exogenously, it produces short term effects in the peripheral nervous system because it is rapidly hydrolyzed (see Chapter 3). Since ACh does not cross the blood-brain barrier readily, it can only be used as a tool for studying cholinergic effects on CNS function if it is administered intracerebrally. Nicotine is a cholinergic agonist at nicotinic receptor sites, and arecoline is a cholinergic agonist at muscarinic receptor sites. Both nicotine and arecoline pass the blood-brain barrier. Methacholine, carbachol and bethanechol are choline esters that act as agonists but do not readily penetrate the blood-brain barrier.

Drugs That Interfere With Synthesis. Hemicholinium interferes with ACh synthesis by blocking the uptake of choline. It does not enter brain, however, and relatively few studies have used it to determine the function of ACh in behavior. A few other compounds interfere with synthesis by inhibiting choline acetylase (or choline acetyltransferase).

Drugs That Interfere With Inactivation. Physostigmine and diisopropyl fluorophosphate (DFP) inhibit acetylcholinesterase in the CNS. Physostigmine is a reversible inhibitor, while DFP is irreversible.

Reuptake Blockers. Acetylcholine does not seem to be inactivated by a reuptake process; however, hemicholinium interferes with the uptake of choline, thereby limiting the synthesis of ACh.

Receptor Blockers. There are two types of cholinergic receptors in the peripheral cholinergic system: muscarinic and nicotinic (see Chapter 3). Atropine and scopolamine block muscarinic receptors, and mecamylamine blocks nicotinic receptors. All three compounds enter the brain.

Drugs That Interfere With Storage. There are none.

Neurotoxins. Botulinus toxin inhibits the release of ACh from nerve. It is lethal because of its peripheral effects. A number of other ACh toxins have been identified, but they are not usually employed in behavioral studies (see O'Brien *et al.*, 1972; Cohen and Changeux, 1975).

In addition, it should be noted that other drugs (see Chapter 6) also affect ACh metabolism. While the relationship between these drugs and their effects on behavior may well involve cholinergic mechanisms of considerable importance, behavioral studies in relation to ACh are not extensive enough to warrant discussion; however, the interested reader might consult the references cited for the following classes of drugs: psychomotor stimulants (Vasko *et al.*, 1974; Sethy and Van Woert, 1974b); antianxiety agents (Rawat, 1974; Consolo *et al.*, 1974); antipsychotic agents (Trabucchi *et al.*, 1974; Sethy and Van Woert, 1974a,b); antidepressants (Aprison *et al.*, 1975); narcotic analgesics and antagonists (Labrecque and Domino, 1974; Wilson and Domino, 1973; Bramwell and Bradley, 1974; Mullin and Phillis, 1974; Merali *et al.*, 1974; Mullin, 1974).

ROLE OF ACETYLCHOLINE IN BEHAVIOR

General Approach

The question as to whether a drug's effects are mediated by a particular chemical system in brain has been examined in Chapters 4, 5 and 6. It was noted that in order to attribute drug-induced modifications in behavior to a specific chemical system, extensive collateral evidence is necessary. In the absence of adequate collateral experimental work, incorrect assumptions about the role of a drug in brain function and behavior may be made. The same caution must be exercised in attributing drug-induced modifications in behavior to the cholinergic system.

The procedures used to establish a causal relationship between a drug, a behavioral effect and cholinergic function are different from the procedures used to examine drug-behavior-chemical interactions in catecholaminergic and serotonergic systems, since different chemical and pharmacological agents are available. For example, if a behavioral effect is thought to be me-diated by catecholamines, there are a number of ways to deplete or replace catecholamines. It is very difficult to reduce or elevate ACh levels through the administration of specific depletors or endogenous chemicals; however, the function of cholinergic systems can be altered by administration of (1) cholinesterase inhibitors, (2) cholinergic agonists or (3) cholinergic blockers.

Elevation of Acetylcholine Levels. Acetylcholine levels can be increased in brain by administration of an AChE inhibitor such as physostigmine, which increases ACh in those areas where it is released. While AChE inhibitors may affect other systems, they do not elevate ACh in areas where ACh does not normally exist.

Agonists/Antagonists. Acetylcholine function can be altered by administra-tion of specific agonists and antagonists. Nicotine is the most commonly used cholinergic agonist. The muscarinic agonist arecoline is also frequently used. Other agonists such as carbachol are administered intracerebrally and intra-ventricularly, because they do not readily pass the blood-brain barrier. Atro-pine and scopolamine block muscarinic cholinergic receptors, and mecamyl-amine blocks nicotinic receptors.

In order to determine whether the behavioral effect produced by a partic-ular drug such as an AChE inhibitor is mediated by the cholinergic system, the following procedure is often employed. First of all, the AChE inhibitor is administered, and behavioral effects are observed. Then a cholinergic blocking agent such as atropine or scopolamine is administered, and behavioral effects are again observed. If the AChE inhibitor affects behavior by increasing the concentration of ACh, a cholinergic blocking agent would be expected to antagonize these behavioral effects.

Procedures used to examine drug-behavior interactions in the cholinergic system usually employ drugs that are assumed to have a certain action in the central nervous system by virtue of their effects in the peripheral cholinergic system. Since most of these drugs have both peripheral and central effects, their peripheral effects must be considered before attributing a behavioral ef-fect to central cholinergic systems. For example, in order to determine whether the behavioral effects of an acetylcholinesterase inhibitor is peripheral or cen-tral, a compound which only inhibits peripheral AChE is administered, and the effect is compared to that of a compound which presumably has both peripheral and central effects.

Electrophysiological Correlates

In 1952, Wikler found that certain cholinergic drugs produced a dissociation between the electrical pattern recorded from the brain of unanesthetized dogs and their behavior. Recall from Chapter 1 that a low voltage fast (14 cycles/sec

and above) electroencephalogram (EEG) is normally associated with wakefulness and behavioral activity while an EEG with high voltage slow waves (1–3
cycles/sec) is associated with sleep. A more detailed account of the EEG and
its behavioral correlates can be found in Chapter 1 (pp. 8–9). The low voltage
fast electrical activity is often referred to as *desynchronized*, while higher
voltage slow activity is referred to as *synchronized*. This nomenclature stems
from the notion that the high voltage electrical activity recorded from macro-
electrodes on the cortex represents a summation of many individual neurons
firing at the same time; when they fire at different times, the voltages do not
form a sum, and therefore the amplitude is lower but the periodicity more
rapid.

Dogs treated with atropine or other cholinergic blocking agents showed a
high voltage slow EEG normally associated with sleep but appeared active;
moreover, their activity levels were somewhat above normal. On the other
hand, physostigmine (an AChE inhibitor) produced a low voltage fast EEG
that was often associated with the typical postures and behavioral signs of
sleep; however, at other times the dogs appeared alert. This early work stimulated further research relating cholinergic drugs to behavior and EEG patterns
(see Bradley and Elkes, 1957; Bradley and Hance, 1957; Bradley, 1958, 1964).

Motor Behavior

Drugs affecting the central cholinergic system cause alterations in locomotor
activity in various species. For example, scopolamine increases locomotor
activity in a jiggle cage over a broad range of doses, but the increase does not
appear to be dose-dependent. Methylscopolamine, which does not penetrate
the blood-brain barrier readily, does not increase locomotor activity, indicating
that the effects of scopolamine on locomotor activity are due to its action in
the CNS (Meyers *et al.*, 1964). Atropine also produces increases in locomotor
activity in the rat (Fig. 7-2), while methylatropine, which does not penetrate
the blood-brain barrier, does not increase locomotor activity (Aquilonius *et al.*,
1972).

Nicotine, a cholinergic agonist, has been reported both to increase and decrease locomotor activity. For example, in rats low doses of nicotine increased
locomotor activity while high doses decreased locomotor activity (Fig. 7-3;
Pradhan, 1970; Morrison and Lee, 1968). On the other hand, in mice nicotine
decreased locomotor activity (Morrison and Armitage, 1967). The effects of
nicotine on locomotor activity have been shown to depend on pre-drug activity
levels. Nicotine decreased the activity in rats which had a high pre-drug level
of activity and increased the activity of rats that had a low pre-drug level of
activity. Thus, the effects of nicotine seem to depend on the dose of the drug
as well as on pre-drug activity levels (see Chapter 9). The fact that mice show

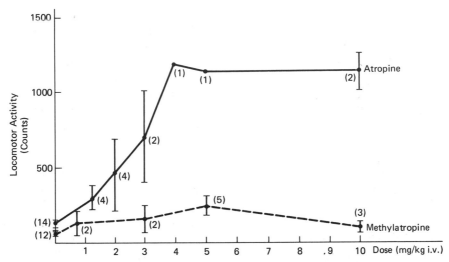

Fig. 7.2. Dose response relationships for locomotor activity 30–60 min after iv injection of atropine or methylatropine.   Mean ± SEM; (N) = number of experiments.   (From Aquilonius *et al.*, 1972.)

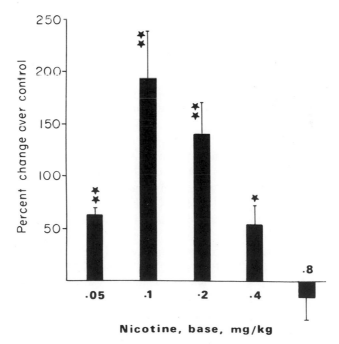

Fig. 7-3. Effect of nicotine on the spontaneous motor activity measured in 12 rats.   Each dose was given to 6 rats.   (*Indicates $P < .05$; **indicates $P < .01$.)   (From Pradhan, 1970.)

only a decrease in locomotor behavior in response to nicotine may be due to pre-drug levels of activity as well as to species differences in response to nicotine.

While cholinergic blockers increase locomotor activity, cholinesterase inhibitors such as physostigmine decrease locomotor behavior. Moreover, decreases in locomotor activity are correlated with decreases in brain AChE activity. Malathion, a peripheral cholinesterase inhibitor, does not affect locomotor activity, nor does it inhibit brain AChE. These results indicate that inhibition of AChE in the CNS leads to reduction of motor activity (Pradhan and Mhatre, 1970).

Other types of motor activity are affected by drugs that exert their action through the acetylcholine system. Cholinergic blocking drugs were the first drugs useful in the treatment of the tremor and, to a certain extent, the dyskinesia that accompanies Parkinson's disease. Acetylcholine is present in high concentration in the striatum. The relationships between the dopaminergic and cholinergic systems in the striatum have not been worked out (see Beani and Bianchi, 1973; Bak *et al.*, 1972), but it is of interest to recall that DA in the striatum is affected by Parkinson's disease (see Chapter 5, p. 135).

In summary, drugs that act on the central cholinergic system affect motor behavior. Although pre-drug activity levels and dose are important variables, nicotinic and muscarinic blockers tend to increase activity, while the AChE inhibitors tend to decrease locomotor activity.

Food and Water Intake

Drugs that have cholinergic effects modify both food and water intake. The degree of modification, as well as the direction of change in intake, depends on several factors including the route of drug administration, the species examined, the extent of deprivation and the type of consummatory response. The range of physiological, biochemical and environmental factors that control the ingestion of both food and water is highly complex; and in spite of many studies on neural, neuropharmacological and environmental aspects of this problem, mechanisms involved in control of ingestive behavior are not well understood. The system is difficult to understand because its representation in brain involves many different anatomical loci. For an excellent and extensive review of the physiological and behavioral parameters involved in the regulation of food and water intake, see Morgane, 1969; Myers, 1974; Fisher, 1973; and Wayner, 1974.

A few representative studies which demonstrate that acetylcholine is involved in drinking and feeding will be reviewed here as a background to research endeavors. Data in this area are often inconsistent, and so a good deal of controversy exists as to their interpretation.

Intracranial Chemical Stimulation. Grossman (see 1969 review) showed that direct cholinergic stimulation of the lateral hypothalamus elicited drinking in sated rats and increased the drinking response in water-deprived rats. Grossman placed small quantities of crystalline cholinergic agonists in a specific locus in the brain of rats through a permanently indwelling cannula. A few minutes following an injection of acetylcholine, the animals began drinking. Drinking could be blocked by either topical or systemic treatment with atropine, but not by systemic injection of methylatropine, which does not cross the blood-brain barrier. This evidence is consistent with the idea that these effects are mediated by central cholinergic systems.

In addition, cholinergic (muscarinic) stimulation of the dorsal hippocampus, posterior hypothalamus, anterior thalamus, medial thalamus, cingulate gyrus, septal nuclei, certain portions of the midbrain and the lateral hypothalamus elicit drinking in sated rats (Fisher and Coury, 1962, 1964). These results have been confirmed with the muscarinic agonist carbachol in several of these areas (Leibowitz, 1972; Spencer and Holloway, 1972). Other chemicals such as 5-HT and histamine do not elicit drinking. It is not surprising that the effects of muscarinic agonists in the rat are similar to the effects of acetylcholine, and the same sites that elicit drinking in response to ACh also elicit drinking in response to intracerebral administration of muscarinic agonists.

While this evidence suggests a role for cholinergic involvement in drinking, it should be noted that some of the sites in which cholinergic agents elicit drinking are also related to feeding. Since drinking usually accompanies the ingestion of food, it is difficult to separate effects on these two behaviors. Moreover, a variety of factors have been shown to affect endogenous release of ACh, including amount of deprivation, activity of the animal, availability of alternative sources of food and water, blood sugar, blood salts and blood volume, as well as hormone balance. Any or all of these factors may determine the way in which ACh affects drinking behavior. For example, when animals are sated, atropine blocks drinking elicited by cholinergic stimulation (carbachol) (Levitt, 1970; Levitt and Fisher, 1967), but when animals are deprived, the effects of atropine are variable; some investigators report that atropine does not block cholinergic-induced drinking in deprived animals (Blass and Chapman, 1971; Singer and Kelly, 1972), while others have reported that drinking produced by deprivation is partially attenuated by atropine (Antunez-Rodriguez and Covian, 1971; Block and Fisher, 1970). These variable effects appear to be related to the dose of atropine, degree of water deprivation and the way in which drinking is elicited (see Gentil et al., 1971).

In addition, the anatomical site examined is an important variable (Sommer et al., 1967). When carbachol is injected in the supraoptic nucleus of the hypothalamus of the rabbit, it elicits eating first and drinking several minutes later. When carbachol is placed in the lateral hypothalamus, lateral preoptic area and the area dorsal and anterior to the medial preoptic area, carbachol elicits drinking at low doses that do not affect eating, while at higher doses, drinking is decreased and eating is increased.

The extent to which cholinergic involvement in drinking occurs in other species has also been examined. Myers (1969) studied chemical mediation of drinking and feeding in monkeys. Compounds were introduced at various sites in the brain, and their effects on drinking and feeding were recorded. While Myers (1969) found that NE increased food and water intake in sated monkeys when injected into the lateral hypothalamus, a small dose of carbachol did not elicit eating or drinking in sated monkeys, nor did it interfere with ingestion of either food or water in deprived monkeys. With larger doses, carbachol inhibited food and water intake in the deprived monkey. This effect could be antagonized by atropine. Acetylcholine produced effects similar to those of carbachol, although the duration of the effect was shorter. Experiments in other anatomical areas and under other behavioral conditions are necessary before these conclusions can be drawn, but at present it appears that the cholinergic mediation of food and water intake differs in the monkey and the rat.

Systemic Administration. Generally, administration of scopolamine and atropine, as well as methylscopolamine and methylatropine, causes a dose-dependent decrease in feeding. The fact that both peripherally and centrally active compounds produce similar effects indicates that the decrease in feeding may be due to effects in the periphery (e.g., dryness of mouth). On the other hand, only centrally active cholinergic blockers interfere with drinking (Stein, 1963; Pradhan and Dutta, 1971; Block and Fisher, 1975). Moreover, both short-term and long-term inhibition of AChE have been reported to increase drinking (Glow *et al.*, 1966); however, pilocarpine (a tertiary muscarinic agonist) decreases drinking in deprived rats. This is not consistent with the conclusion that cholinergic stimulation increases drinking, but the reason for the discrepancy is not clear.

These results suggest that the cholinergic system, particularly in hypothalamic and limbic system structures, plays a role in the modulation of water intake; however, peripheral as well as central mechanisms appear to be important.

Schedule-Controlled Behavior

Negative Reinforcement. The effects of cholinergic blocking agents such as atropine or scopolamine, and cholinesterase inhibitors such as physostigmine, have been examined extensively to determine their effect on the maintenance of avoidance behavior. A number of avoidance procedures have been used, including passive avoidance, one- or two-way active avoidance in a shuttle box and discrete trial or continuous avoidance in an operant chamber. Cholinergic drugs have been shown to have a variety of effects under these conditions. The nature of the drug effect, however, has been shown to depend to a large extent upon the method used to examine avoidance. Therefore, it is difficult to generalize about the role of the cholinergic system in the maintenance of avoidance behavior *per se*. We will review a small portion of a rather extensive literature in this area with a special emphasis on the problems involved in interpreting the results generated by these studies (see Russell, 1969).

Inhibition of acetylcholinesterase by reversible inhibitors disrupts the maintenance of a previously acquired avoidance response. This disruption can be blocked by pretreatment with atropine (Pfeiffer and Jenney, 1957; Goldberg *et al.*, 1963, 1965). By measuring the degree of acetylcholinesterase inhibition produced by the various inhibitors examined and by comparing the effects of AChE inhibitors to the effects of drugs that do not have cholinergic involvement, it was concluded that cholinergic neurons play an important role in the mediation of avoidance responses.

Three questions arise out of the finding that cholinesterase inhibitors disrupt performance of an avoidance response: (1) Are the effects of cholinesterase inhibitors relatively specific to avoidance behavior? (2) Are the effects due to disruption of other chemical systems? (3) Is the effect mediated by the central nervous system, the peripheral nervous system or both? These questions will be brought up repeatedly in our discussion of cholinergic involvement in avoidance behavior.

Goldberg *et al.* (1963, 1965) found that the reversible cholinesterase inhibitor N-methyl-3-isopropylphenylcarbamate (Compound 10854) interfered with a pole jump avoidance response at doses that did not interfere with the escape response. Furthermore, decreases in avoidance could be blocked by atropine (Table 7-1). Atropine did not affect avoidance when given alone. The

TABLE 7-1. Effect of compound 10854 and atropine and their interaction on discrete avoidance behavior in rats

Treatment	Dose mg/kg	Avoidance Behavior[1]	
		% Efficiency ± S.E.	n/N[2]
Controls	—	95 ± 1.3	0/10
Compound 10854	1.0	53 ± 10.3[3]	10/10
Atropine	0.5	98 ± 1.8	0/10
Atropine 30 min before	0.5	89 ± 8.9	3/10
Compound 10854	1.0		

[1]First 30 min after ip injection.
[2]Number of rats with decrease in avoidance efficiency ($P < .01$)/number in group.
[3]$P < .001$.
From Goldberg *et al.* (1963).

effective dose of 10854 which disrupted avoidance behavior by 50% of control values (referred to as the ED50) was about three times less than the ED50 for disrupting escape behavior. Furthermore, the ED50 for escape behavior was 10 times lower than the LD50 (i.e., the dose required to kill 50% of rats treated with this anticholinesterase), indicating that the behavioral results are probably not due to the drug's toxic effects.

Moreover, while the cholinesterase inhibitor 10854 interfered with motor activity, it did so at doses which interfered with avoidance behavior and below those that interfered with escape. If the effect of 10854 on avoidance responding was simply due to its effect on motor activity, one would expect avoidance behavior and escape behavior to be affected at the same dose.

The correlation between avoidance behavior and the degree of AChE inhibition has also been examined. While a correlation between these two events would not establish a causal relationship between them, lack of such a correlation would severely question the role of the cholinergic system in the mediation of this behavior. Goldberg *et al.* (1963) demonstrated a high correlation between 10854-induced inhibition of cholinesterase and disruption of avoidance behavior (Fig. 7-4). They found that avoidance behavior was not disrupted until cholinesterase was inhibited by 50%. When AChE was inhibited by 50% or more, suppression of avoidance behavior was directly proportional to the amount of AChE inhibited. Atropine, a compound which blocks muscarinic cholinergic receptors, blocked the effects of 10854 on avoidance behavior,

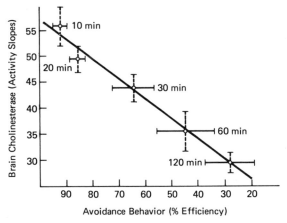

Fig. 7-4. Effect of Compound 10854 dust inhalation on discrete trial avoidance behavior and brain cholinesterase in rats. Regression equation $Y = 18.47 + 0.30X$. Coefficient of correlation = + 0.980. Vertical bars represent ± standard error of mean for enzyme ($N = 6$). Control activity slope ± S.E. = 122 ± 1.3 ($N = 12$). Horizontal bars represent ± standard error of mean for behavior ($N = 10$). Control % avoidance efficiency ± S.E. = 95 ± 0.8 ($N = 10$). (From Goldberg *et al.*, 1963.)

indicating that the mechanism of action is related to increases in ACh produced by the 10854-induced inhibition of AChE. Moreover, methylatropine, which does not pass the blood-brain barrier, did not block the effect of 10854, indicating that the 10854 effects are central. If the effects were peripheral, one would expect atropine and methylatropine to be equally potent in antagonizing the behavioral effects of 10854.

In a similar study, Rosecrans *et al.* (1968) found that the effects of physostigmine (another AChE inhibitor) on both rat brain cholinesterase and acetylcholine were correlated with the effects of physostigmine on a pole jump avoidance procedure. Physostigmine interfered with avoidance responding more than it interfered with escape responding. The time course and extent of the increase in acetylcholine and the decrease in cholinesterase activity roughly corresponded to the effects on avoidance conditioning, although chemical recovery lagged behind the behavioral recovery. Atropine blocked the effect of physostigmine, but methylatropine (which does not readily cross the blood-brain barrier) did so to a far lesser extent. Therefore, the work of both Goldberg and Rosecrans suggests that the central cholinergic system is involved in the mediation of avoidance behavior.

A number of drugs including tetrabenazine, reserpine, chlorpromazine and haloperidol have also been shown to interfere with avoidance responding (see Chapters 5, 6 and 9). The effects of many of these drugs can be antagonized by cholinergic blockers such as scopolamine and atropine (Hanson *et al.*, 1970). The fact that cholinergic blocking agents can antagonize a variety of drugs which are thought to act through catecholaminergic mechanisms suggests that there is an important cholinergic link in the maintenance of avoidance behavior and also indicates that cholinergic systems may be involved in an interaction with catecholaminergic systems. Interactions between different chemical systems in brain are difficult to examine because of the numerous variables that must be considered; however, research in this area is important and certainly will receive greater attention in the future.

Nicotine has been shown to enhance avoidance responding in rats trained on a continuous avoidance procedure (Fig. 7-5). Rate of avoidance responding increased with increasing doses of nicotine (Pradhan, 1970; see also Bovet *et al.*, 1966). Avoidance behavior has also been shown to increase when levels of ACh in brain (particularly the telencephalon) are reduced by a combination of iproniazid and tetrabenazine. Recall that iproniazid inhibits MAO, and tetrabenazine interferes with storage of catecholamines and serotonin. A combination of iproniazid-tetrabenazine also decreases ACh (see Aprison *et al.*, 1968). Rats were trained to avoid shock on a continuous avoidance schedule. Then they were injected with iproniazid 16 hours before the test session, and tetrabenazine approximately one hour before the test session. Avoidance increased following iproniazid-tetrabenazine treatment. Enhancement of

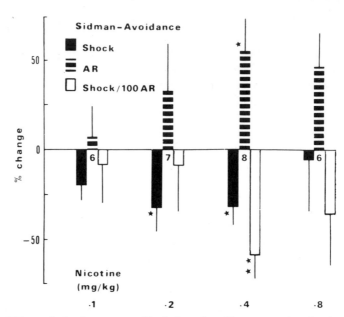

Fig. 7-5. Effects of nicotine on a nondiscriminated avoidance procedure in nine rats. AR: the percent change in the number of avoidance responses from pre-drug baseline control. A positive value on the ordinate indicates that the rat made more avoidance responses, and a negative value indicates that the rat received fewer shocks. Abscissa is mg/kg of nicotine. (From Pradhan, 1970.)

avoidance behavior was correlated with the decrease in ACh in the telencephalon (Fig. 7-6). Neither serotonin nor norepinephrine reductions in telencephalon, midbrain or pons-medulla showed any correlation with the enhancement of avoidance. Furthermore, the enhancement of avoidance behavior elicited by pretreatment with iproniazid followed by tetrabenazine could be attenuated if atropine (0.8 mg/kg) was given 60 minutes before tetrabenazine. This finding provides further evidence that the increase in avoidance behavior is mediated through acetylcholine (Toru *et al.*, 1966; Aprison *et al.*, 1968; Hingtgen and Aprison, 1970; Aprison *et al.*, 1975); however, it does not eliminate catecholamine involvement in avoidance. The fact that a transmitter is important in the mediation of a certain behavior does not mean that other transmitters are not involved in the same behavior (see Beani *et al.*, 1974; Richardson *et al.*, 1971).

In summary, these experiments present evidence that the cholinergic system is involved in the maintenance of avoidance behavior. However, a simple model of whether cholinergic excitation or inhibition enhances or depresses maintenance of avoidance behavior is not yet clearly delineated. What is clear is that additional experiments using similar species, strains, drug regimens and

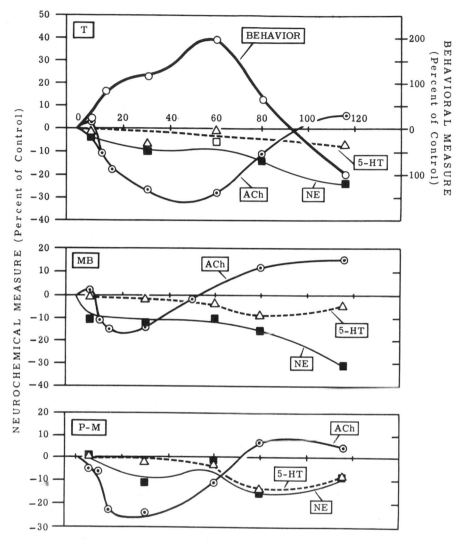

Fig. 7-6. Temporal variations in ACh, 5-HT and NE content in the telencephalon (T), diencephalon plus mesencephalon (MB) and the pons-medulla (P-M) and avoidance rates in rats injected with 50 mg/kg of iproniazid 16 hr before being injected with 2 mg/kg of tetrabenazine. Each point represents the biochemical or behavioral measure obtained from the same group of rats killed at a specified time after injection. The abscissa refers to time in minutes after the tetrabenazine injection. Acetylcholine levels in the telencephalon are most closely related to the increased rate of responding. (From Aprison and Hingtgen, 1970.)

experimental designs must be made to identify sources of apparent contradictions.

Additional information on the involvement of the cholinergic system in avoidance behavior has been derived from neuroanatomical structure-function studies. It has been shown that the septal and hippocampal areas of the brain play a role in habituation, memory and learning. These areas have also been shown to have a cholinergic component. The structure-function aspects are highly relevant to the material discussed in this section; however, a complete review of this literature goes beyond the scope of this book.

Positive Reinforcement. Schedules of positive reinforcement engender a variety of rates and patterns of responding. Drugs that act through the cholinergic system affect schedule-controlled behavior in a manner which depends on the pre-drug rates and patterns of responding engendered by the particular schedule. For a more thorough discussion of the relationship between a drug effect and rate of responding, see Chapter 9. In general, cholinergic blocking agents and cholinergic agonists increase low rates and decrease high rates of responding maintained by food presentation (see Chapter 9). In addition, scopolamine and atropine increase low rates of behavior which occur in the absence of reinforcement.

Since very few attempts have been made to correlate the behavioral effects of cholinergic agents with changes in cholinergic activity, the reader is referred to Chapter 9, Table 9-1, for a summary of the effects of cholinergic agents on behavior maintained by positive reinforcement. The relationship between cholinergic function and behavior maintained by intracranial brain stimulation has been examined and is discussed here.

Recall from Chapter 6 that Wise and Stein (1970) suggested that norepinephrine mediates the positive reinforcing aspects of electrical brain stimulation. Nicotine also enhances responding maintained by intracranial electrical stimulation to the medial forebrain bundle, suggesting that mediation of reinforcement by intracranial electrical stimulation may have a cholinergic as well as a noradrenergic component (Pradhan and Bowling, 1971). Rats were trained to respond for several intensities of intracranial stimulation (ICS). Nicotine (37.5–200 µg/kg) increased the rate of responding when the current level was set slightly above the threshold required to maintain responding. This effect depended on baseline rates of responding as well as on the current intensity of intracranial stimulation. At low rates of responding, nicotine facilitated self-stimulation, while at high rates of responding, it depressed self-stimulation. Similarly, nicotine increased responding maintained by low current intensities and decreased responding maintained at higher current intensities.

While nicotine increases responding maintained by intracranial stimulation, the cholinesterase inhibitor physostigmine decreases responding maintained by ICS.

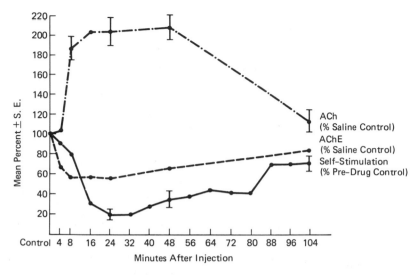

Fig. 7-7. The correlation of self-stimulation behavior, brain ACh levels and AChE after physostigmine. Each point represents a mean of at least six animals. The animals were sacrificed at various time periods after a dose of physostigmine (100 μg/kg sc). Note that increases in ACh correlated with the decreases in self-stimulation behavior. (From Domino and Olds, 1968.)

Moreover, decreases in responding were correlated with an increase in ACh levels and a decrease in brain AChE (see Fig. 7-7). While this study provides direct evidence that ACh levels rise as a result of physostigmine treatment, it should be noted that while a correlation between an increase in ACh and a decrease in responding does not establish causality, it does provide an important link in the search for functional relationships between the regulation of behavior and the utilization of acetylcholine (Domino and Olds, 1968; Olds and Domino, 1969a,b).

Learning

The relationship between cholinergic drugs and behavior in animals has centered around issues related to learning. Therefore, although drug effects on learning and memory are discussed in Chapter 8, the question of cholinergic involvement in learning will be discussed here. There are widespread differences among investigators as to how the term learning should be defined. For the purpose of this presentation, learning will be defined operationally, i.e., as a modification of behavior as a result of prior experience. Learning is often investigated by examining acquisition of some response.

Studies involving facilitation or depression of the rate of acquisition or extinction of a conditioned response such as an avoidance response are in a general sense related to learning. Herz (1960) showed that the effect of a cholinergic blocking drug such as scopolamine is "highly dependent on the state of acquisition of the response at the moment the drug is applied." Herz trained rats on a pole jump avoidance response. One group received minimal training (i.e., they received two hours of training); another group was overtrained (i.e., they received six two-hour training sessions). When scopolamine (1 mg/kg) was injected, the minimally trained group showed inhibition of the avoidance response even at the lowest doses of scopolamine. These results are consistent with those of Meyers *et al.* (1964), which showed that scopolamine disrupted acquisition of an avoidance response when scopolamine was given before training. Scopolamine did not disrupt the response when it was given after training.

In addition, mecamylamine (a nicotinic blocker) interfered with acquisition of a shuttle box avoidance response in which multiple trails were given each day over a five-day period (Oliverio, 1966), while nicotine (a cholinergic agonist) facilitated acquisition of the avoidance response. This effect could be antagonized by mecamylamine. Mecamylamine did not interfere with an avoidance response that was previously established; moreover, the quaternary derivatives of mecamylamine (which do not readily enter the brain) did not affect behavior, suggesting that the effects of mecamylamine were produced by its action on central nicotinic receptors.

Cholinergic agents have also been reported to interfere with the acquisition of a passive avoidance response. The passive avoidance task is designed along the following lines: an animal is placed in one location (for example, in a small open chamber or on a platform). If the animal moves from this position onto a grid floor, shock is delivered. Generally, after the animal has been shocked in this situation, its latency for stepping onto the grid is increased. Since no "performance" other than not moving from the initial position is required of the animal, this paradigm has been referred to as the "passive avoidance technique" (see Chapter 1, p. 21).

Meyers (1965) placed rats on a platform in a modified operant chamber. The rat avoided shock by remaining on the platform. Sessions lasted for 30 minutes and the number of descents from the platform was taken as an index of acquisition and retention. Scopolamine administration resulted in a dose-dependent increase in the number of descents made by the rat during acquisition (especially on the first day of training; Fig. 7-8). The quaternary derivative of scopolamine, which does not readily enter brain, caused no change in avoidance responding, suggesting that the drug effect is centrally mediated. Scopolamine also interfered with the maintenance of a passive avoidance response that had been established prior to drug administration. These effects were dose-dependent (Fig. 7-9).

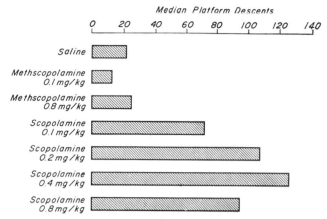

Fig. 7-8. Effects of various doses of scopolamine on the acquisition of a passive avoidance response. (From Meyers, 1965.)

While these data suggest a role for acetylcholine in avoidance acquisition, it should be noted that scopolamine might interfere with passive avoidance by virtue of its effects on motor activity. For example, scopolamine might increase the number of platform descents by virtue of increasing general activity levels. Unless the experiment provides controls for these effects, results from passive avoidance must be interpreted with caution.

Bohdanecký and Jarvik (1967) also found that cholinergic drugs interfere with the acquisition of passive avoidance in mice. Mice were given either scopolamine, physostigmine or saline shortly before being placed into a two-chambered box.

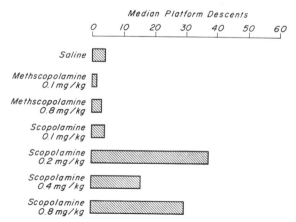

Fig. 7-9. Effects of various doses of scopolamine on the retention of a passive avoidance response. (From Meyers, 1965.)

When they crossed from one chamber to the other (in this instance, usually within a matter of seconds), they were shocked. After a single trial, the mice were removed from the apparatus and returned the following day for testing. It was found that the control mice remained in the original "safe" compartment for a period of greater than five minutes, while mice treated with either scopolamine or physostigmine crossed to the other compartment in about one minute, suggesting that both scopolamine and physostigmine blocked learning that took place on the first trial (Table 7-2). Furthermore, the effects of physostigmine and scopolamine could be antagonized when both drugs were given in combination. Since scopolamine blocks cholinergic receptor sites and physostigmine blocks AChE, the combination of the two drugs would tend to normalize the amount of receptor activation. This evidence strongly suggests that the mechanism of action of these two drugs on passive avoidance acquisition is cholinergic. Furthermore, since the quaternary analogues, methylscopolamine and neostigmine, were without effect on passive avoidance, a *central* cholinergic mode of action is indicated. This result is interpreted by the authors as being due to an effect of the cholinergic drugs on the learning process rather than an effect on performance, since there is no evidence that the effects of the drug carry over to the testing day.

Dilts and Berry (1967) obtained similar results with cholinergic drugs using a slightly different version of the one-trial passive avoidance techniques. They demonstrated that drugs which block muscarinic receptors (i.e., atropine and scopolamine) or nicotinic receptors (mecamylamine) retard the learning of a passive avoidance response. Similarly, the AChE inhibitor, physostigmine, interfered with the acquisition of a one-trial passive avoidance response. For each of the drugs tested, it was found that the drug-response occurred over a wide range of doses. Analogues of these drugs which do not enter brain were without effect. These results are similar to those described above and are consistent

TABLE 7-2. Retest scores of animals drugged before learning
(all values expressed as medians)

Drug	Dose (mg/kg)	Punished Group	Punished Latency (sec)	Unpunished Group	Unpunished Latency (sec)
Saline	—	A	> 300.0	B	3.4
Scopolamine methylbromide	1.0	C	> 300.0	D	1.7
Scopolamine	1.0	E	77.0	F	3.9
Physostigmine	0.5	G	37.0	H	3.2
Neostigmine	0.5	I	> 300.0	J	2.0
Neostigmine	0.25	K	> 300.0	L	2.2

From Bohdanecký and Jarvik, 1967.

with the idea that the cholinergic system in brain plays a role in the learning of an avoidance response.

Another way to measure the rate of learning a new response is to train an animal to perform a response and then extinguish the response by withholding reinforcement (see Chapter 1). Measurement of the rate of extinction has been used as a baseline from which to measure drug effects on learning. Glow and his colleagues (1966, 1967) investigated the effect of cholinesterase inhibition on resistance to extinction following training on an FR schedule for food. Diisopropyl fluorophosphate (DFP) was used to inhibit cholinesterase. Extinction of FR responding took longer when whole-body cholinesterase was inhibited by DFP. When DFP was given with a compound that antagonized peripheral cholinesterase inhibition, extinction rates were again longer, but not so long as with DFP alone. With repeated extinction sessions, the rate of extinction in the control rats was much more rapid than in the cholinesterase-inhibited animals (Fig. 7-10). While rats treated with DFP reached an asymptote more quickly than controls, the asymptotic level was higher in DFP rats than in controls. Rats with both central and peripheral cholinesterase inhibition showed the largest effects. An analysis of the percent of cholinesterase reduction in muscle and brain following DFP treatment demonstrated that the enzyme must be lowered to about 40% of normal before extinction is prolonged.

When cholinesterase was inhibited for 18 or 36 days, the resistance to extinc-

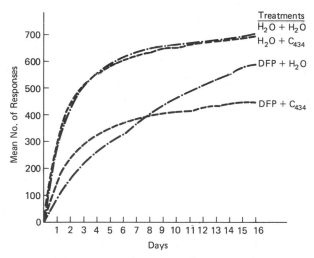

Fig. 7-10. Mean cumulative number of responses during extinction. Note that when the curves reach an asymptote, the rats have stopped responding (i.e., extinction). This happens sooner in the animals treated with water or water plus a peripheral AChE inhibitor (C434). Animals treated with DFP, a central and peripheral AChE inhibitor, do not extinguish as rapidly. (From Glow and Rose, 1966.)

tion was greater than after acute administration. Cholinesterase activity is reduced more with daily DFP treatments than with a single administration. Since DFP is an irreversible inhibitor, AChE recovery must be due to the synthesis of new enzyme. Therefore, daily injections of DFP cause greater reduction in enzyme levels than a single injection, because new enzyme that has been synthesized in the interval between the two injections is inhibited by the next injection of DFP. Whether the effects of cholinesterase inhibition are specific to FR extinction, or whether the effects can be extended to include extinction in other schedules as well as acquisition, has not been investigated.

Other work on the question of cholinergic involvement in learning has been done by Whitehouse and his colleagues (Whitehouse, 1964; Whitehouse et al., 1964). Whitehouse found that atropine impaired the acquisition of a t-maze discrimination in rats and cats. Animals were presented with multiple cues (visual, auditory and tactual) on which to make a discrimination. The animals showed a decrement in the rate of acquisition of the discrimination following atropine. Further research (Whitehouse, 1967) demonstrated that the acquisition of the discrimination was dependent on the number of cues present. With several cues present, atropine caused a distinct deficit in acquisition, but with only one cue present, no deficit was seen. The cholinesterase inhibitor physostigmine enhanced acquisition over a limited range of doses (Whitehouse, 1966).

Carlton (1968) also suggested that cholinergic mechanisms influence learning. According to Carlton, cholinergic blockers "lead to an intrusion of unrewarded responses into the animals' repertoire." These unrewarded responses are inhibited under normal circumstances (i.e., in the absence of a cholinergic blocker). Inhibition of responding to irrelevant (i.e., nonreinforced or nonrewarded) stimuli is referred to as habituation. For example, consider a rat in a chamber. Pressing a lever turns on a flash of light. Typically, the animal will press the lever for a while, but eventually the rat stops lever pressing; at this point the response is considered habituated. Similarly, if a rat is placed into a novel maze environment, it will ordinarily spend a considerable amount of time exploring the maze. After a period of time, exploratory behavior decreases and habituation is said to occur. Carlton contends that the acquisition of new responses involves habituation. For example, when a rat learns to press a lever for food, it also learns not to engage in a variety of other behaviors that would interfere with this response, such as exploring the stimulus lights in the cage, biting the grids, grooming, and so on. If the inhibition of these competing responses (i.e., habituation) is absent, then the acquisition and maintenance of learned behavior will be disrupted.

Evidence that cholinergic blockers interfere with the inhibition of behavior as a result of nonreinforcement has been reviewed extensively by Carlton. A few examples will suffice to illustrate the type of data on which this analysis is based. In one experiment, rats were divided into four groups: two of the groups were allowed to explore a chamber and two were not. Later, the four groups were water-deprived, and one of the groups previously exposed to the chamber and one of the unexposed groups were injected with scopolamine. The other two groups received saline. All rats were then put into the same chamber, which now contained a water bottle. The group that was injected with saline and had previous experience in the chamber went to the water bottle and drank sooner than the saline-treated rats which had no experience in the chamber. Inexperienced rats that were injected with scopolamine or saline spent a good deal of time exploring the chamber, presumably because they had not habituated to the novel stimuli earlier. Similarly, rats that had prior experience in the chamber but were injected with scopolamine took a long time before drinking and behaved as if this were their first experience in the chamber.

In another experiment, rats were placed in a situation in which pressing a lever caused a light to flash. After the rat responded several times on the lever, responding stopped. When these animals were injected with scopolamine, they resumed responding. If scopolamine simply increased activity, one would not expect to see behavior directed only at lever pressing. Since responding was directed at lever pressing, these results indicate that cholinergic stimulation does not simply produce diffuse undirected motor activity. Eventual habituation to irrelevant stimuli is consistent with learning to respond to reinforced stimuli.

In summary, there is evidence that the cholinergic system is involved in the acquisition of new responses. In this sense we can say that the cholinergic system plays a role in learning. As we have seen, however, other factors not related to learning, such as changes in locomotor activity, may account for these effects.

SUMMARY

In this chapter, the behavioral action of drugs that affect the cholinergic system was examined. The evidence that the behavioral effects of these drugs is mediated by the cholinergic system is inferential. Assay techniques for measuring the concentrations or turnover rate of acetylcholine have not been widely used or are not available. Therefore, the cholinergic system is examined with drugs that either block cholinergic receptors or inhibit acetylcholinesterase. Drugs affecting the cholinergic system were found to have effects on a variety of behaviors, including motor behavior and consummatory behavior, as well as behavior maintained by negative and positive reinforcement. In addition, the role of acetylcholine in learning was examined.

REFERENCES

Antunez-Rodriguez, J. and M. R. Covian. 1971. Water and sodium chloride intake following microinjection of carbachol into the septal area of the rat brain. *Experientia* **27**: 784–785.

Aprison, M. H. and J. N. Hingtgen. 1970. Neurochemical correlates of behavior. *Int. Rev. Neurobiol.* **13**: 325–341.

Aprison, M. H., J. N. Hingtgen and W. J. McBride. 1975. Serotonergic and cholinergic mechanisms during disruption of approach and avoidance behavior. *Fed. Proc.* **34**: 1813–1822.

Aprison, M. H., T. Kariya, J. N. Hingtgen and M. Toru. 1968. Neurochemical correlates of behaviour: Changes in acetylcholine, norepinephrine and 5-hydroxytryptamine concentrations in several discrete brain areas of the rat during behavioural excitation. *J. Neurochem.* **15**: 1131–1139.

Aquilonius, S. M., B. Lundholm and B. Winbladh. 1972. Effects of some anticholinergic drugs on cortical acetylcholine release and motor activity in rats. *Eur. J. Pharmacol.* **20**: 224–230.

Bak, I. J., R. Hassler, J. S. Kim and K. Kataoka. 1972. Amantadine actions on acetylcholine and GABA in striatum and substantia nigra of rat in relation to behavioral changes. *J. Neural. Transm.* **33**: 45–61.

Beani, L. and C. Bianchi. 1973. Effect of amantadine on cerebral acetylcholine release and content in the guinea pig. *Neuropharmacology* **12**: 283–289.

Beani, L., C. Bianchi and A. Castellucci. 1974. Correlation of brain catecholamines with cortical acetylcholine outflow, behaviour and electrocorticogram. *Eur. J. Pharmacol.* **26**: 63–72.

Blass, E. M. and H. W. Chapman. 1971. An evaluation of the contribution of the cholinergic mechanism to thirst. *Physiol. Behav.* **7**: 679–686.

Block, M. L. and A. E. Fisher. 1970. Anticholinergic central blockade of salt-aroused and deprivation-induced drinking. *Physiol. Behav.* **5**: 525–527.

Block, M. L. and A. E. Fisher. 1975. Cholinergic and dopaminergic blocking agents modulate water intake elicited by deprivation, hypovolemia, hypertonicity and isoproterenol. *Pharmacol. Biochem. Behav.* **3**: 251–262.

Bohdanecký, Z. and M. E. Jarvik. 1967. Impairment of one-trial passive avoidance learning in mice by scopolamine, scopolamine methylbromide and physostigmine. *Int. J. Neuropharmacol.* **6**: 217–222.

Bovet, D., F. Bovet-Nitti and A. Oliverio. 1966. Effects of nicotine on avoidance conditioning of inbred strains of mice. *Psychopharmacologia* **10**: 1–5.

Bradley, P. B. 1958. The central action of certain drugs in relation to the reticular formation of the brain. *In* H. H. Jasper, L. D. Proctor, R. S. Knighton, W. C. Noshay and R. T. Costello (eds.), *The Reticular Formation of the Brain.* Little, Brown and Co., Boston, pp. 123–149.

Bradley, P. B. 1964. EEG correlates of drug effects. *In* H. Steinberg, A. V. S. DeReuck, J. Knight (eds.), *Animal Behaviour and Drug Action.* Little, Brown and Co., Boston, pp. 119–131.

Bradley, P. B. and J. Elkes. 1957. The effects of some drugs on the electrical activity of the brain. *Brain.* **80**: 77–117.

Bradley, P. B. and A. J. Hance. 1957. The effect of chlorpromazine and methopromazine on the electrical activity of the brain in the cat. *EEG Clin. Neurophysiol.* **9**: 191–215.

Bramwell, G. J. and P. B. Bradley. 1974. Actions and interactions of narcotic agonists and antagonists on brain stem neurones. *Brain Res.* **73**: 167–170.

Butcher, S. G. and L. L. Butcher. 1974. Origin and modulation of acetylcholine activity in the neostriatum. *Brain Res.* **71**: 167–171.

Carlton, P. L. 1968. Brain-acetylcholine and habituation. *In* P. B. Bradley and M. Fink (eds.), *Progress in Brain Research* **28**: 48–60. Elsevier, New York.

Cohen, J. B. and J. Changeux. 1975. The cholinergic receptor protein in its membrane environment. *Ann. Rev. Pharmacol.* **15**: 83–103.

Consolo, S., H. Ladinsky, G. Peri and S. Garattini. 1974. Effect of diazepam on mouse whole brain and brain area acetylcholine and choline levels. *Eur. J. Pharmacol.* 27: 266–268.

Cooper, J. R., F. E. Bloom and R. H. Roth. 1974. *The Biochemical Basis of Neuropharmacology.* Oxford University Press, New York.

Dilts, S. L. and C. A. Berry. 1967. Effect of cholinergic drugs on passive avoidance in the mouse. *J. Pharmacol. Exp. Ther.* 158: 279–285.

Domino, E. F. and M. E. Olds. 1968. Cholinergic inhibition of self-stimulation behavior. *J. Pharmacol. Exp. Ther.* 164: 202–211.

Fisher, A. E. 1973. Relationships between cholinergic and other dipsogens in the central mediation of thirst. *In* A. N. Epstein, H. R. Kissileff and E. Stellar (eds.), *The Neuropsychology of Thirst.* Winston and Sons, Washington, D.C., pp. 243–278.

Fisher, A. E. and J. N. Coury. 1962. Cholinergic tracing of central neural circuit underlying the thirst drive. *Science* 138: 691–693.

Fisher, A. E. and J. N. Coury. 1964. Chemical tracing of neural pathways mediating the thirst drive. *In* M. J. Wayner (ed.), *Thirst: Proceedings of the First International Symposium on Thirst in the Regulation of Body Water.* Pergamon Press, New York, pp. 515–531.

Fonnum, F. 1973. Recent developments in biochemical investigations of cholinergic transmission. *Brain Res.* 62: 497–507.

Gentil, C. G. and J. A. F. Stevenson and G. J. Mogenson. 1971. Effect of scopolamine on drinking elicited by hypothalamic stimulation. *Physiol. Behav.* 7: 639–641.

Glow, P. H., A. Richardson and S. Rose. 1967. Effect of reduced cholinesterase activity on the maintenance of an operant response. *J. Comp. Physiol. Psychol.* 63: 155–157.

Glow, P. H., A. Richardson and S. Rose. 1966. Effects of acute and chronic inhibition of cholinesterase upon body weight, food intake and water intake in the rat. *J. Comp. Physiol. Psychol.* 61: 295–299.

Glow, P. H. and S. Rose. 1966. Cholinesterase levels and operant extinction. *J. Comp. Physiol. Psychol.* 61: 165–172.

Goldberg, A. M. and R. E. McCaman. 1973. The determination of picomole amounts of acetylcholine in mammalian brain. *J. Neurochem.* 20: 1–8.

Goldberg, M. E., H. E. Johnson and J. B. Knaak. 1965. Inhibition of discrete avoidance behavior by three anticholinesterase agents. *Psychopharmacologia* 7: 72–76.

Goldberg, M. E., H. E. Johnson, J. B. Knaak and H. F. Smyth, Jr. 1963. Psychopharmacological effects of reversible cholinesterase inhibition induced by N-methyl-3-isopropyl phenyl carbamate (Compound 10854). *J. Pharmacol. Exp. Ther.* 141: 244–252.

Grossman, S. P. 1969. A neuropharmacological analysis of hypothalamic and extrahypothalamic mechanisms concerned with the regulation of food and water intake. *Ann. N.Y. Acad. Sci.* 157: 902–917.

Hanson, H. M., C. A. Stone and J. J. Witoslawski. 1970. Antagonism of the antiavoidance effects of various agents by anticholinergic drugs. *J. Pharmacol. Exp. Ther.* 173: 117–124.

Harvey, J. A. 1973. Discussion: Use of the ablation method in the pharmacological analysis of thirst. *In* A. N. Epstein, H. R. Kissileff and E. Stellar (eds.), *The Neuropsychology of Thirst.* Winston and Sons, Washington, D.C., pp. 293–306.

Hebb, C. 1972. Biosynthesis of acetylcholine in nervous tissue. *Physiol. Rev.* 52: 918–957.

Herz, A. 1960. Die Bedeutung der Bahnung für die Wirkung von Scopolamin und ähnilchen Substanzen auf bedingte Reaktionen. *Z. Biol.* 112: 104–112.

Hingtgen, J. N. and M. H. Aprison. 1970. Increased duration of neuropharmacologically induced behavioral excitation by atropine. *Neuropharmacology* 9: 419–425.

Hoskin, F. C. G. 1972. Acetylcholine. *In* R. W. Albers, G. J. Siegel, R. Katzman and E. W. Agranoff (eds.), *Basic Neurochemistry.* Little, Brown Co. Boston, pp. 105–130.

Hrdina, P. D. 1974. Metabolism of brain acetylcholine and its modification by drugs. *Drug Metab. Rev.* 3: 89–129.

Hubbard, J. I. 1970. Mechanism of transmitter release. *Prog. Biophys. Mol. Biol.* 21: 33–124.

Katz, B. 1969. *The Release of Neurotransmitter Substances.* C. C Thomas, Springfield, Illinois.

Koelle, G. B. 1969. Significance of acetylcholinesterase in central synaptic transmission. *Fed. Proc.* 28: 95–100.

Krnjevic, K. 1974. Chemical nature of synaptic transmission in vertebrates. *Physiol. Rev.* 54: 418–540.

Labrecque, G. and E. F. Domino. 1974. Tolerance to and physical dependence on morphine: Relation to neocortical acetylcholine release in the cat. *J. Pharmacol. Exp. Ther.* 191: 189–200.

Leibowitz, S. F. 1972. Central adrenergic receptors and the regulation of hunger and thirst. *Res. Publ. Assoc. Res. Nerv. Ment. Dis.*, Ch. 15, 50: 327–358.

Levitt, R. A. 1970. Temporal decay of the blockade of carbachol drinking by atropine. *Physiol. Behav.* 5: 627–628.

Levitt, R. A. and A. E. Fisher. 1967. Failure of central anticholinergic brain stimulation to block natural thirst. *Physiol. Behav.* 2: 425–428.

Loewi, O. 1921. Über humorale Übertragbarkeit der herznervenwirküng. *Plüger's Arch. Ges. Physiol.* 189: 239–242.

Merali, Z., P. K. Ghosh, P. D. Hrdina, R. L. Singhal and G. M. Ling. 1974. Alterations in striatal acetylcholine, acetylcholine esterase and dopamine after methadone replacement in morphine-dependent rats. *Eur. J. Pharmacol.* 26: 375–378.

Meyers, B. 1965. Some effects of scopolamine on a passive avoidance response in rats. *Psychopharmacologia* 8: 111–119.

Meyers, B., K. H. Roberts, R. H. Riciputi and E. F. Domino. 1964. Some effects of muscarinic cholinergic blocking drugs on behavior and the electrocorticogram. *Psychopharmacologia* 5: 289–300.

Morgane, P. J. (ed.), 1969. Neuroregulation of food and water intake. *Ann. N.Y. Acad. Sci.* 157: 531–1216.

Morrison, C. F. and A. K. Armitage. 1967. Effect of nicotine upon the free operant behavior of rats and spontaneous motor activity of mice. *Ann. N.Y. Acad. Sci.* 142: 268–276.

Morrison, C. F. and P. N. Lee. 1968. A comparison of the effects of nicotine and physostigmine on a measure of activity in the rat. *Psychopharmacologia* 13: 210–221.

Mullin, W. J. 1974. Central release of acetylcholine following administration of morphine to unanesthetized rabbits. *Canad. J. Physiol. Pharmacol.* 52: 369–374.

Mullin, W. J. and J. W. Phillis. 1974. Acetylcholine release from the brain of unanesthetized cats following habituation to morphine and during precipitation of the abstinence syndrome. *Psychopharmacologia* 36: 85–99.

Myers, R. D. 1974. *Handbook of Drug and Chemical Stimulation of the Brain.* Van Nostrand Reinhold Co., New York.

Myers, R. D. 1969. Central mechanisms in the hypothalamus mediating eating and drinking in the monkey. *Ann. N.Y. Acad. Sci.* 157: 918–933.

O'Brien, R. D., M. E. Eldefrawi and A. T. Eldefrawi. 1972. Isolation of acetylcholine receptors. *Ann. Rev. Pharmacol.* 12: 19–34.

Olds, M. E. and E. F. Domino. 1969a. Comparison of muscarinic and nicotinic cholinergic agonists of self-stimulation behavior. *J. Pharmacol. Exp. Ther.* 166: 189–204.

Olds, M. E. and E. F. Domino. 1969b. Differential effects of cholinergic agonists on self-stimulation and escape behavior. *J. Pharmacol. Exp. Ther.* 170: 157–167.

Oliverio, A. 1966. Effects of mecamylamine on avoidance conditioning and maze learning of mice. *J. Pharmacol. Exp. Ther.* 154: 350–356.

Pepeu, G. 1973. The release of acetylcholine from brain: an approach to the study of the central cholinergic mechanisms. *Prog. Neurobiol.* 2: 259–288.

Pepeu, G., A. Mulas and M. L. Mulas. 1973. Changes in the acetylcholine content in the rat brain after lesions of the septum, fimbria and hippocampus. *Brain Res.* 57: 153–164.

Pfeiffer, C. C. and E. H. Jenney. 1957. The inhibition of the conditioned response and the counteraction of schizophrenia by muscarinic stimulation of the brain. *Ann. N.Y. Acad. Sci.* 66: 753–764.

Pradhan, S. N. 1970. Effects of nicotine on several schedules of behavior in rats. *Arch. Int. Pharmacodyn.* 183: 127–138.

Pradhan, S. N. and C. Bowling. 1971. Effects of nicotine on self-stimulation in rats. *J. Pharmacol. Exp. Ther.* 176: 229–243.

Pradhan, S. N. and S. N. Dutta. 1971. Central cholinergic mechanism and behavior. *Int. Rev. Neurobiol.* 14: 173–231.

Pradhan, S. N. and R. M. Mhatre. 1970. Effects of two anticholinesterases on behavior and cholinesterase activity in rats. *Res. Comm. Chem. Path. Pharmacol.* 1: 682–690.

Rawat, A. K. 1974. Brain levels and turnover rates of presumptive neurotransmitters as influenced by administration and withdrawal of ethanol in mice. *J. Neurochem.* 22: 915–922.

Richardson, J. S., P. D. Stacey and M. O. De Camp. 1971. A possible synaptic mechanism underlying the similar behavioural effects of adrenaline-like and acetylcholine-like drugs. *J. Pharm. Pharmacol.* 23: 884–886.

Rosecrans, J. A., A. T. Dren and E. F. Domino. 1968. Effects of physostigmine on rat brain acetylcholine, acetylcholinesterase and conditioned pole jumping. *Int. J. Neuropharmacol.* 7: 127–134.

Russell, R. W. 1969. Behavioral aspects of cholinergic transmission. *Fed. Proc.* 28: 121–131.

Sethy, V. H. and M. H. Van Woert. 1974a. Brain acetylcholine and cholinesterase: Effect of phenothiazines and physostigmine interaction in rats. *J. Neurochem.* 23: 105–109.

Sethy, V. H. and M. H. Van Woert. 1974b. Modification of striatal acetylcholine concentration by dopamine receptor agonists and antagonists. *Res. Comm. Chem. Path. Pharmacol.* 8: 13–28.

Sethy, V. H., M. J. Kuhar, R. H. Roth, M. H. Van Woert and G. K. Aghajanian. 1973. Cholinergic neurons: Effect of acute septal lesion on acetylcholine and choline content of rat hippocampus. *Brain Res.* 55: 481–484.

Shute, C. C. D. and P. R. Lewis. 1967. The ascending cholinergic reticular system: neocortical, olfactory and subcortical projections. *Brain* 90: 497–540.

Singer, G. and J. Kelly. 1972. Cholinergic and adrenergic interaction in the hypothalamic control of drinking and eating behavior. *Physiol. Behav.* 8: 885–890.

Sommer, S. R., D. Novin and M. LeVine. 1967. Food and water intake after intrahypothalamic injections of carbachol in the rabbit. *Science* 156: 983–984.

Somogyi, G. T. and J. C. Szerb. 1972. Demonstration of acetylcholine release by measuring efflux of labelled choline from cerebral cortical slices. *J. Neurochem.* 19: 2667–2677.

Spencer, J. and F. A. Holloway. 1972. Differentiation between carbachol and eserine during deprivation-induced drinking in the rat. *Psychon. Sci.* 28: 16–18.

Stavinoha, W. B., S. T. Weintraub and A. T. Modak. 1973. The use of microwave heating to inactivate cholinesterase in the rat brain prior to analysis for acetylcholine. *J. Neurochem.* 20: 361–371.

Stein, L. 1963. Anticholinergic drugs and the central control of thirst. *Science* 139: 46–48.

Toru, M., J. N. Hingtgen and M. H. Aprison. 1966. Acetylcholine concentrations in brain areas of rats during three states of avoidance behavior: normal, depression and excitation. *Life Sci.* 5: 181–189.

Trabucchi, M., D. Cheney, G. Racagni and E. Costa. 1974. Involvement of brain cholinergic mechanisms in the action of chlorpromazine. *Nature* 249: 664–666.

Vasko, M. R., L. E. Domino and E. F. Domino. 1974. Differential effects of *d*-amphetamine on brain acetylcholine in young, adult and geriatric rats. *Eur. J. Pharmacol.* 27: 145–147.

Weiss, B. and A. Heller. 1969. Methodological problems in evaluating the role of cholinergic mechanisms in behavior. *Fed. Proc.* 28: 135–146.

Warburton, D. M. 1969. Behavioral effects of central and peripheral changes in acetylcholine systems. *J. Comp. Physiol. Psychol.* 68: 56–64.

Wayner, M. J. 1974. Specificity of behavioral regulation. *Physiol. Behav.* 12: 851–869.

Whitehouse, J. M. 1964. Effects of atropine on discrimination learning in the rat. *J. Comp. Physiol. Psychol.* 57: 13–15.

Whitehouse, J. M. 1966. The effects of physostigmine on discrimination learning. *Psychopharmacologia* 9: 183–188.

Whitehouse, J. M. 1967. Cholinergic mechanisms in discrimination learning as a function of stimuli. *J. Comp. Physiol. Psychol.* 63: 448–451.

Whitehouse, J. M., A. J. Lloyd and S. A. Fifer. 1964. Comparative effects of atropine and methyl-atropine on maze acquisition and eating. *J. Comp. Physiol. Psychol.* 58: 475–476.

Wikler, A. 1952. Pharmacologic dissociation of behavior and EEG—"Sleep patterns" in dogs: morphine, N-allylnormorphine, and atropine (19345). *Proc. Soc. Exp. Biol.* 79: 261–265.

Wilson, A. E. and E. F. Domino. 1973. Verification of rat brain acetylcholine antidepletion by morphine using gas chromatography. *Biochem. Pharmacol.* 22: 1943–1944.

Wise, C. D. and L. Stein. 1970. Amphetamines: facilitation of behavior by augmented release of norepinephrine from the medial forebrain bundle. *In* E. Costa and S. Garattini (eds.), *International Symposium on Amphetamines and Related Compounds.* Raven Press, New York, pp. 463–485.

8
Pharmacological and Biochemical Aspects of Learning and Memory

The mechanisms by which learning occurs and information is stored (i.e., memory) have been of vital interest to scientists interested in behavior and the central nervous system. A large amount of research has been directed at localizing the so-called memory trace within the CNS, as well as examining the chemical or physiological *mechanism* by which the trace is initially recorded in the CNS and subsequently preserved. While the investigation of memory involves a number of disciplines, including psychology, anatomy, physiology, chemistry and pharmacology, this chapter will focus on *pharmacological agents* implicated in either facilitation or inhibition of memory, and on *macromolecular systems* [ribonucleic acid (RNA) and protein] believed to be involved in the storage of the memory trace. (For further references, the interested reader should consult the following texts and reviews: McGaugh, 1972; Ansell and Bradley, 1973; Bowman and Datta, 1970; Albers *et al.*, 1972; Byrne, 1970a,b; Deutsch, 1973; Uphouse *et al.*, 1974).

In general, experimental evidence relating to the pharmacological and biochemical aspects of learning and memory is not strong. Evaluation of the data has often been questioned because of inappropriate use of statistics, testing procedures and biochemical methods. In addition, many experiments reported over the past 10 to 15 years have not been successfully replicated by other scientists. Consistent, independent replication of experimental data is one of the more important precepts in science. Failure to replicate suggests artifact or nonsystematic occurrence of uncontrolled but important variables. Unless the basis for the failure of replication can be determined, the original data are open to serious question. Moreover, failure to replicate results in confusion; for in spite of these failures, theory and further experimentation based on the unreplicated data often proceed with little attempt to identify crucial factors responsible for the lack of replicability. This is not to say that all the experiments performed in this area are open to all of these criticisms. There are however, very few experiments that are not subject to at least one of the criticisms mentioned above.

BASIC CONSIDERATIONS

Historical Background

In the late 1700s and early 1800s, it was thought that nerves conducted electrical impulses to and from the brain and that the impulse (afferent) to the brain constituted sensation and perception (see Brazier, 1959). The integration of sensory information with stored information was thought to lead to nerve discharge from the brain (efferent) toward muscles to execute muscle movement involved in both simple and complex responses. The experimental findings and theories of Muller, Helmholz, Bernard, Bell, Fritch, Hitzig and Sherrington contributed greatly to understanding the organization of sensory and motor areas in the cerebral cortex. The localization of specific sensory and motor functions in discrete cortical areas led to the notion that integration of sensory input and motor output occurred in the cortex and, furthermore, that information (memory) was stored in various cortical areas.

In the early 1900s, K. S. Lashley attempted to locate the memory trace (or engram) in the visual system of the rat. In a research career that spanned three decades, Lashley developed behavioral procedures that consisted of training and testing rats on visual discrimination problems of varying degrees of complexity. Either before or after training of a visual discrimination, part of the visual cortex was lesioned. The rat was retested after the lesioning to assess impariment of discrimination function and recovery of function (see Lashley, 1950). Lashley's research into learning deficits produced by brain lesions set the foundation for current research in the pharmacological and biochemical basis of learning and memory.

Lashley found that lesions of the visual cortex of rats produced deficits when lesions were large enough to destroy more than 95% of the visual cortex. If the lesion spared at least 5% of the visual cortex of the rat, a rather complex visual discrimination (e.g., discriminating a circle from a triangle) remained intact. Similar results were obtained in work with more difficult discriminations. For example, when a very complex visual discrimination was examined (e.g., discriminating between two different-sized circles), more cortex was needed to maintain the visual discrimination. Lashley found that there was a *direct relationship* between the *amount* of deficit produced on a discrimination task and the amount of neocortical tissue extirpated. He referred to this as *mass action*.

Lashley also found that it did not matter which part of the visual cortex was left intact as long as there was sufficient quantity of tissue for a given visual discrimination. From these data, Lashley suggested that, at least within a given sensory modality, all cells were equally capable of storing information, i.e., the cells were *equipotential*. Moreover, Lashley (1950) concluded that it was not possible to localize the memory trace in a discrete region of a given sensory area of the brain nor was it possible to localize the memory trace in any discrete area of the nervous system. Nevertheless, with more sophisticated lesioning techniques, better anatomical localization, more sensitive behavioral testing techniques and experimentation on subhuman primates, investigators have been able to find some localization of memory in discrete cortical areas (see Iversen, 1973). Within the last 30 years, the question of localization of memory traces has been examined by a variety of investigators. There is evidence that the frontal cortex and the temporal cortex, including the underlying structures (amygdala and hippocampus), play a role in memory (Iversen, 1973).

Current Views

According to current views, memory is divided into three processes, i.e., registration, consolidation and retrieval (see Fig. 8-1). While these distinctions are useful in discussing memory, it should be noted that these distinctions are not operationally defined.

1. *Registration:* the process of sensory perception and the ability to act on the information perceived (i.e., a behavioral response). In theory, this process involves a change in brain activity (possibly electrical), and is often referred to as *short-term memory*.

2. *Consolidation:* the process of conversion of registered short-term information to a *long-term memory* trace. There is evidence that consolidation is a process in which physical-chemical changes occur in CNS neurons.

3. *Retrieval:* the process that makes long-term memory accessible. After consolidation takes place, the long-term changes in the CNS due to consolidation must be accessible.

Recent work on memory storage follows two lines of investigation: electrophysiological and chemical. The first stage of memory (i.e., short-term memory) is thought to be electrophysiological (Hebb, 1949). Evidence for this view stems from findings that electroconvulsive shock* and other events (e.g., a blow on the skull) that grossly interfere with the electrical activity of the brain inhibit memory of recent events (retrograde amnesia). Typically, events that took place several hours before the event are forgotton while events that occurred days or years before are recalled. The fact that recent events are forgotton while distant

---

*Electroconvulsive shock: a procedure in which convulsions are produced by the passage of electric current through the brain. In small animals this is usually done by placing electrodes on the corneas or the ears.

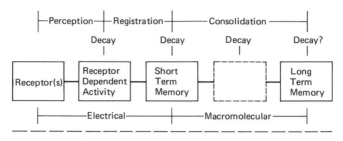

Consolidation and Macromolecules
A. Physical changes e.g. conformation
B. Chemical changes (New molecules)
  1. DNA   4. Lipid
  2. RNA   5. Glycoprotein
  3. Protein   6. Glycolipid

Fig. 8-1. Multiple stages in learning. Learning may be considered as a multiple-stage process. It would appear that the initial learning (short-term memory) does not require the synthesis of new molecules; this is indicated as an electrical (electrochemical) process. Consolidation may involve conformational changes in macromolecules (postulate *A*) or it may involve the synthesis of new molecules (postulate *B*). It should be noted that the arrow indicating decay of long-term memory is given with a question mark. Direct experimental attempts to induce permanent amnesia following consolidation have failed. If long-term memory has a molecular basis involving specific anatomical sites, this suggests that there is a finite limit to long-term memory capacity, and this finite capacity could conceivably become a significant (limiting) variable in behavior. (From Byrne, 1970b.)

events are not, led to the suggestion that short-term memory is related to changes in brain electrical activity.

Electroconvulsive shock has been used extensively to investigate short-term memory in animals. An experiment from Luttges and McGaugh (1967) exemplifies a typical experiment in learning and memory in which ECS is used. First, mice were each given a single training trial on a passive avoidance procedure. The mice were shocked when they stepped through a door that separated two chambers. Learning on the passive avoidance task was measured by latencies to step into the second chamber following training. Short latencies were taken as an indicator of failure to learn, and long latencies were thought to indicate learning. Immediately following single-trial training, mice were removed from the chamber and ECS was administered. Mice were retested 12 hours, one week or one month after the first trial. Control groups of mice received either (1) no foot shock and ECS, (2) foot shock and no ECS or (3) neither foot shock nor ECS. The foot shock but no ECS group learned the passive avoidance response in one trial, while the control group which received no foot shock and no ECS and the experimental group (foot shock and ECS) did not learn the passive avoidance response, as evidenced by short step latencies at 12 hours, 1 week and one month. Since ECS was administered a few seconds after training, it was suggested that

ECS interfered with the consolidation phase of memory and thereby caused amnesia of events that occurred shortly before the experience.

It has been estimated that the optimum time between the training trial and ECS for producing retrograde amnesia is between 10 seconds and 24 hours (Quartermain et al., 1965; Chorover and Schiller, 1965; Kopp et al., 1967; McGaugh, 1966). This interval is thought to correspond to the period during which consolidation is labile. In addition, some investigators maintain that ECS temporarily interferes with, but does not permanently block, memory consolidation. While Luttges and McGaugh (1967) report complete amnesia a month after ECS, others (Hunt, 1965) report no memory deficit one month after the shock treatments. Differences such as these are not surprising since behavioral procedures, ECS parameters and species often vary (Hunt and Brady, 1961; Hunt, 1965; Robbins and Meyer, 1970).

While short-term memory is thought to be related to changes in brain electrical activity, long-term memory is thought to be due to chemical changes. In 1950, Katz and Halstead suggested that an alteration of the structure of proteins contained in neurons may be the chemical change responsible for the long-term memory encoding. Currently, research has focused on structural changes in ribonucleic acid (RNA) and polypeptides as well as proteins. All of these are long chain polymers which are capable of maintaining complex structural configurations. It is by virtue of this complexity that they have been investigated as likely candidates for the transmission and storage of information in cells (Fig. 8-1).

In this chapter we shall be concerned with: (1) registration (i.e., short-term memory) and processes reported to enhance or disrupt it; and (2) various aspects of consolidation, including the formation of long-term memory traces as well as the chemical nature of the memory trace. By and large we will consider short-term memory from a pharmacological point of view, i.e., that of drugs which can modify it; long-term memory will be considered from a pharmacological and biochemical point of view.

DRUG EFFECTS

Some drugs have been reported to facilitate memory, in particular strychnine, amphetamine and related compounds. While a good deal of evidence has been presented that these drugs affect some aspect of performance, whether these changes in performance can be attributed to changes in learning or memory is still open to question.

Methods

In most investigations of drug effects on learning and memory, discrete trial maze procedures are used (see Chapter 1). The rat is said to have learned a maze when he proceeds down the maze without making cul-de-sac errors. A standard procedure is to regard 90% error-free performance as learning the maze. Learning is measured by the number of errors the animal makes in reaching the criterion (i.e., errors to criterion). Usually there is a great deal of variability in the speed at which different animals acquire this task. If an animal learns a maze faster following drug administration than vehicle-injected control animals learn it, it is often suggested that improvement is due to more rapid and efficient consolidation of the memory trace as a result of the drug; however, other interpretations are also possible. For example, improvement might be independent of changes in learning or memory, and may be the result of an alteration in spontaneous motor activity or in sensitivity to reinforcing stimuli (motivational variables) or other relevant sensory stimuli. We have seen in previous chapters that a single experimental result rarely, if ever, isolates the biochemical or behavioral changes that are responsible for a drug effect. A drug's effect on behavior can only be attributed to changes in learning and memory when other factors such as drug-induced changes in sensory perception or motor function are eliminated.

One experimental design that partially circumvents some of these problems is the method of post-trial injections. In the post-trial injection procedure, the drug is given following training trials. Therefore, drug effects that might be operative during conditioning such as increased sensitivity to the reinforcing stimuli or increases in spontaneous motor activity do not confound interpretation of the data. Presumably, administration of the drug post-trial still affects consolidation processes in the CNS.

Strychnine

Strychnine (and related compounds) produces convulsions when given in high doses. Interest in strychnine and its effects on memory is partially based on this neurophysiological effect. Strychnine is also known to block inhibitory synapses in the spinal cord (Goodman and Gilman, 1970), and thereby facilitate transmission of nerve impulses through the cord. Since strychnine presumably acts the same way in the brain as in the spinal cord, it has been suggested that strychnine facilitates learning and memory consolidation through enhanced neurophysiological activity.

In 1917 Lashley reported that young rats treated with strychnine 10 minutes prior to a training session reached criterion in a maze (three consecutive trials without an error) in 40% fewer trials than vehicle controls. No changes occurred following a lower dose of strychnine, nor was the effect replicated in slightly older rats.

Following Lashley's initial work with strychnine on learning and memory, investigation of the effects of strychnine was not continued until McGaugh (1959) examined the effect of strychnine on learning. McGaugh and Petrinovich (1959) reported that learning was facilitated slightly in rats receiving pre-trial administration (19 minutes) of strychnine; however, there was no relationship between the dose of strychnine (0.33, 0.66 and 1.0 mg/kg) and the amount of facilitation. Subsequent investigation (McGaugh, 1961) of the effects of low (0.33 mg/kg) and high (1.0 mg/kg) doses of strychnine administered 10 minutes before each training trial, revealed no facilitation except when animals were separated into two groups—worst performers and best performers. Strychnine facilitated maze learning in the best performers at low doses, while strychnine (Fig. 8-2) had no effect on the worst performers.

Post-trial injections of strychnine have been shown to facilitate learning in mice of a visual discrimination in a Y maze in a dose-dependent manner (McGaugh, 1968). Facilitation of learning occured at doses around 0.10 and 1.0 mg/kg of strychnine; intermediate doses had little effect (Fig. 8-3). While biphasic dose-response relationships are not typical, the effect was reliable in that there was relatively small variation in the mean number of errors to criterion at the doses examined.

McGaugh (1968) also investigated the relationship between *time* of strychnine administration and facilitation of visual discrimination. Strychnine (1.0 mg/kg) was administered between 5 and 60 minutes before daily training trials and at different times after the trials. Learning was facilitated when strychnine was injected between 60 minutes before and 60 minutes after training (Fig. 8-4). McGaugh found that strychnine was most effective in facilitating learning when

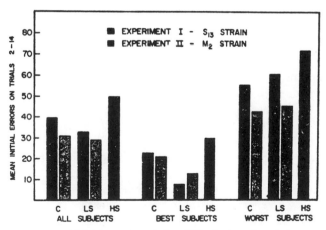

Fig. 8-2. Mean number of initial errors made by all Ss, the best Ss and the worst Ss on trials 2 to 14 in the 14-unit maze. Repetitive errors were not recorded since multiple pushes on the doors and re-entries could not be separately recorded. LS = 0.33 mg/kg strychnine; C = control; HS = 1.0 mg/kg strychnine. (From McGaugh, 1961.)

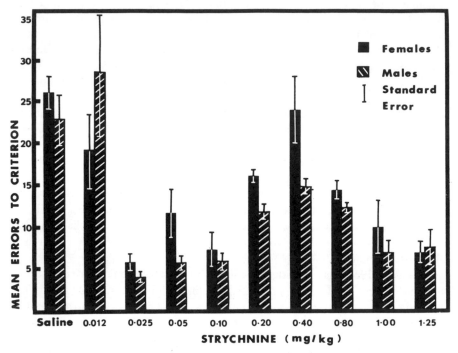

Fig. 8-3. The effect of post-training administration of strychnine on visual discrimination learning in mice. (From McGaugh, 1968.)

injections were close to training trials. Longer post-trial injections of strychnine (two and four hours) did not affect learning.

Two important points emerge from this study. First, both pre-trial and post-trial injections of strychnine facilitated learning. Second, strychnine facilitated learning when injected between 60 minutes before and 60 minutes after training but had no effect when injected two or four hours after training, suggesting that strychnine does not remain in brain or other tissue to exert its effect on the next trial 24 hours later (see Fig. 8-4). In view of these data, McGaugh concluded that strychnine enhances memory consolidation occurring during the first hour after learning.

On the other hand, Schaeffer (1968) reported that strychnine did not facilitate learning in rats. Rats were tested in a four-alley maze. Strychnine sulfate was injected immediately after training trials. When a single dose of strychnine (0.33 mg/kg) was given, there was no difference in latency, cul-de-sac entries and total number of errors between the strychnine-injected rats and vehicle-injected controls. Similarly, no differences were found when several doses of strychnine (0.08–0.64 mg/kg) were injected immediately post-trial; however, strychnine had

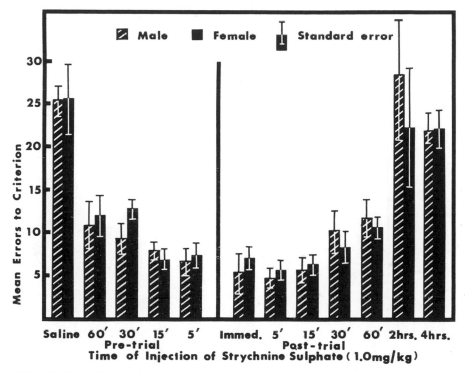

Fig. 8-4. The effect of time of administration of strychnine (1.0 mg/kg ip) on visual discrimination learning in mice. (From McGaugh, 1968.)

a small but significant effect when rats were separated by their running speed in preliminary testing procedures into groups of slow and fast rats. In this case, the two lowest doses of strychnine facilitated learning in the slow rats and impaired learning in the fast rats.

Oglesby and Winter (1974) found that strychnine did not facilitate learning in the rat. They examined the effects of several pre-trial (15 minutes) and post-trial (immediate) injections of strychnine (0.005 to 0.60 mg/kg) on the acquisition of a discrimination between a continuous light and a flashing light. Avoidance acquisition was not facilitated in rats following post-trial strychnine administration, although others (Bovet et al., 1966) have reported facilitation in avoidance acquisition. Until factors accounting for these different results can be identified, the generality of the finding that learning can be facilitated by strychnine sulfate is limited.

Table 8-1 lists the effects of strychnine on learning in a variety of situations. Facilitation occurs in some experiments but not in others. Lack of generality across species, behavioral task, dose range and treatment times suggests that more research is necessary.

TABLE 8-1. Summary of findings of strychnine effects on learning and memory

Author(s)	Task	Pre- or Post-Trial	Dose[1]	Species	Comments
		POSITIVE RESULTS—FACILITATION OF LEARNING			
Lashley (1917)	circular maze	10 min pre-trial	0.1 mg/150 g	rat	also obtained negative results in slightly older rats
McGaugh and Petrinovich (1959)	four-unit maze; spatial discrimination	pre-trial injection	0.22–1.0[1]	rat	obtained facilitation but no dose-response
Keleman and Bovet (1962)	escape response to shock and heat	20 min pre-trial	0.3	rat	
McGaugh (1961)	14-unit spatial maze	10 min pre-trial	0.33 and 1.00	rat	
McGaugh et al. (1962)	maze, spatial discrimination	pre- and post-trial, 6 min before to 19 min later	1.0	rat	
Petrinovich (1963)	maze, visual discrimination	pre-trial 10 min	1.0	rat	
Hudspeth (1964)	oddity problem: brightness discrimination reversal	30 sec post-trial injection	0.2	rat	
Irwin and Benuazizi (1966)	modified passive avoidance	pre- and post-trial injections	0.25–0.8	mice	
Petrinovich (1967)	spacial maze	10 min pre-trial	0.125–1.75	rat	
Krivanek and Hunt (1967)	maze, visual discrimination	immediate, post-trial	0.33	rat	
Franchina and Moore (1968)	modified passive avoidance	15 min post-trial	0.25–0.2	rat	
McGaugh and Krivanek (1970)	Y maze, visual discrimination	pre- and post-trial	0.012–1.25	mice	
Alpern and Crabbe (1972)	maze, spacial discrimination	long-term effects	0.2–1.0	mice	

NEGATIVE AND CONFLICTING RESULTS

			Dose[1]		
Prien et al. (1963)	32-unit spacial discrimination maze	20 min pre-trial 1 min post-trial	0.75–1.0	rat	did not observe facilitation in any measure
Schaeffer (1968)	spacial maze	immediate post-trial before training for a 7-day period, post-trial	0.08–0.64	rat	little, if any, effect
Cholewiak et al. (1968)	classically conditioned eye blink	pre- and post-trial injection	0.3	rabbit	pre-injection facilitates post-injection inhibits
Carlini et al. (1972)	maze and shuttle box reinforced with food	post-trial	0.02–0.3	rat	negative results, similar results with other drugs
Cooper and Krass (1963)	Hebb-Williams maze	injected 24–72 hr before testing	1.25	rat	facilitation of learning not consistent with McGaugh's ideas, vis à vis consolidation
Livecchi and Dusewicz (1969)	spacial maze	pre-trial	0.6	rat	facilitates massed practice, no effect with spaced practice
Le Boeuf and Peeke (1969)	maze learning	given drug as weanlings for 30 days, tested at 107 days	1.0	rat	proactive positive effect in cage-reared but not in animals reared in enriched environment
Oglesby and Winter (1974)	discrimination, avoidance acquisition	pre- and post-trial	0.005–0.60	rat	no facilitation

[1] Dose in mg/kg except as noted.

Other Drugs

A number of drugs have been reported to facilitate or interfere with learning and memory; however, as with strychnine, reports are conflicting. Table 8-2 lists the drugs examined most extensively. The effects of cholinergic drugs on learning and memory are discussed in Chapter 7. Strychnine-like drugs, amphetamine and magnesium pemoline will be discussed here.

Strychnine-like Drugs. Drugs that resemble strychnine in facilitating CNS transmission (e.g., picrotoxin, bemegride and pentalenetrazol) have also been examined for their effects on learning and memory in designs similar to those used with strychnine. Generally, studies reporting facilitation in learning and memory following strychnine, also report facilitation when other drugs are examined. Similarly, studies reporting no effect with strychnine usually report no effect with other compounds (see McGaugh, 1972).

Amphetamine. The effects of amphetamine and related compounds have been extensively studied with regard to their biochemical and behavioral mode of action (see Chapters 6 and 9). Amphetamine-induced facilitation or inhibition of ongoing behavior is thought to be mediated by actions on CA-containing neurons in the brain. Amphetamine is often classified as a central stimulant, capable of decreasing fatigue and improving learning. It has been suggested that amphetamine-produced improvement in learning may relate to its ability to decrease fatigue (Weiss and Laties, 1962). If this is the case, amphetamine might facilitate memory and/or learning without facilitating neuronal processes in-

TABLE 8-2. Pertinent review articles—drug effects on learning and memory

Compound	Review
Convulsant drugs:	Dawson and McGaugh (1973)
strychnine, pentylenetetrazol, picrotoxin	Jarvik (1972)
	Essman (1971)
Cholinergic drugs:	Carlton (1968)
nicotine, scopolamine, atropine, physostigmine	Deutsch (1971)
	Essman (1971)
	Deutsch (1973)
Catecholaminergic drugs:	Dawson and McGaugh (1973)
amphetamine, methamphetamine, reserpine, L-dopa,	Essman (1971)
alpha-methyltyrosine	Weiss and Laties (1962)
Serotonergic drugs:	Jarvik (1972)
parachlorophenylalanine, reserpine,	Essman (1971)
5-hydroxytryptophan	
Magnesium pemoline	Weiss and Laties (1969)
Caffeine	Essman (1971)

volved in the memory trace. As Jarvik (1972) has pointed out, however, the ability of a drug to facilitate learning by disinhibiting or arousing a subject should not be disparaged.

There is evidence that amphetamine both facilitates (Doty and Doty, 1966; Krivanek and McGaugh, 1969) or has no effect (e.g., Wolthuis, 1971) on learning in a variety of situations. Since it has been suggested that the effect of amphetamine on learning may be related to its effects on performance, it is interesting to distinguish the effect of a drug such as amphetamine on performance of a response from its effect on learning that response. Thompson (1973) utilized a modification of a procedure that was initially developed by Boren (1963) for rhesus monkeys. Thompson's procedure consisted of the following paradigm in which pigeons repeatedly acquired a new response sequence: pigeons pecked a key in a chamber containing three response keys; all keys were illuminated at the same time by one of four colors. For each session, the pigeon's task was to learn a new four-response sequence by pecking the correct key in the presence of each color. For example, a sequence might be the following: left key, center key, right key, center key. Which response sequence was correct was signaled by the key light color—i.e., in the presence of yellow key lights, a left key response was correct; in the presence of green key lights, a right key response was correct; in the presence of red key lights, a center key response was correct; in the presence of white key lights, a right key response was correct. The sequence was varied daily so that the acquisition of a sequence could be measured in a single session. The average number of errors it took each pigeon to learn a new sequence was referred to as the pigeon's steady-state learning behavior. Drug effects were examined on this steady-state behavior.

d-Amphetamine increased the total number of errors in a session, as well as increasing the total session time, i.e., both learning and performance were impaired by amphetamine. While these results do not agree with previous reports that amphetamine improves learning in other species (Weiss and Laties, 1962; Jarvik, 1972), this procedure is unique in that it can separate a drug's effect on learning from its effect on performance.

Magnesium Pemoline. Initial work (Plotnikoff, 1966) suggested that magnesium pemoline enhanced learning and memory. Rats were placed in a box, and after 15 seconds had elapsed a buzzer sounded for 5 seconds, during which time the rat was shocked. Rats could avoid shock by jumping out of the box during the 15-second preshock interval or escape it by jumping after the shock was presented. Rats ("slow learners") that did not jump from the box during the preshock interval on the first three trials were used in the study. They were divided into a magnesium pemoline group and a vehicle control group. The magnesium pemoline group learned the response more rapidly and was more resistant to extinction.

The results of this experiment and its interpretation have been controversial. Weiss and Laties (1969) point out some objections. First of all control rats received more trials and shocks than rats treated with magnesium pemoline. Since the magnesium pemoline rats learned the avoidance response more rapidly, they received less shock; however, they were also reinforced more often for avoiding successfully. When Frey and Polidora (1967) held frequency of shock constant across groups, rats treated with magnesium pemoline did not acquire the response more quickly than control rats. It was also pointed out that magnesium pemoline could have facilitated acquisition of avoidance by virtue of its effects on locomotor activity. Magnesium pemoline is thought to facilitate performance on a variety of tasks; this facilitation might affect learning and memory indirectly (see p. 254; also see Essman, 1971; Goldberg and Ciofalo, 1967; Beach and Kimble, 1967).

MACROMOLECULES

In 1950, Katz and Halstead suggested that long-term memory traces might be encoded in protein. Since then, there has been a great deal of research and interest in the macromolecular basis of memory. This interest was given added impetus by data which clearly demonstrated that the macromolecule deoxyribonucleic acid (DNA) contained the genetic code. Research over the past 15 years has elucidated the relationships between DNA, RNA (ribonucleic acid) and protein synthesis. RNA, protein and polypeptides are considered to be the molecules most likely to store nongenetic information in the nervous system. Three approaches have been used to study the role of macromolecules in learning and memory:

1. *Measurement of RNA and protein*: RNA and protein can be measured by (a) direct measurement of total RNA and/or protein content in specific cells or cell groups; (b) indirect measurement of changes in the rate of RNA or protein synthesis; and (c) measurement of changes in the shape of protein molecules, i.e., conformational changes. These measurements are usually made before and after an animal is trained to perform some task.

2. *Inhibition of RNA or protein synthesis*: RNA or protein synthesis is inhibited by certain antibiotics. Antibiotics are usually administered after an animal has been trained to perform some task, and subsequent deficits in his ability to recall the task are measured.

3. *Transfer of training*: A chemical fraction of the nervous system (RNA and/ or polypeptide of a trained animal) is isolated and injected into a naive (i.e., untrained animal. If the untrained animal then shows evidence of training, "chemical transfer of training" is said to occur.

In the following pages, we will review and evaluate data obtained from each of these approaches; however, no approach has conclusively demonstrated that the memory trace is contained in a certain type of molecule. In evaluating these data, the following criteria for establishing a permanent memory trace should be considered: (1) it should undergo a change of state in response to the experience to be remembered; (2) the altered state should persist as long as the memory can be demonstrated; and (3) specific destruction of the altered state should result in permanent destruction of the memory (Dingham and Sporn, 1964).

Basic Biochemistry

In the last 15 years, research on the structure, metabolism and function of DNA, RNA and protein has been one of the most productive areas in biochemical research. Since current knowledge of RNA and protein synthesis is extensive, a complete review of this subject goes beyond the scope of this book and is not necessary for an understanding of material covered in the following pages (see Albers *et al.*, 1972; Watson, 1970). Nevertheless, a brief summary of RNA and protein synthesis is given here.

DNA is a genetic material that is involved in the synthesis of specific cellular proteins including structural proteins and enzymes. Except for mutations, DNA is relatively unalterable. In order for DNA to regulate protein synthesis in the cytoplasm, an intermediate compound must be transferred from the cell nucleus where DNA is found to the cytoplasm. This compound is messenger RNA (*mRNA*), and the bulk of mRNA is associated with structures that are visible with the electron microscope. These structures form a series of tubules called the *endoplasmic reticulum*. Attached to these tubules are numerous dense spherical granules called *ribosomes*, which contain about 80% of the RNA. Protein synthesis occurs at the ribosomes. In most cases, the mRNA is transcribed from DNA; however, mRNA may also be altered by the cellular environment. For example, chemicals (and drugs) of various types as well as stimulation of the cell can apparently alter the quantity and/or the type of protein synthesized from a particular type of mRNA.

RNA is a long chained polymer composed of a series of four nucleotides. The four nucleotides can be differentiated from one another by the characteristic base that they contain. Two of these bases are called *purines*, and the naturally occurring purines in RNA are *adenine* and *guanine*; the other two are called *pyrimidines*, and the naturally occurring pyrimidines are *uracil* and *cytosine*. A nucleotide consists of the base plus an attachment of a sugar called *ribose* plus the attachment of *phosphoric acid*. The following nucleotides occur in RNA and can be arranged in a wide variety of sequences to form a specific RNA polymer:

> Adenylic acid: adenine + ribose + phosphoric acid
> Guanylic acid: guanine + ribose + phosphoric acid
> Cytidylic acid: cytidine + ribose + phosphoric acid
> Uridylic acid: uridine + ribose + phosphoric acid

In the synthesis of a particular protein, the constituent amino acids are arranged in a given sequence. This sequencing of amino acids is referred to as the primary structure of the protein. Small protein molecules may contain a sequence of as few as 20 amino acids, while larger proteins may contain several thousand. There are 20 different commonly occurring amino acids in living organisms, and the unique structure of a protein is determined by the number of amino acids in a polypeptide chain as well as their sequential order. mRNA contains the code for both the sequencing and the number of amino acids. The position of each amino acid in the chain is determined by three nucleotides sequentially arranged on the mRNA molecule. These three bases are referred to as a *codon*. For example, the codon for the amino acid leucine is cytidylic acid followed by uridylic acid followed by adenylic acid. There are also codons for initiating and terminating the polypeptide chain (see Fig. 8-5). The codon for each amino acid is now known.

The utilization of the amino acids for protein synthesis requires three steps. First, the amino acid is activated by attachment to a molecule capable of combining with a certain type of transfer RNA (tRNA). This process is shown in Fig. 8-6. Then the activated amino acid combines with transfer RNA (tRNA) (Fig. 8-7) in the cytoplasm. There is a specific tRNA for each amino acid.

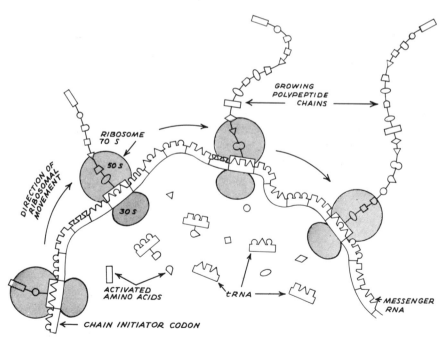

Fig. 8-5. Relationship of messenger RNA to ribosomes in protein synthesis. (From Harper, 1971.)

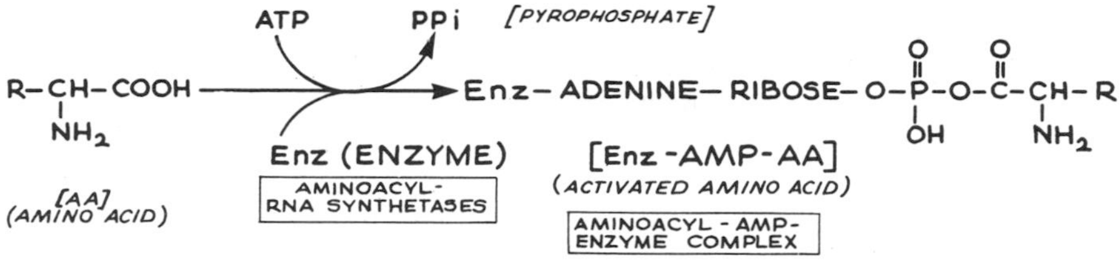

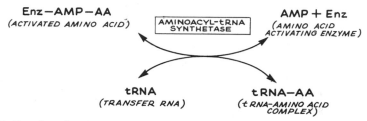

Fig. 8-6. Activation reaction in the utilization of amino acids for protein synthesis. (From Harper, 1971.)

Fig. 8-7. Transfer of activated amino acids to form tRNA amino acid complexes. (From Harper, 1971.)

Like the codon for amino acids, it consists of a unique set of three nucleotides called the *anticodon*. In the third step, the tRNA–amino acid complex combines with the codon of the mRNA. By proceeding from the codon that initiates the sequence (called the chain activator) along the mRNA, the polypeptide (or protein) is synthesized (Fig. 8-5).

Certain compounds interfere with these processes. Actinomycin D prevents the formation of messenger RNA. Tetracycline, streptomycin and chloramphenicol (antibiotics) inhibit activity at the ribosomes, thereby preventing protein synthesis. Puromycin attaches to transfer RNA and prevents the addition of amino acids to the peptide. As we shall see, alterations in the mRNA and the proteins produced by it may be related to modification of nerve cell function. When the modifications of mRNA and protein occur as a result of a learning experience, these changes are believed to show some relationship to memory.

Measurement of RNA and Protein Synthesis

In 1960, Hydén proposed that memory was stored in RNA or in protein in the central nervous system. He based this proposal on experiments showing that RNA synthesis and protein synthesis were correlated with changes in neuronal function. Furthermore, it was postulated that altered RNA caused altered electrical activity and concomitant changes in sensory and motor activity.

Subsequently, Hydén showed that increases in total RNA content and changes in base ratios (i.e., the ratio between the concentration of purines and pyrimidines) occurred in Dieters' nerve cells as a result of a learning experience in the rat, which involved acquisition of a difficult motor coordination task involving balance. Dieters' cells were examined because they are in the vestibular nuclei (which is involved in balance) and are directly involved in the maintenance of balance. Food-deprived rats were placed in a large chamber with a small platform mounted on a pole 45 cm from the floor. A 90-cm wire (1.5 mm in diameter) was stretched between the floor of the cage and the platform in such a way that the wire formed an inclined plane reaching between the floor and the platform. The rat could reach the food by balancing on the wire and climbing to the platform. Hydén found that rats took about four days of training to make one successful trip in a 45-minute session. After reaching the platform, the rat took the food in his mouth and walked down the wire before consuming it. On the first day of a successful trip, the rat usually accomplished three or four more trips; but after four more days of trials, rats made about 20 trips in the 45-minute session. Two control groups were used; one control group consisted of littermate rats with free access to food and water and normal motor activity in the cage. Another control group consisted of rats subjected to passive vestibular stimulation by swinging in a pendulum.

At the end of this procedure, rats were killed and single Dieters' cells were dissected from the brain-stem. The nucleus was separated from the rest of the cell, and the cytoplasm and nucleus were analyzed separately for total RNA content and base ratios. Hydén and Egyházi (1962) found that rats that had been trained to climb the wire had an increased concentration of RNA in the Dieters' cells and a change in the RNA base ratios in the nucleus but not in the cytoplasm (see Table 8-3). (Small changes in cytoplasm may have gone undetected because of the large quantity of RNA in cytoplasm.) The relative proportion of adenine increased and uracil decreased. Rats that received passive stimulation of the vestibular system also showed an increase in the total RNA present in the cell, but unlike the rats that learned to climb the wire, this group showed no change in the base ratios of RNA (Table 8-3). Recall that nuclear RNA is transcribed from DNA. Since DNA usually is not altered by environmental conditions, one might expect nuclear RNA also to be unaltered; however, these experiments demonstrate a change in nuclear RNA. Hydén speculates that learning activates sites on the DNA in the chromosome and thereby changes the composition of nuclear RNA.

Changes in RNA content and base composition in cortical neurons have also been demonstrated in rats learning transfer of "handedness" (Hydén and Egyházi, 1964). Food-deprived rats were placed in a chamber with a glass

TABLE 8-3. Change in RNA content or base ratio composition in the Dieters' cells of rats learning to climb a wire (*experimental*) as opposed to *caged controls* or controls subjected to passive stimulation, *passive stimulation controls*

	Caged controls	Experimental	Passive stimulation controls
I. Total amount of RNA/Dieters' cell compared to caged controls			
RNA/Dieters' cell $\mu\mu$g/cell ± S.E.M.	683 ± 17	751[1] ± 10	722[1]
II. Composition of nuclear RNA of Dieters' nerve cells (base ratios expressed as molar proportions in the percent of the sum)			
Adenine	21.4	24.1[1]	21.3
Guanine	26.2	26.7	25.7
Cytosine	31.9	31.0	31.3
Uracil	20.5	18.2[1]	21.7
III. Composition of cytoplasmic RNA (base ratios expressed as molar proportions in the percent of the sum)			
Adenine	20.5	20.9	
Guanine	33.7	34.0	
Cytosine	27.4	26.8	
Uracil	18.4	18.3	

[1]P less than 0.05.
From Hydén and Egyházi (1962).

cylinder from which they could retrieve food by placing one paw through a small opening. First the rat's preferred paw was determined. Rats that preferred the right paw continued in the experiment. After experience with obtaining their total daily food ration from the cylinder, the situation was changed in such a way that the rat could reach food only with the nonpreferred left paw. Over a period of six days, the frequency of reaches with the nonpreferred left paw increased (Fig. 8-8). Each animal was used as its own control. Neurons were removed from the left side (controls) and the right side (learning-experimental) of the motor cortex. Recall that the right side of the brain contains neurons controlling the left paw and vice versa. The total RNA con-

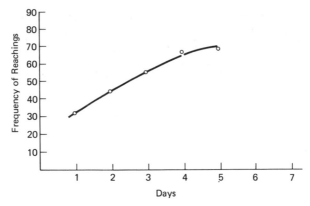

Fig. 8-8. Number of reaches of six rats during a 25-min experimental session, for five days. Each symbol represents one rat. (From Hydén and Egyházi, 1964.)

tent in cells taken from the right side of the brain increased when the rats learned to reach with their left paw (Table 8-4). In addition, there was a difference in RNA base composition between the right and left sides. As a result of learning, adenine, guanine and uracil increased, and cytosine decreased (Table 8-4). These shifts in base characteristics indicate that the new RNA synthesized is of the mRNA variety.

TABLE 8-4.   RNA and base composition changes in cortical neurons of rats transferring "handedness" from the right to the left paw

	Control side (left)	Experimental side (right)
I. RNA content per cell		
RNA ($\mu\mu$g/cell)	22 ± 2.3	27 ± 2.5[1]
II. Changes in RNA base composition (base ratios expressed as molar proportions in the percent of the sum)		
Adenine	18.4	20.1[1]
Guanine	26.5	28.7[1]
Cytosine	36.8	31.5[1]
Uracil	18.3	19.6[1]

[1]P less than 0.05.
From Hydén and Egyházi (1964).

In summarizing these quantitative and qualitative changes in brain protein as a result of learning, McEwen and Hydén (1966, p. 823), stated: "In view of the well established relationship between RNA and protein synthesis, these changes in brain cell RNA suggest that the genetic material of neurons and glia is called upon to make adjustments to physiological changes by elaborating information for the formation of new and perhaps different protein molecules which may themselves be directly involved in nervous activity."

Further impetus in the search for protein molecules related to learning and memory was provided by the isolation of a protein (S-100) that is unique to brain (Moore, 1965). The isolated protein was called S-100 because it is soluble at neutral pH in a 100% saturated solution of ammonium sulfate; other proteins tend to precipitate at much lower ammonium sulfate concentrations. The S-100 protein is present in the central nervous system of all animals tested, including cattle, hogs, rats, hamsters, guinea pigs, mice, dogs, cats, humans, turkeys, eagles, alligators, turtles and monkeys. The amino acid composition of S-100 protein is similar in all species tested. Moreover, the S-100 antiserum shows cross reactions in various species. It has a molecular weight of 21,000, three distinct subunits, and a high content of glutamic and aspartic acids (Kessler et al., 1968). The S-100 protein has been shown to occur in cell bodies of glia and in the nucleus of neurons. The S-100 fraction comprises about 0.1% of the total brain protein (Mihailović and Hydén, 1969). Several fractions of the S-100 protein can be obtained with gel electrophoresis. The S-100 protein binds calcium and, as a result, undergoes conformational changes (Calissano, 1973).

Hydén and his colleagues have observed quantitative changes in the S-100 protein as a result of learning. Rats were trained to use the nonpreferred left paw to reach for food (as outlined above). The rats were trained in three sessions: 4 days of initial training; 14 days rest; 2 days of training; 14 days rest; 2 days of training. Each training session involved two 25-minute sessions. Rats were killed, and a portion of the hippocampus was analyzed for the S-100 protein fraction.

Training produced an increase in the total amount of S-100 protein in the hippocampal cells. Moreover, during the second training session, two bands appeared in the S-100 fraction of trained rats, whereas only one band appeared in the S-100 fraction of untrained rats (Table 8-5). One of two bands was found to have a higher calcium content, suggesting a conformational change.

Therefore, since the S-100 protein changes in response to a training experience, it fills one of the criteria set forth by Dingman and Sporn (1964) for establishing a molecular memory trace (see p. 257). Alteration is the S-100 fraction did not persist as long as the animal performed the task; therefore, it is questionable whether S-100 fits Dingman and Sporn's second criterion, i.e.,

TABLE 8-5.   Frequency of single- and double-frontal anodal proteins in the electrophoretic pattern of 75-polyacrylamide gels from 23 rats (7 controls, 4 resumed training on the 14th day, 12 resumed training on the 14th day and on the 30th day)

Controls−7		Resumed training on day 14−4		Resumed training on day 30−12	
1 fraction	2 fractions	1 fraction	2 fractions	1 fraction	2 fractions
20	0	5	10	20	20

From Hydén (1973).

that the change be permanent. Failure of the S-100 protein to persist may be explained in two ways. First, the S-100 protein may be an intermediate molecule, and its presence may lead to the formation of another molecule. Second, and more likely, the S-100 protein may have been absorbed into the cell wall where it would be undetectable. While changes in S-100 appear to be temporary, destruction of S-100 does lead to destruction of memory, thereby filling Dingman and Sporn's third criterion for establishing molecular encoding of a memory trace. Hydén and Lange (1970) report that injection of an S-100 antiserum disrupted acquisition. Note that an antiserum contains antigen which is capable of complexing with a specific protein and thereby inactivating it. The S-100 antiserum was injected on the fourth day of training on the handedness task. Rats continued to perform the task, but no improvement was seen. The specificity of this chemical reaction to the S-100 antigen was shown by injecting gamma globulins which are nonspecific antigens and which enter the brain like the S-100 antigen. No change in acquisition was seen following gamma globulin injection (see Fig. 8-9).

On the basis of this evidence, Hydén (1973) has concluded that learning produces specific changes in mRNA within the central nervous system. These changes in turn alter the type of protein synthesized from the changed mRNA. In this case, Hydén speculated that changes in the S-100 fraction occurred as a result of learning. Proteins of the S-100 type could be part of synaptic nerve cells. The selective uptake of calcium in nerve cells could have a dual effect: it could induce a conformational change in the S-100 protein and increase the impulse activity (Rasmussen, 1970), thereby inducing protein synthesis (Rasmussen and Nagata, 1970) and possibly regulating the release of transmitters (Banks, 1970).

Changes in the synthesis of RNA have also been shown in mice following acquisition of an avoidance task (Zemp et al., 1966). Following learning,

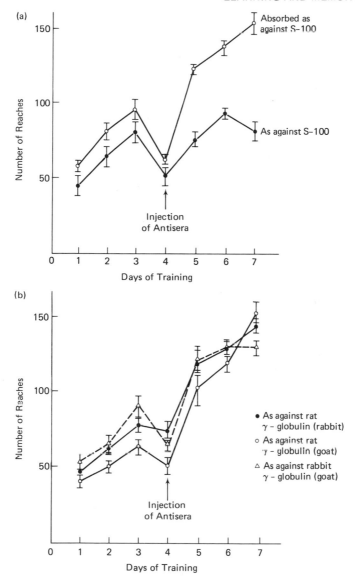

Fig. 8-9. Performance curves of rats injected intraventricularly on day 4 with 2 × 30 μg of antiserum: (a) against S-100 protein and against S-100 absorbed with S-100 protein; (b) against rat gamma globulin from rabbit and from goat, and rabbit gamma globulin from goat. (From Hydén, 1973.)

the incorporation of uridine into ribosomal, polysomal and nuclear RNA increased. Increased incorporation of uridine into RNA suggests an increased synthesis of RNA. Mice were trained to avoid or escape a shock by jumping from a grid floor onto a shelf. The preshock stimulus was a light, a buzzer or a combination of the two. Shock was delivered through the grid floor. One group (the learning group) was trained with a shelf present in the chamber. Three control groups were examined, including: (1) *a yoked control*—a group exposed to the preshock stimulus and the shock along with the learning group, but with no shelf in the box for escape; (2) *a shock control group*—a group exposed to intermittent shocks for the same time interval in the same box as the learning group but with neither preshock stimulus nor shelf present in the box; (3) *a quiet control group*—a group kept in their home cages. Mice were lightly anesthetized with ether, and radioactively labeled uridine was injected directly into the frontal lobes of the brain 30 minutes before exposure to one of the four conditions (learning, yoked, shock or quiet). They were killed after the experimental session, their brains were quickly removed, and the amount of labeled uridine incorporated into the RNA was determined (see Chapter 2).

Both ribosomal and nuclear incorporation of uridine into RNA increased as a result of learning, suggesting that the learning experience caused an increase in the metabolism of RNA. Increased metabolism was observed in trained animals as compared to yoked controls, or quiet controls. No difference in incorporation was observed between any of the control groups (Table 8-6). No differences were seen in kidney or liver, suggesting that the changes were specific to brain (Table 8-7).

It is of interest to note that the differences in brain RNA were only observed if the mice were killed immediately after training. Mice killed 30 minutes after training did not show differences. At this time, changes in a specific RNA fraction may be obscured by the very heavy radioactive labeling of RNA (Zemp

TABLE 8-6.   Effects of 15 minutes experience on the incorporation of uridine into RNA from mouse brain

Paired experiences	Number of pairs	Change in RNA radioactivity
Trained vs. yoked	18	+ (Trained)
Trained vs. quiet	7	+ (Trained)
Yoked vs. quiet	4	0
Shocked vs. quiet	4	0

From Zemp *et al.* (1970).

TABLE 8-7. Changes in incorporation of uridine into RNA from brain, liver and kidney of trained and yoked mice sacrificed immediately after training

Tissue	Number of pairs	Average percentage increase in trained mouse (Corrected for radioactivity in UMP)	
		Ribosomal RNA	Nuclear RNA
Liver	5	−2.2	−2.2
Kidney	4	1.8	1.9
Brain	10	40.2	29.2

From Zemp *et al.* (1970).

et al., 1966) that occurs during the 30-minute time interval after the mice are removed from the experimental situation.

Subsequent experiments (Zemp *et al.*, 1970) demonstrated that acquisition of an avoidance response caused an increased incorporation of ^{3}H-uridine into polysomes (polysomes are ribosomes plus mRNA). RNA synthesis increased when the preshock stimulus was a light, buzzer, or light and buzzer or when no preshock stimulus was used. In addition, further changes in RNA uridine incorporation did not occur as a result of further exposure to the conditioning situation. For example, a group of mice were trained for several days until they avoided shock on over 90% of the trials. They were then injected with tritiated uridine and given further trials in the box; uridine incorporation into polysomes did not change as a result of further training.

The results of the above experiments suggest that changes in the synthesis of RNA occur as a result of acquiring an avoidance response. These changes do not occur as a result of exposure to the various stimuli (light, buzzer or shock) present in the box. However, it cannot be discerned from these data how acquisition of the avoidance response correlated with the increased incorporation of uridine into RNA. In the absence of this information, it is difficult to judge the role of learning in this chemical response. Because observable RNA changes are short-lived, it is difficult to determine what the role of these changes is on memory formation (Glassman and Wilson, 1973). Nevertheless, this work, along with that of Hydén, represents the beginning of what to date has been a most formidable and elusive problem: the correlation of central nervous system changes with learning and memory.

Inhibition of Protein Synthesis

The administration of drugs that inhibit protein synthesis is a common approach for assessing the role of protein synthesis in the maintenance of memory. Typically, antibiotics that inhibit a specific phase of protein synthesis (see p. 259) are administered. The experimental paradigm usually involves first training an animal on some task and injecting a protein synthesis inhibitor either shortly before or after the animal undergoes training. At a later time the animal is tested, and deficits in performance are taken as an index of memory interference. Control subjects receive the same treatment except that they are not injected with protein inhibitors. In general, work in this area suggests that the inhibition of protein synthesis interferes with memory.

For example, Flexner *et al.* (1963, 1964) found that short-term memory and, to a lesser extent, long-term memory formation were inhibited when puromycin was injected into the brain of a mouse trained to avoid shock. Mice were trained in a Y maze to avoid shock until individual mice achieved 9 correct responses out of 10 attempts. Following training, puromycin (30 to 90 μg) was injected once 24 hours after training, or daily between 11 and 60 days after the initial training.

When puromycin was injected 24 hours after training, deficits in short-term memory were reported. Deficits in long-term memory occurred only when daily injections of puromycin were made into several areas of the brain (temporal lobe, the ventricular system and the frontal lobe) at the same time. The latter result suggests that long-term memory is more diffusely localized in the brain than short-term memory.

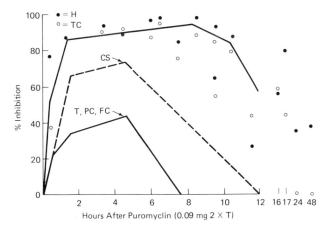

Fig. 8-10. Changes with time in the incorporation of radiovaline into protein of the hippocampus (H), temporal cortex (TC), corpus striatum (CS), thalamus (T), parietal cortex (PC) and frontal cortex (FC) after bitemporal injections each with 90 μg of puromycin in 12 μl. (From Flexner *et al.*, 1967.)

Flexner *et al.* (1967) also measured the effect of puromycin on protein synthesis. Puromycin was injected into the temporal lobes of a mouse, and protein synthesis was estimated by measuring incorporation of labeled valine into protein. They found that the greatest inhibition of incorporation occurred in the hippocampus (Fig. 8-10). The time course of inhibition suggested that puromycin acted on the hippocampus. Flexner *et al.* also reported that long-term memory was only inhibited when protein synthesis was inhibited in several brain areas. Their conclusion is consistent with evidence that massive lesions of the CNS affect long-term memory, while lesions restricted to the temporal region affect short-term memory (Table 8-8).

While this work suggests that puromycin interferes with memory by inhibiting protein synthesis, Flexner *et al.* (1967) reported that the protein synthesis inhibitor, acetoxycycloheximide, did not interfere with short-term memory.

TABLE 8-8. Effects of different sites of injection of puromycin on short- and long-term memory. L, lost; I, impaired; R, retained; Days, days after learning. T, V and F refer, respectively, to temporal, ventricular and frontal injections, all given bilaterally. For the mice with loss of memory, the means and standard deviations for percentages of savings of trials and of errors were, respectively, 1 ± 3 and 2 ± 6; for those with impaired memory, 26 ± 29 and 39 ± 12; for those with retention of memory, 90 ± 14 and 90 ± 9.

Puromycin injections			Number of mice in which memory was		
Site	Days	Dose (mg)	L	I	R
Short-term memory					
T + V + F	1	.03–.06	7	0	0
T	1	.09	10	0	0
V	1	.09	0	0	5
F	1	.09	0	0	5
V + F	1	.09	0	1	2
Longer-term memory					
T + V + F	11–60	.03	17	2	0
T	11–35	.06–.09	0	0	7
V	12–38	.06–.09	0	0	3
F	16–27	.06–.09	0	0	3
V + F	28	.06–.09	0	2	2
V + T	28–43	.09	1	1	2
V + F	28	.09	0	0	3

From Flexner *et al.* (1967).

Moreover, acetoxycycloheximide administration prevented the effects of puromycin. It should be noted that acetoxycycloheximide and puromycin have different biochemical mechanisms of action. Acetoxycycloheximide suppresses the formation of the peptide bonds between the amino acids in a protein, while puromycin allows peptide bond formation to proceed at a normal rate, but small abnormal peptides are formed. Acetoxycycloheximide might prevent the effects of puromycin on memory by suppressing peptide bond formation.

On the other hand, Barondes and Cohen (1967) found deficits in long-term memory but not in short-term memory when acetoxycycloheximide was injected about five hours before training. Five hours following acetoxycycloheximide treatment, mice were trained to escape shock by running to the left alley of a Y maze. Acetoxycycloheximide did not interfere with its retention three hours after training; however, when acetoxycycloheximide was injected six hours after training, large deficits in memory appeared. The deficits persisted until testing was discontinued, with no evidence of recovery (Fig. 8-11). Similar results were obtained when a larger dose of acetoxycycloheximide was injected systemically (Barondes and Cohen, 1968a). Moreover, acetoxycycloheximide produced memory deficits if administered between 30 minutes prior to and 5 minutes after training (Fig. 8-12).

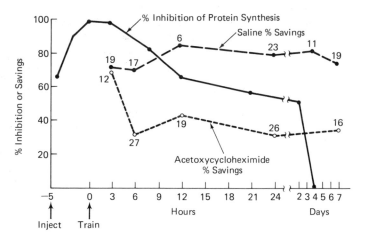

Fig. 8-11. Effect of intracerebral acetoxycycloheximide on cerebral protein synthesis and memory. Mice were injected in both temporal regions of the brain with a total of 20 μl of 0.15 M NaCl with or without 20 μg of acetoxycycloheximide. Five hours later they were trained to escape shock by choosing the correct limb of a one-choice maze to a criterion of three out of four consecutive correct responses. Retention was determined at the indicated times. Protein synthesis inhibition was estimated in three to six mice at the indicated times. There was no significant difference in the savings of the two groups three hours after training, but thereafter acetoxycycloheximide-injected mice had significantly poorer savings ($P < .05$, or less) than saline-injected mice. (From Barondes and Cohen, 1967.)

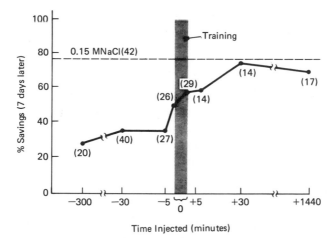

Fig. 8-12. Effect of subcutaneous administration of acetoxycycloheximide at various times before or after training on memory. Mice were injected subcutaneously with 240 μg of acetoxycycloheximide at the indicated time relative to training. They were trained to escape shock by choosing the lighted limb of a t-maze to a criterion of five out of six correct responses. Training took an average of 8 min. Approximately 90% of cerebral protein synthesis was inhibited within 10-15 min of subcutaneous injection of acetoxycycloheximide. All mice were tested for retention seven days after training, long after they had recovered from the drug. The mice injected before or within 5 min after training all had significantly less savings ($P < .05$ or less, Mann-Whitney U test) than saline controls. The mice injected 5 or more min before training had significantly less savings than those injected immediately after training. Injections 30 min or more after training had no effect on memory. (From Barondes and Cohen, 1968b.)

These studies have shown that inhibition of protein synthesis can cause inhibition of memory. Studies by Flexner suggested that the effect was on short- rather than long-term memory, whereas experiments by other investigators (Barondes and Cohen, 1967; Barondes and Squire, 1972; Barondes, 1970) suggested that protein synthesis inhibition mainly affects long-term memory. Differences in species, procedures and definitions of long- and short-term memory could well account for the differences in the interpretation of the results. The most important point is that inhibition of protein synthesis affects memory in different species with different experimental drugs and in different experimental situations.

While the inhibition of protein synthesis has been reported to interfere with memory, the following points should be considered in evaluating research in this area. First, memory deficits are usually only seen following an 80% inhibition of protein synthesis. A dose of a drug that produces 80% synthesis inhibition also has toxic effects including lethargy, incoordination and in some cases death. Second, protein synthesis inhibitors are usually injected directly into the brain.

In an organism with a small brain (e.g., the mouse, whose average brain weight is 300 mg) it is possible that CNS damage could occur because of the injection.

Transfer of Training

Over the past 15 years, several investigators have reported that brain extract (usually RNA, but more recently polypeptides) taken from a trained organism (usually planaria or rodents) and introduced into an experimentally naive organism facilitates the acquisition of the same task in naive organisms. From this work it has been suggested that learning induces changes in RNA which can, in turn, influence the performance of other animals. In this section a few of these experiments will be reviewed, and the logical and experimental problems of this work will be discussed.

The first transfer experiments were carried out with planaria (see review by Chapouthier, 1973). Thompson and McConnell (1955) classically conditioned planaria by pairing a light with shock. After a certain number of pairings, the planaria reacted (i.e., moved) to the light in a manner similar to shock-induced reactions. When the planaria were cut in two and both halves allowed to regenerate, the two regenerated planaria retained the classically conditioned response. McConnell et al. (1959) postulated that the memory was stored in the RNA which was now contained in both planaria. When the halved planaria were incubated in RNase (an RNA catabolizing enzyme), the memory was lost. Further experiments (McConnell, 1962) showed that when naive planaria were fed conditioned planaria, the conditioning was transferred. Further work, however, failed to replicate these studies—both the regeneration and the transfer by cannabalism.

In 1965, investigators from four different laboratories (Reinis, 1965; Fjerdingstad et al., 1965; Ungar and Oceguera-Navarro, 1965; Babich et al., 1965) reported transfer of an acquired conditioned response from trained animals by injecting RNA extracts into untrained animals. The experiment by Babich et al. (1965) will serve as an example of this early work. In this experiment, rats were trained to approach a food cup whenever the food magazine clicked. Rats were given 200 trials per day of the click delivered with food for four days. After the fourth day, the trained rats were killed and RNA was extracted from their brains. Untrained rats served as control donors. A new batch of rats were injected with RNA extracted from either trained or untrained control rats and then given 25 trials in which the number of approaches to the food cup in response to the magazine click was measured. Rats injected with RNA from trained rats made significantly more approaches to the cup than rats injected with RNA extracted from the brains of untrained rats (see Table 8-9). Babich et al. (1965) speculated that changes in either the configuration or the quantity of RNA occur as the result of learning. Other possible behavioral mechanisms such as in-

TABLE 8-9. Total number of responses per animal on the 25 test trials

Experimental rats	Control rats
1	0
3	0
7	0
8	1
9	1
10	1
10	2
	3

From Babich *et al.* (1965).

creased arousal or increased motor activity were also considered, as well as the possibility that the active ingredient in their extract was a chemical other than RNA.

The initial work of Babich *et al.* (1965) stimulated investigation of transfer of training. While several investigators attempted to replicate this work, many failures to replicate were reported (Gross and Carey, 1965; Luttges *et al.*, 1966). Indeed, 23 investigators collaborated in a single paper to report that they had all obtained negative results (Byrne *et al.*, 1966). Transfer of training has been examined in a variety of behavioral tests including avoidance, escape and habituation, as well as behavior maintained by positive reinforcement. While positive results are often reported, the basic transfer phenomenon remains elusive, since failure to replicate is common (see Chapouthier, 1973). Possible reasons for these failures include inadequate dose of the donor material, insufficient time between training of donor animals and extraction of the material and inadequate training of the donor animals, suggesting that it takes a certain time for material to form in the brain of the donor. Little systematic work has been done to verify which, if any, of these factors is crucial to positive transfer effects. Moreover, no procedure has been specified in sufficient detail to guarantee that the phenomenon can be replicated.

Transfer was also reported (Ungar and Fjerdingstad, 1971) when a polypeptide isolated from the brains of rats conditioned to avoid a dark chamber was injected into naive mice which ordinally preferred a dark chamber. Following transfer the naive mice also avoided the dark chamber.

Ungar *et al.* (1972) purified and determined the amino acid sequence of the polypeptide thought to be responsible for this effect. They named the molecule scotophobin—meaning fear of the dark. Ungar and his group postulate that polypeptides (rather than RNA) are responsible for transfer of learning effects.

While crude preparations of RNA contain polypeptides that are closely attached to the ribosomal RNA, the attached polypeptides are removed if RNA is sufficiently purified. Therefore, if the active compound is removed from the transfer extract, transfer of training would not be expected to occur. In crude RNA preparations however, the polypeptide remains attached to the RNA and therefore transfer occurs.

Although these results are appealing, it has been pointed out (Stewart, 1972) that these experiments are difficult to reproduce since details as to the exact training and testing procedures are not presented. In addition, the effect has not always been reproduced in other laboratories even when the transfer material has been supplied by Ungar. Moreover, the purity of the substance used and the determination of its chemical properties, as well as the details of the chemical isolation techniques, have been questioned (Stewart, 1972).

In summary, transfer of training has been reported with a variety of behavioral procedures, including avoidance and escape paradigms (see Chapouthier, 1973). Despite some generality, failure to replicate these findings is common. Since little systematic work has been done to date to determine what factors are crucial to the positive transfer effect, the transfer phenomenon remains elusive. In addition, numerous variables, including handling, deprivation, locomotor activity, habituation and sensory changes, have not been adequately controlled, making interpretation of this work difficult (Smith, 1974).

Controversy about transfer of training has also centered around the implausibility of the phenomenon. Many scientists find it difficult to envision the notion that macromolecules could be extracted from the brain of a trained animal and injected into or fed to another animal and find their way essentially unchanged into the proper neurons of the receiver animal. The question of what happens to a complex molecule when it is extracted from the brain of one animal and injected into another has been tentatively examined. Luttges *et al.* (1966) found that radioactive RNA from trained rats injected ip into naive rats did not reach the brain (see also Smith, 1974; Gaito, 1974; Weinstein, 1973; Guttman, 1973).

The fact that this work presents difficulty in replication and in interpreting behavioral results suggests that future experimentation in this complex area should proceed with caution.

SUMMARY

The historical background of learning and memory and their relationship to brain function was reviewed in this chapter. Memory is considered to involve three processes: registration, consolidation and retrieval. Short-term memory is believed to be related to registration and to early phases of the consolidation process, while long-term memory involves the entire consolidation process as well as the physical changes that occur in the central nervous system as a result of the consolidation process. The chapter has focused on two main issues: (1) the effects of drugs on memory and (2) changes in macromolecules in the brain which may be responsible for encoding and storing learned information.

Evidence was reviewed that strychnine interferes with short-term memory. Experimental results were variable. McGaugh and his co-workers found that post-trial injection of strychnine and other convulsants facilitates learning in mice and rats. Other scientists have not been able to replicate some of McGaugh's work: thus the generality of the finding is questionable. Other drugs were also discussed.

Physical changes in brain macromolecules are thought to occur as a result of learning and are presumably responsible for long-term storage of memory. The criteria for identifying such a molecule were discussed, and it was noted that none of the macromolecules investigated thus far meet all of the criteria. Three macromolecules were discussed in terms of their role in long-term memory storage: RNA, protein and polypeptides. Although some of the experimental evidence is suggestive, additional experimental work must be done before a definite role for any of these macromolecules can be firmly designated.

REFERENCES

Albers, R. W., G. J. Siegel, R. Katzman and B. Agranoff. 1972. *Basic Neurochemistry*. Little, Brown and Co., Boston.

Alpern, H. P. and J. C. Crabbe. 1972. Facilitation of the long-term store of memory with strychnine. *Science* **177**: 722–724.

Ansell, G. B. and P. B. Bradley. 1973. *Macromolecules and Behavior*. University Park Press, Baltimore.

Babich, F. R., A. L. Jacobson, S. Bubash and A. Jacobson. 1965. Transfer of a response to naive rats by injection of ribonucleic acid extracted from trained rats. *Science* **149**: 656–657.

Banks, P. 1970. Involvement of calcium in secretion of catecholamines. *In* A. W. Cuthbert (ed.), *A Symposium on Calcium and Cellular Function*. St. Martin's Press, N.Y., pp. 148–162.

Barondes, S. H. 1970. Cerebral protein synthesis inhibitors block long-term memory. *Int. Rev. Neurobiol.* **12**: 177–205.

Barondes, S. H. and H. D. Cohen. 1967. Delayed and sustained effect of acetoxycycloheximide on memory in mice. *Proc. Nat. Acad. Sci. U.S.A.* **58**: 157–164.

Barondes, S. H. and H. D. Cohen. 1968a. Arousal and the conversion of "short-term" to "long-term" memory. *Proc. Nat. Acad. Sci. U.S.A.* **61**: 923–929.

Barondes, S. H. and H. D. Cohen. 1968b. Memory impairment after subcutaneous injection of acetoxycycloheximide. *Science* **160**: 556–557.

Barondes, S. H. and L. R. Squire. 1972. Slow biological processes in memory storage and "recovery" of memory. *In* J. McGaugh (ed.), *The Chemistry of Mood, Motivation and Memory*. Plenum Press, New York, pp. 207–216.

Beach, G. and D. P. Kimble. 1967. Activity and responsivity in rats after magnesium pemoline injections. *Science* **155**: 698–701.

Boren, J. J. 1963. Repeated acquisition of new behavioral chains. *Am. Psychologist* **18**: 421.

Bovet, D., J. L. McGaugh and A. Oliverio. 1966. Effects of post trial administration of drugs on avoidance learning of mice. *Life Sci.* **5**: 1309–1315.

Bowman, R. E. and S. P. Datta (eds.). 1970. *Biochemistry of Brain and Behavior*. Plenum Press, New York.

Brazier, M. A. 1959. The historical development of neurophysiology. *In* J. Field, H. W. Magoun and V. E. Hall (eds.), *Handbook of Physiology*, Section 1, Neurophysiology, Vol. 1. Waverly Press, Baltimore, pp. 1–58.

Byrne, W. L. (ed.). 1970a. *Molecular Approaches to Learning and Memory*. Academic Press, New York.

Byrne, W. L. 1970b. Introduction. *In* W. L. Byrne (ed.), *Molecular Approaches to Learning and Memory*. Academic Press, New York, pp. xi–xxiii.

Byrne, W. L., D. Samuel, E. L. Bennett, M. R. Rosenzweig, E. Wasserman, A. R. Wagner, F. Gardner, R. Galambos, B. D. Berger, D. L. Margules, R. L. Fenichel, L. Stein, J. A. Corson, H. E. Enesco, S. L. Chorover, C. E. Holt, III, P. H. Schiller, L. Chiappetta, M. E. Jarvik, R. L. Leaf, J. D. Dutcher, Z. P. Horovitz and P. L. Carlson. 1966. Memory transfer. *Science* **153**: 658–659.

Calissano, P. 1973. Specific properties of the brain-specific protein S-100. *In* D. J. Schneider, R. H. Angeletti, R. A. Bradshaw, A. Grasso and B. W. Moore (eds.), *Proteins of the Nervous System*. Raven Press, New York, pp. 13–26.

Carlini, E. L. A., R. M. T. de Lorenzo and E. T. de Almeida. 1972. A suggested aversive effect in rats of post-trial administration of central nervous system stimulants. *Behav. Biol.* **7**: 391–400.

Carlton, P. L. 1968. Brain acetylcholine and habituation. *In* P. B. Bradley and M. Fink (eds.), *Progress in Brain Research* **28**: 48–60. Elsevier, New York.

Chapouthier, G. 1973. Behavioral studies of the molecular basis of memory. *In* J. A. Deutsch (ed.), *The Physiological Basis of Memory*. Academic Press, New York, pp. 1–25.

Cholewiak, R. W., R. Hammond, I. C. Seigler and J. D. Papsdorf. 1968. Effects of strychnine sulphate on classically conditioned nictitating membrane responses of rabbits. *J. Comp. Physiol. Psychol.* **66**: 77–81.

Chorover, S. L. and P. H. Schiller. 1965. Short-term retrograde amnesia in rats. *J. Comp. Physiol. Psychol.* **59**: 73–78.

Cooper, R. M. and M. Krass. 1963. Strychnine: Duration of effects on maze learning. *Psychopharmacologia* **4**: 472–475.

Dawson, R. G. and J. L. McGaugh. 1973. Drug facilitation of learning and memory. *In* J. A. Duetsch (ed.), *The Physiological Basis of Memory*. Academic Press, New York, pp. 77–111.

Deutsch, J. A. 1971. The cholinergic synapse and the site of memory. *Science* **174**: 788–794.

Deutsch, J. A. 1973. Electroconvulsive shock and memory. *In* J. A. Deutsch (ed.), *The Physiological Basis of Memory*. Academic Press, New York, pp. 113–124.

Dingman, W. and M. B. Sporn. 1964. Molecular theories of memory. *Science* **144**: 26–29.

Doty, B. A. and L. A. Doty. 1966. Facilitating effects of amphetamine on avoidance conditioning in relation to age and problem difficulty. *Psychopharmacologia* **9**: 234–241.

Essman, W. B. 1971. Drug effects and learning and memory processes. *Adv. Pharmacol. Chemother.* **9**: 241–330.

Fjerdingstad, E. J., T. Nissen and H. H. Roigaard-Peterson. 1965. Effect of ribonucleic acid (RNA) extracted from the brain of trained animals on learning in rats. *Scand. J. Psychol.* **6**: 1–6.

Flexner, J. B., L. B. Flexner and E. Stellar. 1963. Memory in mice as affected by intracerebral puromycin. *Science* **141**: 57–59.

Flexner, L. B., J. B. Flexner and R. B. Roberts. 1967. Memory in mice analyzed with anti-biotics. *Science* **155:** 1377–1383.

Flexner, L. B., J. B. Flexner, R. B. Roberts and G. de la Haba. 1964. Loss of recent memory in mice as related to regional inhibition of cerebral protein synthesis. *Proc. Nat. Acad. Sci.* **52:** 1165–1169.

Franchina, J. J. and M. H. Moore. 1968. Strychnine and the inhibition of previous performance. *Science* **160:** 903–904.

Frey, P. W. and V. J. Polidora. 1967. Magnesium pemoline: Effect on avoidance conditioning in rats. *Science* **155:** 1281–1282.

Gaito, J. 1974. A biochemical approach to learning and memory: Fourteen years later. *Adv. Psychobiol.* **2:** 225–239.

Glassman, E. and J. E. Wilson. 1973. RNA and brain functions. *In* G. B. Ansell and P. B. Bradley (eds.), *Macromolecules and Behavior.* University Park Press, Baltimore, pp. 81–92.

Goldberg, M. E. and V. B. Ciofalo. 1967. Failure of magnesium pemoline to enhance acquisition of the avoidance response in mice. *Life Sci.* **6:** 733–737.

Goodman, L. S. and A. Gilman (eds.). 1970. *The Pharmacological Basis of Therapeutics.* Macmillan Co., New York.

Gross, C. G. and F. M. Carey. 1965. Transfer of learned response by RNA injection: failure of attempts to replicate. *Science* **150:** 1749.

Guttman, H. N. 1973. Letters: Requirements for testing of hypotheses about molecular coding of experience: Transfer studies. *Psychopharmacol. Bull.* **9:** 6–12.

Harper, H. A. 1971. *Review of Physiological Chemistry.* Lange Medical Publications, Los Angeles, California.

Hebb, D. O. 1949. *The Organization of Behavior.* Wiley, New York.

Hudspeth, W. J. 1964. Strychnine: Its facilitating effect on the solution of a simple oddity problem by the rat. *Science* **145:** 1331–1333.

Hunt, H. F. 1965. Electro-convulsive shock and learning. *Trans. N.Y. Acad. Sci.* **27:** 923–945.

Hunt, H. F. and J. V. Brady. 1961. Some effects of electro-convulsive shock on a conditioned emotional response ("anxiety"). *J. Comp. Physiol. Psychol.* **44:** 88–98.

Hydén, H. 1960. The neuron. *In* J. Brachet and A. E. Mirsky (eds.), *The Cell: Biochemistry, Physiology, Morphology.* Vol. 4. Academic Press, New York. pp. 215–323.

Hydén, H. 1973. Changes in brain protein during learning. *In* G. D. Ansell and P. B. Bradley (eds.), *Macromolecules and Behavior.* University Park Press, Baltimore, pp. 3–26.

Hydén, H. and E. Egyházi. 1962. Nuclear RNA changes of nerve cells during a learning experiment in rats. *Proc. Nat. Acad. Sci.* **48:** 1366–1373.

Hydén, H. and E. Egyházi. 1964. Changes in RNA content and base composition in cortical neurons of rats in a learning experiment involving transfer of handedness. *Proc. Nat. Acad. Sci.* **52:** 1030–1035.

Hydén, H. and P. W. Lange. 1970. Do specific biochemical correlates to learning processes exist in brain cells? *Adv. Biochem. Psychopharmacol.* **2:** 317–338.

Irwin, S. and A. Benuazizi. 1966. Pentylenetetrazol enhances memory function. *Science* **152:** 100–102.

Iversen, S. D. 1973. Brain lesions and memory in animals. *In* J. A. Deutsch (ed.), *The Physiological Basis of Memory.* Academic Press, New York, pp. 305–364.

Jarvik, M. E. 1972. Effects of chemical and physical treatments on learning and memory. *Ann. Rev. Psychol.* **23:** 457–486.

Katz, J. J. and W. C. Halstead. 1950. Protein organization and mental function. *Comp. Psychol. Monog.* **20:** 1–38.

Keleman, K. and D. Bovet. 1962. Effect of drugs upon the defensive behavior of rats. *Acta Physiol.* **19**: 143–154.

Kessler, D., L. Levine and G. Fasman. 1968. Some conformational and immunological properties of a bovine brain acidic protein (S-100). *Biochemistry* **7**: 758–764.

Kopp, R., Z. Bohdanecky and M. E. Jarvik. 1967. Proactive effect of a single ECS on step-through performance on naive and punished mice. *J. Comp. Physiol. Psychol.* **64**: 22–25.

Krivanek, J. and E. Hunt. 1967. The effects of posttrial injections of pentylenetetrazol, strychnine and mephenesin on discrimination learning. *Psychopharmacologia* **10**: 189–195.

Krivanek, J. and J. L. McGaugh. 1969. Facilitating effects of pre- and post-trial amphetamine administration on discrimination learning in mice. *Agents Act.* **1**: 92–98.

Lashley, K. S. 1917. The effects of strychnine and caffeine upon the rate of learning. *Psychobiology* **1**: 141–170.

Lashley, K. S. 1950. In search of the engram. *S.E.B. Symp.* **4**: 454–482.

Le Boeuf, B. J. and H. V. S. Peeke. 1969. The effect of strychnine administration during development on adult maze learning in the rat. *Psychopharmacologia* **16**: 49–53.

Livecchi, S. G. and R. A. Dusewicz. 1969. Effects of pretrial strychnine on maze learning. *Psychol. Rep.* **24**: 735–736.

Luttges, M. W. and J. L. McGaugh. 1967. Permanence of retrograde amnesia produced by electroconvulsive shock. *Science* **156**: 408–410.

Luttges, M., T. Johnson, L. Buck, J. Holland and J. McGaugh. 1966. An examination of "transfer of learning" by nucleic acid. *Science* **151**: 834–837.

McConnell, J. V. 1962. Memory transfer through cannibalism in planarians. *J. Neuropsychiat.* **3** (Suppl. 1): 42–48.

McConnell, J. V., A. L. Jacobson and D. P. Kimble. 1959. The effects of regeneration upon retention of a conditioned response in the planarian. *J. Comp. Physiol. Psychol.* **52**: 1–5.

McEwen, B. and H. Hydén. 1966. A study of specific brain proteins on the semi-micro scale. *J. Neurochem.* **13**: 833.

McGaugh, J. L. 1959. Some neurochemical factors in learning. Unpublished doctoral dissertation. University of California, Berkeley.

McGaugh, J. L. 1961. Facilitative and disruptive effects of strychnine sulfate on maze learning. *Psychol. Rep.* **8**: 99–104.

McGaugh, J. L. 1966. Time-dependent processes in memory storage. *Science* **153**: 1351–1358.

McGaugh, J. L. 1968. Drug facilitation of memory and learning. *In* D. H. Efron (ed.), *Psychopharmacology: A Review of Progress*. Washington, D.C., Public Health Service Publ. No. 1836. U.S. Government Printing Office, Washington, D.C., pp. 891–904.

McGaugh, J. L. 1972. *The Chemistry of Mood, Motivation, and Memory. Advances in Behavioral Biology*, Vol. 4. Plenum Press, New York.

McGaugh, J. L. and J. A. Krivanek. 1970. Strychnine effects on discrimination learning in mice: Effects of dose and time of administration. *Physiol. Behav.* **5**: 1437–1442.

McGaugh, J. L. and L. L. Petrinovich. 1959. The effect of strychnine sulphate on maze-learning. *Am. J. Psychol.* **72**: 99–102.

McGaugh, J. L., C. W. Thomson, W. H. Westbrook and W. J. Hudspeth. 1962. A further study of learning facilitation with strychnine sulphate. *Psychopharmacologia* **3**: 352–360.

Mihailović, L. and H. Hydén. 1969. On antigenic differences between nerve cells and glia. *Brain Res.* **16**: 243–256.

Moore, B. W. 1965. A soluble protein characteristic of the nervous system. *Biochem. Biophys. Res. Comm.* **19**: 739–744.

Oglesby, M. W. and J. L. Winter. 1974. Strychnine sulfate and piracetam. Lack of effect on learning in the rat. *Psychopharmacologia* **36**: 163–173.

Petrinovich, L. 1963. Facilitation of successive discrimination learning by strychnine sulphate. *Psychopharmacologia* 4: 103–113.

Petrinovich, L. 1967. Drug facilitation of learning: strain differences. *Psychopharmacologia* 10: 375–378.

Plotnikoff, N. 1966. Magnesium pemoline: Enhancement of learning and memory of a conditioned avoidance response. *Science* 151: 703–704.

Prien, R. F., M. J. Wayner, Jr. and S. Kahan. 1963. Lack of facilitation in maze learning by picrotoxin and strychnine sulfate. *Am. J. Physiol.* 204: 488–492.

Quartermain, D., R. M. Paolino and N. E. Miller. 1965. A brief temporal gradient of retrograde amnesia independent of situational change. *Science* 149: 1116–1118.

Rasmussen, H. 1970. Cell communication, calcium ion, and cyclic adenosine monophosphate. *Science* 170: 404–411.

Rasmussen, H. and N. Nagata. 1970. Renal gluconeogenesis. Effects on parathyroid hormone and dibutyryl $3',5'$-AMP. *Biochem. Biophys. Acta* 215: 17–28.

Reinis, S. 1965. The formation of conditioned reflexes in rats after parenteral administration of brain homogenate. *Activitas Nervosa Superior* 7: 167–168.

Robbins, M. J. and D. R. Meyer. 1970. Motivational control of retrograde amnesia. *J. Exp. Psychol.* 84: 220–225.

Schaeffer, B. H. 1968. Strychnine and maze behavior: Limited effects of varied concentrations and injection times. *J. Comp. Physiol. Psychol.* 66: 188–192.

Smith, L. T. 1974. The interanimal transfer phenomenon: A Review. *Psychol. Bull.* 81: 1078–1095.

Stewart, W. W. 1972. Comments on the chemistry of scotophobin. *Nature* 238: 202–210.

Thompson, D. M. 1973. Repeated acquisition as a behavioral baseline for studying drug effects. *J. Pharmacol. Exp. Ther.* 184: 506–514.

Thompson, R. and J. McConnell. 1955. Classical conditioning of the planarian, Dugesia dorotocephala. *J. Comp. Physiol. Psychol.* 48: 65–68.

Ungar, G. and E. J. Fjerdingstad. 1971. Chemical nature of the transfer factors: RNA or protein? Proceedings of the Symposium on Biology of Memory (Tihany, Hungary, 1969). *In: Biology of Memory.* Plenum Press, New York, pp. 137–143.

Ungar, G. and C. Oceguera-Navarro. 1965. Transfer of habituation by material extracted from brain. *Nature* 207: 301–302.

Ungar, G., D. M. Desiderio and W. Parr. 1972. Isolation, identification and synthesis of a specific-behaviour-inducing brain peptide. *Nature* 238: 198–202.

Uphouse, L. L., J. W. MacInnes and K. Schlesinger. 1974. Role of RNA and protein in memory storage: A review. *Behav. Genet.* 4: 29–81.

Watson, J. D. 1970. *The Molecular Biology of the Gene.* W. A. Benjamin, New York.

Weinstein, B. 1973. Letters: Requirements for testing of hypotheses about molecular coding of experience: Transfer studies. *Psychopharmacol. Bull.* 9: 4–5.

Weiss, B. and V. G. Laties. 1962. Enhancement of human performance by caffeine and the amphetamines. *Pharm. Rev.* 14: 1–36.

Weiss, B. and V. G. Laties. 1969. Behavioral pharmacology and toxicology. *Ann. Rev. Pharmacol.* 9: 297–326.

Wolthuis, O. L. 1971. Experiments with UCD 6215, a drug which enhances acquisition in rats: Its effects compared with those of metamphetamine. *Eur. J. Pharmacol.* 16: 283–297.

Zemp, J. W., L. B. Adair, J. E. Wilson and E. Glassman. 1970. The effect of training on the incorporation of radioactive precursors into RNA of brain. *In* W. L. Byrne (ed.), *Molecular Approaches to Learning and Memory.* Academic Press, New York.

Zemp, J. W., J. E. Wilson, K. Schlesinger, W. O. Boggan and E. Glassman. 1966. Brain function and macromolecules, I. Incorporation of uridine into RNA of mouse brain during short-term training experience. *Proc. Nat. Acad. Sci. U.S.A.* 55: 1423–1431.

III
DRUG-BEHAVIOR
INTERACTIONS

While there has been a long-standing interest in behaviorally active drugs, extensive investigation of drug-behavior interactions did not really begin until the 1950s when research and discovery in both clinical and preclinical pharmacology and psychology resulted in the application of operant conditioning procedures to the examination of drug effects. Several drugs were found to be effective in the treatment of psychosis, including chlorpromazine. In addition, meprobamate was found to be effective in the treatment of anxiety, although new drugs have since replaced it (see Chapter 6). At the same time, the neurochemical action of a number of drugs (e.g., reserpine, amphetamine, monoamine oxidase inhibitors) was being elucidated (see Section II).

The simultaneous discovery of clinically effective drugs and some notions of their neuropharmacological actions led to a need for a methodology to bring behavior under precise experimental control so that behavioral assessments of drug action could be made. The procedures of operant conditioning offered such a methodology. The development of new clinically active drugs coupled with the techniques of operant conditioning prompted the beginning of an extensive and systematic investigation of drug-behavior interactions in laboratory animals both in the drug industry and in the academic community.

Operant conditioning procedures offer several advantages for the assessment of the behavioral effects of drugs. First, they provide stable baselines for studying behavior over long periods of time. Not only can these procedures maintain behavior for periods of several hours, but responding can also be maintained over many consecutive experimental sessions. Second, the procedures are adaptable for several species. In addition, rates and patterns of responding can be varied over a wide range. Finally, a reliable and sophisticated technology has been developed that facilitates the accurate programming and recording of experimental data. Therefore, these techniques have been used extensively to examine drug-behavior interactions. In subsequent chapters a variety of drug-behavior interactions will be examined. In addition, the fundamental importance of behavioral variables as determinants of drug action will be stressed. We shall see that the analysis of drug action requires precise specification of the behavior examined and the conditions under which it occurs.

Chapter 9 will examine the effects of drugs on behavior maintained by various schedules of reinforcement (schedule-controlled behavior). While some generalizations will be made about drug effects on the rate and pattern of responding maintained by the various schedules of reinforcement, we will see that the effects of many drugs depend upon the rate of responding maintained by different schedule conditions. Chapter 10 deals with the effects of drugs on sensory systems (discrimination). Practically all behavior is dependent on intact sensory function, and it is reasonable to inquire as to whether a given drug affects sensory function. Since the measurement of sensory function involves the measurement of behavior which occurs at different rates and in different patterns, we shall see that it is exceedingly difficult to describe a drug's effect on sensory functions apart from its effects on these different rates and patterns of responding. Therefore, Chapter 10 will emphasize methodological approaches as well as difficulties in examining drug effects on sensory function.

In Chapters 11 and 12, we will discuss the ability of drugs to serve a variety of stimulus functions, including that of an unconditioned stimulus, a reinforcing stimulus and a discriminative stimulus. We will examine the degree to which the rate and pattern of responding maintained by drug administration depend on the particular drug administered, the drug dose, its availability, the schedule under which it is administered and the organism's past drug history.

We will also examine data which show that animals can be trained to respond differentially in the presence or absence of various drug conditions, suggesting that drugs can act as discriminative stimuli. Generalization between similar drugs and between different doses of the same drug will be examined, as well as discrimination between drugs.

9
Drug Effects on Schedule-Controlled Behavior

The use of operant conditioning techniques in the investigation of drug effects has led to an emphasis on the importance of behavioral variables in drug-behavior interactions. For example, it is now quite clear that the effects of behaviorally active drugs do not depend solely on pharmacological variables such as the type of drug examined, the dose of the drug or the time and route of administration, but they also depend on the nature of the behavior being investigated and on the schedules of reinforcement which maintain the behavior. We saw in Chapter 5 that behavioral and environmental variables modify the distribution and metabolism of catecholamines. It is not unlikely that behavioral variables will influence drug effects as well.

An early experiment by Dews (1955) illustrates the importance of the ongoing behavior in determining a drug effect. Dews trained pigeons to peck a key under two different intermittent schedules of food presentation, a fixed interval and a fixed ratio. Recall from Chapter 1 that schedules of intermittent reinforcement provide a controlled situation in which drug effects can be examined and in which variables important to the maintenance of a behavior can be identified. After responding was stable on both schedules, various doses of pentobarbital were administered. Dews found that fixed ratio responding was depressed by 4.0 or 5.6 mg/bird of pentobarbital. Fixed interval responding was also markedly reduced, but by smaller doses (1.0–4.0 mg/bird). Moreover, fixed ratio responding was *increased* by doses of pentobarbital which *decreased* fixed interval responding. Smaller doses (0.25–0.5 mg/bird) produced increases in rates of responding on both schedules (see Figure 9-1). One important point demonstrated by these data is that the effects of a drug depend on the nature of the ongoing behavior. The ongoing behavior depends on the schedule of reinforcement maintaining that behavior. Second, a drug's effect depends on the dose of the drug. Had Dews examined only one dose of pentobarbital with one

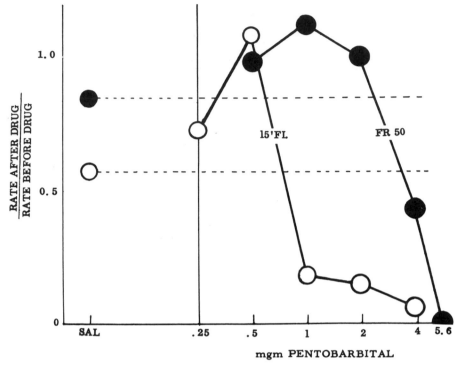

Fig. 9-1. Output ratio (i.e., rate of responding after drug/rate of responding before drug) on an FI 15-min and an FR 50 schedule of food presentation as a function of saline and six doses of pentobarbital in pigeons. Each point represents the arithmetic mean of the ratios for the same four birds at each dosage level on each schedule. Open circles, birds working on FI 15-min. Solid circles, birds working on FR 50. Note that saline had an effect. (From Dews, 1955.)

schedule of reinforcement, the conclusions might have been quite different from those when additional doses and/or schedules were examined.

In this chapter, we will examine drug effects on schedule-controlled behavior with an emphasis on the interaction between drug effects and behavioral variables. The importance of drug dose will also be stressed. We will see that many drugs have an inverted U-shaped dose effect curve, in that behavior is increased at low doses and decreased at higher doses. Obviously, any drug will decrease behavior if given in a sufficiently high dose. Therefore, discussion will generally be limited to a dose range that alters behavior but does not produce anesthesia, ataxia or toxicity.

The following drugs will be examined: psychomotor stimulants; antipsychotics; benzodiazepines, barbiturates (also called antianxiety agents); ethanol; narcotics and tricyclic antidepressants. (See Chapter 6 for a discussion of the clinical utility of these drugs.) In addition, the hallucinogens and tetrahydrocannabinols will be discussed briefly, as well as cholinergic agents (see Chapter 7).

The effects of each of these drugs will be examined on behavior maintained by: (1) positive reinforcement, (2) negative reinforcement and (3) procedures that decrease response rate. A summary statement for each drug class will be given in Table 9-1 (positive reinforcement), Table 9-3 (negative reinforcement) and Table 9-4 (procedures that decrease response rate). Drugs that have received the most emphasis in the investigation of schedule-controlled behavior will be discussed in detail. In a later section of this chapter, a comparison will be made of drug effects on behavior under the control of positive or negative reinforcement. In addition, the importance of variables such as the experimental subject and drug regimen will be examined.

POSITIVE REINFORCEMENT

In this section, the effects of drugs on behavior maintaned by the following four schedules of reinforcement will be reviewed: fixed ratio (FR), fixed interval (FI), variable interval (VI) and differential reinforcement of low rates (DRL). The extent to which these effects depend on pharmacological variables such as the dose of the drug will be examined. The importance of rate of responding as a determinant of a drug's effect will also be discussed. In order to examine the relationship between a drug effect and rate of response, drug effects will be examined in terms of the overall rate of responding generated by particular schedules of reinforcement. Overall rate of responding is a measure of the total number of responses divided by the length of the experimental session. Since schedules of reinforcement do not always generate uniform response rates, it is also necessary to consider different rates of responding generated within a schedule component (i.e., local rates). For example, responding on an FI schedule of reinforcement is characterized by a pause after reinforcement followed by an acceleration in rate. A drug may affect overall response rates on the FI. It may also differentially affect low rates of responding that occur early in the FI interval and high rates of responding that occur at the end of the interval. Moreover, while the effects of many drugs depend on rate of responding (i.e., the effects are rate-dependent), we shall see that rate-dependent effects can be modified by several variables, including discriminative stimuli, punishing stimuli and schedule variables.

General Effects

Table 9-1 presents the effects of a variety of drugs on overall rates of responding maintained by FR, FI, VI or DRL schedules of reinforcement. While generalizations can sometimes be made about drug effects on these schedules of

TABLE 9-1. Drug effects on behavior maintained by positive reinforcement

Schedule	Effect	Reference
PSYCHOMOTOR STIMULANTS (*d*-, *dl*-, *l*-amphetamine, methamphetamine, pipradrol, cocaine, caffeine)		
FI	usually increases response rate; but response rate decreases: (1) with high doses and (2) on FI schedules that generate high response rates	Skinner and Heron (1937); Dews (1958b, 1962); Kelleher *et al.* (1961); Weiss and Laties (1963, 1964); Smith (1964); Kelleher and Morse (1964, 1968); Rutledge and Kelleher (1965); Laties and Weiss (1966); McMillan (1968a,b, 1969); Stitzer *et al.* (1970); Davis *et al.* (1973); Byrd (1973); McKearney (1974); Holtzman (1974a); Barrett (1974); Branch and Gollub (1974); Branch (1975)
FR	usually has no effect at very low doses and decreases response rate at higher doses but response rate increases on FR schedules that generate low response rates	Dews (1958b); Owen (1960); Kelleher *et al.* (1961); Kelleher and Morse (1964); Smith (1964); Rutledge and Kelleher (1965); McMillan (1968a,b, 1969); Davis *et al.* (1973); Byrd (1973); Barrett (1974)
DRL	either has no effect or increases response rate at low doses; decreases response rate at high doses	Sidman (1955); Kelleher *et al.* (1961); Hearst and Vane (1967); McMillan and Campbell (1970); Sanger *et al.* (1974); MacPhail and Gollub (1975)
VI	variable effects	Dews (1958b); Kelleher *et al.* (1961); Hanson *et al.* (1967); MacPhail and Gollub (1975)
ANTIPSYCHOTICS (chlorpromazine, promazine, prochlorperazine, haloperidol, triflupromazine, perphenazine, fluphenazine, trifluoperazine, benzquinamide, tetrabenazine, chlorprothixene)		
FI	usually decreases response rate	Dews (1958a); Waller (1961); Boren (1961b); Cook and Kelleher (1962); Kelleher and Morse (1964); Laties and Weiss (1966); Bignami and Gatti (1969); Clark (1969); McMillan (1971); Leander and McMillan (1974); McKearney (1974); Leander (1975); Byrd (1974)
FR	decreases response rate	Paasonen and Dews (1958); Waller (1961); Kelleher *et al.* (1961); Cook and Kelleher (1962); Kelleher and Morse (1964); Hanson *et al.* (1967); Clark (1969); McMillan (1971); Leander and McMillan (1974); Leander (1975)

Schedule	Effect	Reference
DRL	decreases response rate	Kelleher *et al.* (1961); Sanger and Black-man (1975a)
VI	usually decreases response rate	Waller (1961); Waller and Waller (1962); Hanson *et al.* (1967)

ANTIANXIETY AGENTS (amobarbital, pentobarbital, phenobarbital, chlordiazepoxide, diazepam, oxazepam)

FI	increases response rate at low doses; decreases at high doses	Dews (1955, 1964); Kelleher *et al.* (1961); Richelle *et al.* (1962); Cook and Kelleher (1962); Cook and Catania (1964); Rutledge and Kelleher (1965); Laties and Weiss (1966); Bignami and Gatti (1969); Wuttke and Kelleher (1970); McMillan (1973a)
FR	usually increases response rate at low doses; decreases at high doses	Dews (1955); Kelleher *et al.* (1961); Morse (1962); Cook and Catania (1964); Waller and Morse (1963); Rutledge and Kelleher (1965); Wedeking (1968, 1974)
DRL	increases response rate at low doses; decreases at high doses	Kelleher *et al.* (1961); Morse (1962); Richelle *et al.* (1962); McMillan and Campbell (1970); Sanger *et al.* (1974); Sanger and Blackman (1975a)
VI	increases response rate at low doses; decreases at high doses	Kelleher *et al.* (1961); Morse (1962); Hanson *et al.* (1967); Wedeking (1974)

NARCOTIC ANALGESICS AND NARCOTIC ANTAGONISTS (morphine, nalorphine, methadone, naloxone, naltrexone, cyclazocine, pentazocine)

FI	occasionally increases response rate at low doses; decreases at high doses	McMillan and Morse (1967); Woods (1969); McMillan *et al.* (1970b); Thompson *et al.* (1970); McMillan (1971); Dykstra *et al.* (1974); Mc-Kearney (1974); Goldberg and Morse (1974); Heifetz and McMillan (1971)
FR	decreases response rate	Cook and Kelleher (1962); McMillan and Morse (1967); McMillan *et al.* (1970b); Thompson *et al.* (1970); McMillan (1971); Holtzman and Villarreal (1973); Dykstra *et al.* (1974)
VI	decreases response rate	Thompson *et al.* (1970); Holtzman and Villarreal (1973)

TRICYCLIC ANTIDEPRESSANTS (imipramine, desipramine)

FI	increases response rate in pigeons; decreases in rats	Dews (1962); Smith (1964); Wuttke and Kelleher (1970); McKearney (1968)

TABLE 9-1.   (Continued)

Schedule	Effect	Reference
FR	decreases response rate	Cook and Kelleher (1962); Smith (1964); McKearney (1968)
DRL	increases response rate	Kornetsky (1965)

ETHANOL

FI	increases response rate at low doses; decreases at high doses	Leander *et al.* (1974)
FR	increases response rate at low doses; decreases at high doses	Holloway and Vardiman (1971); Leander *et al.* (1974)
DRL	usually decreases response rate; increases have been reported at low doses	Sidman (1955); Laties and Weiss (1962); Holloway and Vardiman (1971)

HALLUCINOGENS (lysergic acid diethylamide, mescaline, psilocybin)

FI	increases response rate at low doses; decreases at high doses	Tilson and Sparber (1973); Altman and Appel (1975)
FR	decreases response rate	Appel and Freedman (1965)
DRL	increases response rate at low doses; decreases at high doses	Appel (1971)
VI	increases response rate at low doses; decreases at high doses	Jarrard (1963); Appel (1971)

TETRAHYDROCANNABINOLS (Δ^8-THC; Δ^9-THC)

FI	decreases response rate	McMillan *et al.* (1970a); Frankenheim *et al.* (1971); Dykstra *et al.* (1975); Wayner *et al.* (1973); Miller and Drew (1974)
FR	usually decreases response rate	McMillan *et al.* (1970a); Frankenheim *et al.* (1971); Dykstra *et al.* (1975); Ferraro *et al.* (1971)
DRL	variable effects	Frankenheim *et al.* (1971); Ferraro *et al.* (1971); Conrad *et al.* (1972); Manning (1973); Frankenheim (1974)
VI	increases response rate at low doses; decreases response rate at high doses	Grisham and Ferraro (1972); Kosersky *et al.* (1974); Dykstra *et al.* (1975)

CHOLINERGIC BLOCKERS (scopolamine, atropine)

FI	usually decreases response rate; however, increases have been reported at low doses	Herrnstein (1958); Boren and Navarro (1959); Laties and Weiss (1966); Willis and Windland (1968); Bignami and Gatti (1969); McKim (1973, 1974)
FR	usually decreases response rate	Dews (1955); Boren and Navarro (1959); Willis and Windland (1968); Bignami and Gatti (1969)
VI	decreases response rate	Hanson *et al.* (1967); Willis and Windland (1968); Hines *et al.* (1969, 1970)

Schedule	Effect	Reference
CHOLINERGIC AGONISTS (nicotine)		
FI	increases response rate	Morrison (1967); Stitzer *et al.* (1970); Davis *et al.* (1973); Pradhan (1970)
FR	usually decreases response rate; however, increases have been reported with individual animals	Morrison (1967); Pradhan (1970); Davis *et al.* (1973)
DRL	usually increases response rate; however occasional decreases have been reported at high doses	Morrison (1968); Pradhan and Dutta (1970)
VI	increases response rate	Morrison (1967)

reinforcement, it is important to remember that a drug effect depends on the doses examined and the experimental parameters employed in each study.

Psychomotor Stimulants. Increases in overall rates of responding have been observed following amphetamine (*d*, *l*, *dl*), methamphetamine, pipradol, caffeine and cocaine on schedules of reinforcement which generate low rates of responding (e.g., FI and DRL schedules). Moreover, increases in response rate can be observed over a wide range of doses. For example, McMillan (1968b) observed increases in FI responding in pigeons in a dose range of 0.3–10 mg/kg of *d*-amphetamine. The ability of low doses of amphetamine to increase rates of responding while higher doses increase rates less or decrease rates of responding can be demonstrated with both FI and DRL schedules of reinforcement. The shape of the amphetamine dose-response curve is therefore an inverted U. We shall see that the inverted U is a common shape for the dose-response curves of a variety of drugs.

Decreases in response rate are usually observed following amphetamine on schedules which generate high baseline response rates (e.g., FRs). The same dose of amphetamine that increases FI responding will decrease FR responding (McMillan, 1968b) (see Fig. 9-2). These effects have been demonstrated in a variety of species including rats, pigeons and squirrel monkeys.

Antipsychotic Agents. In general, chlorpromazine (the prototypic antipsychotic) decreases responding under FR, FI, DRL and VI schedules. The absence of increases in overall rate following chlorpromazine differentiates it from the psychomotor stimulants and from other drugs. Increases in overall response rates have been reported, however, in a few instances following low doses of chlorpromazine in dogs and chimpanzees on FI schedules (Byrd, 1974; Waller, 1961). Decreases in response rate are observed over a wide range of doses and following a variety of antipsychotic agents. For example, Leander (1975) reports decreases in both FI and FR response rates in pigeons following promazine (3.0–30 mg/kg), chlorpromazine (3.0–100 mg/kg), triflupromazine (1.0–100

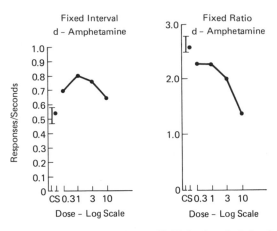

Fig. 9-2. Rate of responding on a multiple FR 30 FI 5-min schedule of food presentation as a function of four doses of d-amphetamine in pigeons. The brackets at C represent the range of control values during sessions just before each drug session, and the points at S show response rates after a saline injection. Each point is the mean of single determinations in each of six birds. (From McMillan, 1968b.)

mg/kg), prochlorperazine (0.3–10 mg/kg), trifluoperazine (0.3–100 mg/kg), benzquinamide (1.0–30 mg/kg), haloperidol (0.03–3.0 mg/kg), chlorprothixene (1.0–17.5 mg/kg) and tetrabenazine (3.0–30 mg/kg). Similar decreases have been reported with chlorpromazine in rats and squirrel monkeys.

Antianxiety Agents. Several drugs are used in the treatment of anxiety, including ethanol, meprobamate, various barbiturates and the benzodiazepines, diazepam and chlordiazepoxide. See Chapter 6 for a discussion of their general clinical effects. Meprobamate is not generally used anymore as an antianxiety agent, and ethanol is only recently receiving attention in this area of psychopharmacological research. Therefore, discussion will be confined to the barbiturates and the benzodiazepines. The effects of ethanol are summarized in Table 9-1.

The effects of the antianxiety agents depend on the dose of the drug and the schedule of reinforcement used to maintain responding. For example, Hanson *et al.* (1967) have shown that overall VI rates are increased at low doses of pentobarbital and chlordiazepoxide, while they are decreased at higher doses. Figure 9-3 illustrates dose effect curves for chlordiazepoxide and pentobarbital on a VI schedule of food presentation in squirrel monkeys. Similar dose-dependent effects have been reported on FI, FR and DRL schedules, indicating an inverted U-shaped dose effect curve.

The effects of the barbiturates and the benzodiazepines on FR schedules of food presentation differ from the effects of most other drugs. For example, amphetamine typically has no effect (low doses) or decreases overall fixed ratio

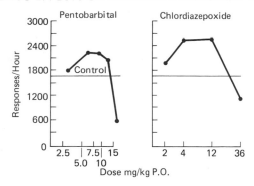

Fig. 9-3. Average number of responses per hour in four animals on a VI 1-min schedule of food presentation as a function of several doses of pentobarbital and chlordiazepoxide. (From Hanson *et al.*, 1967.)

rates of responding. The barbiturates, however, often *increase* FR response rates. Moreover, they increase FR rates at doses that decrease FI rates. Dews (1955) reported that FR rates were increased following 1.0 mg/bird of pentobarbital but decreased at 5.6 mg/bird (see Fig. 9-1). Chlordiazepoxide has also been reported to increase FR rates in rats (Wedeking, 1968, 1974); however, this effect is not always obtained (Cook and Catania, 1964).

Narcotic Analgesics and Narcotic Antagonists. In general, morphine decreases response rates maintained by FI and FR schedules of reinforcement in pigeons, squirrel monkeys and rhesus monkeys; however, increases have sometimes been reported at very low doses on behavior maintained by FI schedules in both pigeons and rhesus monkeys. Similar effects have been reported for methadone and codeine (McMillan *et al.*, 1970b; Woods, 1969). Drugs with narcotic antagonist activity (see Chapter 6, p. 202) have also been reported to increase FI responding at low doses, while higher doses decrease both FI and FR response rates (Goldberg and Morse, 1974; McMillan and Harris, 1972; McMillan *et al.*, 1970b). Figure 9-4 illustrates the effects of naloxone on behavior maintained by FI and FR schedules of food presentation in pigeons.

Both the rate-increasing and rate-decreasing effects of morphine on an FR 30 FI 5-min schedule of food presentation can be blocked with small doses of naloxone, cyclazocine, nalorphine and pentazocine (McMillan *et al.*, 1970b). McMillan first determined dose effect curves for morphine alone. Dose effect curves were then redetermined in the presence of each of the narcotic antagonists. Figure 9-5 illustrates the effect of morphine in the presence and absence of naloxone on responding maintained by a multiple FR FI schedule of food presentation. A dose of 10.0 mg/kg of morphine decreased responding, which was completely blocked by 0.3 mg/kg of naloxone. It is important to note that the dose of naloxone which blocked the effects of morphine on schedule-controlled

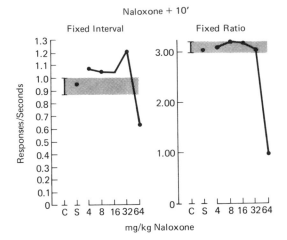

Fig. 9-4. Rate of responding under multiple FR 30 FI 5-min schedule as a function of dose of naloxone. Shaded areas represent the range of non-drug control values, and the points as S show rates of responding after an injection of distilled water. (From McMillan *et al.*, 1970b.)

behavior was much lower than the dose which produced effects on schedule-controlled behavior when given alone (see Fig. 9-4). That is, at low doses naloxone and other narcotic antagonists can antagonize the effects of morphine, while at higher doses these drugs have agonistic effects.

Table 9-1 summarizes the effects of a variety of other drugs on schedule-controlled behavior. Since the tricyclic antidepressants, ethanol, hallucinogens, tetrahydrocannabinols (THC) and cholinergic agents have been examined less extensively than the drugs discussed above, generalizations are difficult to make and must be carefully qualified. Often only one species or a very narrow dose range has been examined.

In summary, it might be concluded that most drugs with the exception of chlorpromazine and THC increase overall FI rates of responding at least at low doses. Higher doses of most drugs usually decrease FI response rates. Similarly, most drugs with the exception of the barbiturates decrease response rates on FR schedules of reinforcement. Effects on DRL or VI schedules are less well documented so that generalizations are difficult to make. While generalizations can be made about drug effects on schedule-controlled behavior, they must always be qualified by a number of factors, including: (1) the dose of the drug; (2) the drug regimen; (3) the species examined. (See the final section of this chapter for a discussion of these variables.) In addition, drug effects on schedule-controlled behavior have been shown to be related to the schedule examined. Since each schedule maintains a characteristic rate and pattern of responding, it has been suggested that a drug's effect is related to the rate of responding generated by these schedules.

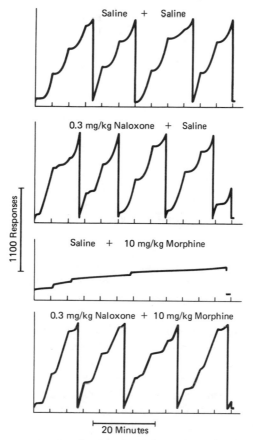

Fig. 9-5. Cumulative response records of one bird showing the effects of (1) a saline injection, (2) 0.3 mg/kg of naloxone, (3) 10.0 mg/kg of morphine and (4) a combination of 0.3 mg/kg of naloxone and 10.0 mg/kg of morphine on patterns of responding in a multiple FR 30 FI 5-min schedule of reinforcement. Abscissa: time. Ordinate: cumulative number of responses. The FI and the FR components are alternated. The components change after each presentation of food, which is indicated by a horizontal line on the bottom event record. If reinforcement is not obtained within 40 sec on the FR component or within 40 sec after 5 min has elapsed on the FI component, the component automatically changes. (From McMillan *et al.*, 1970b.)

Rate-Dependency

Whether a drug increases or decreases responding is very often a function of the schedule of reinforcement examined.   For example, Dews (1958b) trained pigeons on four different schedules of food presentation : VI 1-min, FR 50, a modified FR 900 and FI 15-min. The effect of methamphetamine depended on the schedule examined and the dose of the drug. Methamphetamine produced

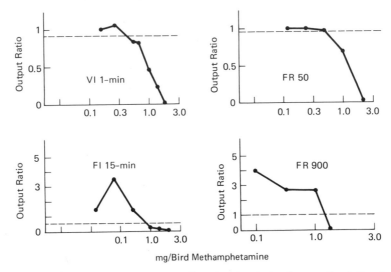

Fig. 9-6. Output ratio (i.e., rate of responding after drug/rate of responding before drug) on four different schedules of reinforcement (VI 1-min, FR 50, FI 15-min, FR 900) as a function of several doses of methamphetamine in pigeons. (From Dews, 1958b.)

an increase in response rates at several doses on the FI 15-min and FR 900 schedules and decreased response rates at the same doses on the VI 1-min and FR 50 schedules (see Fig. 9-6). Overall response rates on the VI and FR 50 schedules were generally high. FR 900 and FI rates were generally low. The overall low rates of responding on the FR 900 schedule were the result of long periods of pausing. (See Chapter 1, p. 16 for a discussion of response patterns on FR schedules with high response requirements.)

From these findings, Dews suggested that the effects of methamphetamine could best be described in terms of the pre-drug rate of responding, since methamphetamine increased rates of responding when pre-drug response rates were low [or when time between responses (IRTs) was long, i.e., 5–10 sec.] and decreased rates of responding when pre-drug response rates were high [or when time between responses (IRTs) was short, i.e., 1 sec or less]. This was the first statement of what has become known as the "rate-dependency hypothesis." It is now known that the effects of several drugs are influenced by the pre-drug rate of responding under a variety of experimental conditions (Kelleher and Morse, 1968).

Clark and Steele (1966) demonstrated the rate-dependent effects of d-amphetamine in rats with a multiple schedule containing three components (S^Δ during which responding was not reinforced, FI 4-min and FR 25). The high rates of responding engendered by the FR 25 schedule were decreased as a function of dose; the intermediate FI rates were slightly increased with low doses, while the very low rates during the S^Δ period increased as a function of dose.

While there have been numerous observations of rate-dependent drug effects on overall rates of responding engendered by different schedules of reinforcement, recall that overall rate of responding is a measure of the total number of responses in an experimental session divided by the length of the experimental session. Response rate is not always constant within a schedule component. For example, FI and FR schedules both generate low rates of responding after reinforcement followed by relatively high rates prior to reinforcement. It has been shown that drugs affect these low and high rates differentially. For example, pentobarbital increases overall rates of responding on FR schedules of food presentation. If the effects of pentobarbital are examined (1) on the pause that occurs immediately after reinforcement on an FR schedule and (2) on the steady high rate of responding that follows the pause, it becomes apparent that pentobarbital increases FR response rates by decreasing the length of the post-reinforcement pause (Weiss and Gott, 1972). Moreover, methamphetamine increased rates of responding on a FR 900 schedule which was characterized by long periods of no responding. Dews (1958b) reported that methamphetamine increased response rate by decreasing the length of these periods of no responding.

Drugs have also been shown to affect differentially responding during FI schedules of reinforcement. One way to analyze drug effects on different rates of responding in an FI component is to examine response patterns. The quarter life statistic is often used to quantify FI response patterns. The quarter life is a measure of the time required for the first 25% of the responses to occur (see Chapter 1, p. 16). If a drug produces an increase in response rate early in the FI component and/or decreases response rate later in the FI, the quarter life might decrease while overall response rates remain unchanged. For example, chlorpromazine has been reported to decrease quarter life at doses (3.0–10 mg/ kg) which do not decrease overall FI rates of responding (Leander, 1975). The decreases in quarter life were due to drug-induced increases in the low rates of responding early in the FI and decreases later in the FI.

Drug effects on different rates of responding during an FI component can also be analyzed by examining drug effects at different times in the FI. Smith (1964) examined the effects of d-amphetamine, pipradrol, cocaine and imipramine in pigeons during the first and last minute of an FI 5-min schedule of food presentation. All drugs increased the low rates of responding during the first minute of the interval, while they decreased the high rates during the last minute of the interval.

Drug effects have also been analyzed on the rate of responding in several segments of an FI schedule. For example, if an FI component is divided into several segments, rates of responding during each segment can be computed, and drug effects can be analyzed in terms of changes in each segment of the FI component. A convenient way to represent these effects is to plot response rates after drug administration as a function of pre-drug rates of responding during each segment of the schedule. Pre-drug control rates are represented on the abscissa and the drug effects are expressed as a percent of pre-drug or control rate on the ordinate. If the drug produced no change in response rate, responding after drug administration is represented at 100% of control rate. Increases in responding following drug administration are represented as greater than 100% of control rate; decreases as less than 100% of control rate. When these values are plotted on logarithmic coordinates, a linear function will appear if there is a rate-dependent relationship between a drug's effect and pre-drug rates of responding. For example, McKearney (1972) observed a rate-dependent effect for amphetamine in successive minutes of an FI 10-min schedule of food presentation. Alterations in response rate following d-amphetamine were an inverse function of pre-drug response rate within each of the ten 1-min segments of the FI. Figure 9-7 illustrates this relationship for d-amphetamine on rates of responding generated in 10 different 1-min segments of an FI 10-min schedule and on overall rate of responding during an FR component. The low control rates engendered during the first few minutes of the FI (0.01–0.1 responses per second) were increased by d-amphetamine, the intermediate rates (0.1–0.3 responses per second) were increased only slightly, and the high rates

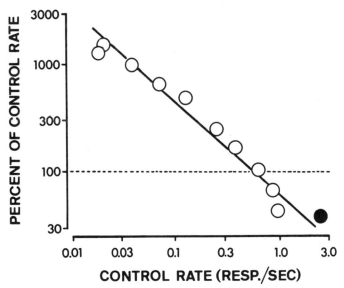

Fig. 9-7. Change in response rate in each 1-min segment of the FI 10-min component (o) and the FR 30 component (•) of a multiple FR FI schedule of food presentation as a function of control rates of responding following d-amphetamine. Coordinates are logarithmic. Each point represents a single observation. Note that there is an inverse linear relationship between control rate and amount of increase after d-amphetamine. (From McKearney, 1972.)

(0.3–1.0 responses per second) were decreased. Responding on the FR 30 schedule which occurred at a rate of 3.0 responses per second was also decreased.

Rate-dependent effects on FI schedules of reinforcement have also been reported for amobarbital (Dews, 1964), pentobarbital (Leander and McMillan, 1974), diazepam, chlordiazepoxide, nitrazepam (Wuttke and Kelleher, 1970; McMillan, 1973a), imipramine (Dews, 1962; Smith, 1964) and scopolamine (McKim, 1973). Chlorpromazine and a variety of phenothiazines also produce rate-dependent effects on FI schedules (Fry *et al.*, 1960; Marr, 1970; Leander and McMillan, 1974; Leander, 1975; Dews, 1962). The fact that these drugs increase very low rates of responding which occur early in an FI while decreasing higher rates that occur later in the interval is interesting in light of the fact that they generally only decrease overall response rates.

Variables Which Modify Rate-Dependent Effects

Schedule of Reinforcement. While available experimental evidence suggests that a drug effect on schedule-controlled behavior is related to the rate of responding generated by a particular schedule of reinforcement, it is not clear whether the drug effect depends on the rate of responding generated by the particular schedule or some other factor related to the schedule such as frequency of reinforcement or response patterning. In an attempt to investigate the role of rate-dependency versus schedule-dependency, McMillan (1969) examined the effects of *d*-amphetamine on several parameters of a multiple FR FI schedule in pigeons. Three different FR components (FR 30, FR 150 and FR 250) and two FI components (FI 5-min and FI 60-sec) were examined. While the FR 30 schedule of food presentation generates high rates of responding (about 3.0 responses per second), the FR 150 and 250 generate much lower rates (1.0 response per second or less). On the other hand, an FI 5-min schedule generates low response rates (0.7 response per second) while an FI 60-sec schedule generates much higher rates (2.0 responses per second). *d*-Amphetamine produced rate-dependent effects under each schedule condition. When FI rates were low (under the FI 5-min), *d*-amphetamine increased the rate of responding at low doses (0.3–1.0 mg/kg). When FI rates were high (FI 60-sec), *d*-amphetamine (3.0 and 5.6 mg/kg) only produced decreases in the rate of responding. In the FR 30 schedule (which produced a high rate of responding), low doses of *d*-amphetamine (0.3 and 1.0 mg/kg) had no effect, while high doses decreased response rates. Larger FR requirements, which produced lower response rates were followed either by amphetamine-induced increases in rate of responding at low doses or decreases at higher doses (see Fig. 9-8 and compare it to Fig. 9-2). Therefore, the effects of amphetamine seem to be more closely related to control rates of responding than to the schedule of reinforcement. Similarly, the effects of amobarbital have been shown to depend on the pre-drug rate of

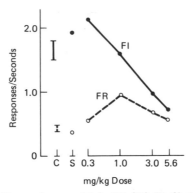

Fig. 9-8. Rate of responding under a multiple FR 250 FI 60 LH 720 schedule of food presentation as a function of four doses of *d*-amphetamine in pigeons. The brackets at *C* represent the range of control values during sessions just before each drug session, and the points at *S* show response rates after a saline injection. Each point is the mean of single determinations in each of four birds. (From McMillan, 1969.)

responding generated by different schedule parameters (Morse, 1962). Pigeons were trained to respond on two different FR schedules of reinforcement (FR 33 and FR 330) and on two different DRL schedules (DRL 10-sec and DRL 100-sec). A dose of 10 mg/kg of amobarbital increased responding on the FR 330 schedule and had little effect on responding on the DRL 100-sec schedule, both of which generated low pre-drug response rates. The same dose of amobarbital decreased responding on the FR 33 schedule and on the DRL 10-sec schedule, both of which generated high pre-drug response rates.

While these studies indicate that drug effects are more closely related to control rates of responding than to the schedule of reinforcement, it should be noted that each schedule produced different frequencies of reinforcement. Therefore, the differences observed may be due to differences in reinforcement frequency rather than response rate. MacPhail and Gollub (1975) developed a procedure in which response rate could be manipulated independently of reinforcement frequency. They examined the effects of *d*-amphetamine and scopolamine on a multiple schedule in which each of three components generated a different response rate but the same frequency of reinforcement. The effects of both *d*-amphetamine and scopolamine were found to depend on pre-drug response rate and on drug dose but not on reinforcement frequency. (See also Sanger and Blackman, 1975b.)

Therefore, these studies all indicate that response rate is a fundamental determinant of a drug effect; however, in a few situations schedule parameters have been shown to determine drug effects even when both schedules maintain the same rate of responding (MacPhail, 1971; Brown and Seiden, 1975).

Discriminative Stimuli.   Recent reports indicate that the rate-dependent effects of a variety of drugs can be modified by the intensity and mode of presentation of environmental stimuli associated with the schedule under which the behavior is maintained.   Laties and Weiss (1966) found that the effects of drugs on an FI schedule of food presentation could be changed by adding an external stimulus (or "clock") to the FI schedule.   They used a multiple FI 5-min FI 5-min schedule.   During one component, different stimuli were presented for each successive minute of the FI clock.   No temporally correlated stimuli were present in the other component.   In the clock component, most responding occurred during the last minute of the interval.   In the conventional, no-clock condition, some responding occurred earlier in the FI.   The effects of five different drugs were examined: amphetamine, scopolamine, pentobarbital, chlorpromazine and promazine.   Laties and Weiss (1966) found that amphetamine, pentobarbital and scopolamine increased low rates of responding less under the FI clock schedule than the low rates under the conventional (no-clock) FI schedule.   While amphetamine, pentobarbital and scopolamine produced only negligible increases in the clock condition, both chlorpromazine and promazine increased response rate during both the clock condition and the no-clock condition (Fig. 9-9).

Similar effects have been reported by Thompson and Corr (1974).   Thompson used a multiple VI 1-min VI 1-min schedule of food presentation.   In one component, a stimulus signaled reinforcement availability.   *d*-Amphetamine did not increase low rates of responding in the signaled component, while it did increase higher response rates in the nonsignaled component.   Similarly, *d*-amphetamine did not increase the low response rates engendered by a DRL schedule when a stimulus was added to signal reinforcement availability.   Rate increases were seen after amphetamine when no signal was present (Carey and Kritkausky, 1972).

While these effects suggest that discriminative stimuli can alter drug effects, this interpretation is confounded by the fact that the schedules examined produced different response rates in the presence and absence of discriminative stimuli.   Nevertheless, in situations in which rate of responding is the same under conditions in which discriminative stimuli are present or absent, drug effects are altered by the presence of discriminative stimuli.   For example, Laties (1972) found that discriminative stimuli can modify the effects of a drug on a consecutive number schedule.   In this schedule the pigeon makes a specified number of consecutive responses on one key.   After the correct number of responses have been made, a response on a second key is reinforced.   Laties used two versions of this schedule.   In one, an external stimulus was presented when the correct number of responses had been made on the first key.   In the other version, no stimulus was presented.   Response rates in the signaled and unsignaled versions were the same, but the schedule with the external stimulus produced more reinforced response sequences.   When a discriminative stimulus was not present, *d*-

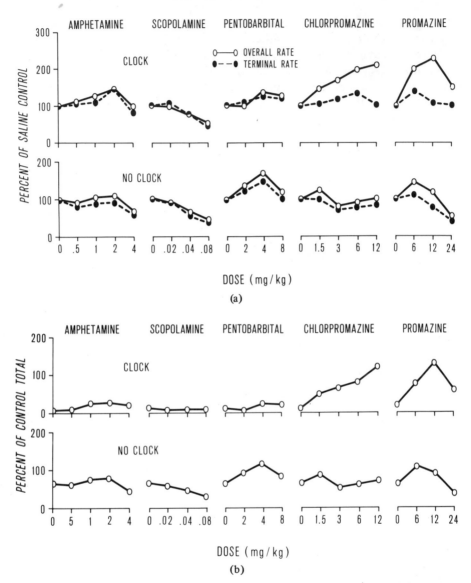

Fig. 9-9. Rate of responding as percent of control on an FI 5-min schedule of reinforcement with or without a stimulus (clock) to signal each minute of the FI as a function of saline (0 dose) and several doses of amphetamine, scopolamine, pentobarbital, chlorpromazine and promazine. Plot (a) represents drug effects on overall response rates (average rate during the entire FI 5-min schedule, and on terminal response rates (rate during the last minute of the FI 5-min). Plot (b) presents drug effects on response rates during the first 4 min of the FI 5-min. (From Laties and Weiss, 1966.)

amphetamine and scopolamine produced increases in premature switching to the reinforcement key. These effects were attenuated somewhat by the addition of the discriminative stimulus. On the other hand, increases in premature switching following chlorpromazine and promazine were not altered by a discriminative stimulus. Wagman and Maxey(1969) report similar effects with scopolamine in a similar procedure with rats. This work suggests that amphetamine and scopolamine are less likely to increase low rates of responding when discriminative stimuli are present, while the effects of chlorpromazine and promazine are not altered by the presence of a discriminative stimulus. On the other hand, Byrd (1974) has shown that the effects of chlorpromazine in chimpanzees on a multiple FR FI schedule of food presentation were different when a brief (20 msec) auditory stimulus followed each response. Responding was examined under two conditions. In one condition, all responses were followed by a brief auditory stimulus; in the other condition, no additional stimuli were present. Chlorpromazine increased responding on the FI component under both conditions; however, the rate-increasing effects of chlorpromazine on the FI component were enhanced when a brief auditory stimulus followed each response.

Other evidence suggests that drug-induced decreases in high rates of responding maintained by FR schedules of food presentation can be modified by discriminative stimuli. Leander and McMillan (1974) compared the effects of chlorpromazine on performance of pigeons under a multiple FR 30 FI 5-min schedule and a mixed FR 30 FI 5-min schedule. On the multiple schedule, external stimuli signal the different schedule components, while in the mixed schedule, discriminative stimuli are not present (see Chapter 1). A dose of 3.0 mg/kg of chlorpromazine decreased FR responding in the mixed schedule, whereas 100 mg/kg of chlorpromazine was required to produce an equivalent decrease in FR responding in the multiple schedule.

Therefore, drug effects may be determined by the degree to which the behavior under investigation is controlled by discriminative stimuli. Unfortunately, we have no way to express the strength of control exerted by discriminative stimuli except to observe differential rates of responding in their presence. Since rate and pattern of responding are often altered by drug administration, it is difficult to separate drug effects on discriminative control from effects on the measure of discriminative control (see Chapter 10 for a more thorough discussion of this problem; see also Branch, 1974; McKearney, 1970 and Laties, 1975, for a review of this literature).

Punishing Stimuli. While a variety of studies have clearly demonstrated that several drugs increase low rates of responding, the low response rates which occur when responding is followed by electric shock (i.e., punished) are not always increased. For example, it has been reported that amphetamine does not

increase low rates of punished responding.   Indeed, it has sometimes been reported that amphetamine further reduces low rates of punsihed responding
(Geller and Seifter, 1960; Morrison, 1969; Hanson *et al.*, 1967).

While these reports indicate that amphetamine does not increase low rates of
responding when responding is suppressed by punishment, McMillan (1973a)
has shown that amphetamine will increase low rates of punished responding
under certain conditions.   McMillan (1973a) trained pigeons under a multiple
FI 5-min FI 5-min schedule of food presentation.   In one component (unpunished) responding was maintained by an FI 5-min schedule of food presentation,
and in the other component (punished) responding was maintained by an FI
5-min schedule of food presentation in which all responses were also followed by
shock.   McMillan then examined the effects of *d*-amphetamine on punished and
unpunished responding which occurred at equal rates.   Low doses of *d*-ampheta-
mine increased the low rates of both punished and unpunished responding; however, low rates of responding in the unpunished component were increased more
than equally low rates in the punished component.   Chlorpromazine, like amphetamine, increased low rates of unpunished responding more than low rates of
punished responding, but diazepam, chlordiazepoxide or pentobarbital tended
to increase low rates of punished responding more than matched rates of unpunished responding.   Therefore, although the effects of a variety of drugs are
clearly rate-dependent in that they increase low rates of both punished and unpunished responding, punishment can modify these rate-dependent effects under
certain conditions.   (See punishment section for further discussion of these
results.)

We might conclude that while pre-drug rate of responding remains one of the
most important determinants of a drug's effect, rate-dependent effects are influenced by a variety of factors, including the presence or absence of discriminative or punishing stimuli and sometimes schedule variables.   In summary, we
have seen that a drug effect on behavior maintained by schedules of positive
reinforcement depends on pharmacological variables such as the particular drug
and the dose.   Moreover, drug effects were shown to be related to the rate of
responding generated by a particular schedule of reinforcement.   As Dews (1971,
p. 41) has written: "Schedules are not the exclusive determinants of behavior
nor of drug effects thereon; but they are ubiquitous as well as powerful and their
effects must always be taken into serious account, from the first, in the analysis
of drug effects on behavior."

NEGATIVE REINFORCEMENT

Negative reinforcement increases the rate or probability of occurrence of a response that terminates or postpones an event such as electric shock.   Generally,
two procedures are used as baselines to access the effects of drugs on behavior

maintained by negative reinforcement. These two procedures—discrete trial avoidance and continuous avoidance—are described in Chapter 1. It has been suggested that drugs which affect behavior maintained by negative reinforcement do so through their actions on internal states of fear and anxiety. For example, behavior in a discrete trial avoidance procedure has been interpreted in the following way: A stimulus paired with the occurrence of an avoidable shock was thought to produce a state of anxiety in the animal since it signaled impending shock. When the animal terminated or avoided this stimulus, he was said to reduce anxiety (Miller *et al.*, 1957; Hunt, 1957). If the animal no longer avoided the shock after drug administration, then the drug was said to produce a state in which the animal no longer feared nor was anxious about the impending shock. We will see in a later section that this interpretation is not viable. When one compares the effects of drugs on various procedures maintained by shock, all of which might be assumed to involve fear or anxiety, it becomes apparent that drug effects depend more on variables related to the experimental design and the behavioral patterns developed in such experiments than to the fact that behavior is maintained by shock. Nevertheless, this interpretation is important historically since drugs that have received most attention in terms of their effects on behavior maintained by negative reinforcement are drugs which traditionally have been thought to modify emotional states—i.e., antipsychotics, benzodiazepines, barbiturates and narcotics.

In 1953 Courvoisier *et al.* examined the effects of chlorpromazine on a pole jump avoidance task. They found that chlorpromazine suppressed the avoidance response at doses that neither produced ataxia nor impaired performance of the escape response. Since the rats were capable of escaping the shock, motor deficits were ruled out as a factor in the chlorpromazine effect. Moreover, since avoidance responding was suppressed while escape responding remained unchanged, chlorpromazine was said to have a "selective" effect on avoidance. Cook and Weidley (1957) confirmed this finding. They showed that a dose of chlorpromazine (40 mg/kg) which blocked avoidance responding in 100% of their rats only blocked escape responding in 15% of their rats. Furthermore, they found that the *selective* blockade of avoidance, although not unique to chlorpromazine (morphine acts similarly), was not a general characteristic of all drugs. Barbital, pentobarbital, secobarbital and chlordiazepoxide have all been reported to block avoidance responses only at doses that blocked escape responses and produced ataxia. These effects contrast with the effects of chlorpromazine, which decreases avoidance responding without affecting escape responding.

Similar effects are reported for chlorpromazine in the continuous avoidance procedure. Recall that in the continuous avoidance procedure, shocks are scheduled to occur at specified intervals (SS interval) in the absence of responding, and responses postpone the occurrence of shock for a specified period of time

(RS interval). It should be noted that the overall rate of responding in a continuous avoidance procedure does not always correlate with the number of shocks received. Since each response postpones shock for a specified interval, and since the timing of the interval starts immediately after each response, a few evenly spaced responses will postpone shock longer than a burst of responses. Therefore, it is important to measure both response rate and shock rate when describing a drug's effect on continuous avoidance, or alternatively to use a procedure in which shock rate, response rate and escape failure can be measured separately. In one such procedure, shocks are avoided by responses on one lever and escaped by responses on another lever. Drugs that increase shock rate in the continuous avoidance procedure at doses which do not decrease overall response rate or produce escape failure are said to have a "selective" effect on avoidance.

Heise and Boff (1962) examined the effects of a variety of drugs in a modified continuous avoidance procedure in which shocks were scheduled to occur every 20 sec (SS interval) and responding postponed shock for 40 sec (RS interval). Rats postponed shock by responding on one lever. If a shock occurred, it could be terminated (escaped) by a response on a second lever. The dose of a drug that increased shock rates and the dose that produced failure to escape the shock were determined. The median effective dose for escape failure was divided by the median effective dose for shock-rate increase, and the resulting number was called the dose-range ratio. For example, if the median effective dose (M.E.D.) of chlorpromazine for increasing shock were 0.20 mg/kg and the M.E.D. for producing failure to escape were 0.60 mg/kg, the dose-range ratio would be 3.0 A ratio of 1.0 would indicate that avoidance and escape responses were affected at the same dose. The dose-range ratios for a variety of drugs are presented in Table 9-2. Morphine has a dose-range ratio similar to that of chlorpromazine, indicating that it has a *selective* effect on avoidance. Both diazepam and chlordiazepoxide increase shock rate at a dose much lower than that which produces escape failure, as indicated by their very high dose-range

TABLE 9-2. Dose-range ratios: Avoidance/escape responding

Drug	Dose-range ratio
Chlorpromazine	3.4
Morphine	2.7
Barbiturates:	
Phenobarbital	2.1
Hexobarbital	1.7
Pentobarbital	1.1
Chlordiazepoxide	3.8
Diazepam	5.5

From Heise and Boff (1962).

ratios (3.8 for chlordiazepoxide and 5.5 for diazepam). Phenobarbital and hexobarbital have similar but less dramatic effects, while pentobarbital affects avoidance and escape responding at about the same dose.

Table 9-3 summarizes the effects of a variety of drugs on discrete trial and continuous avoidance procedures. Interest in drug effects on avoidance has centered around the antipsychotics, narcotics, barbiturates and benzodiazepines. Only these will be discussed in detail in the text, followed by a discussion of some of the variables that have been shown to be important in avoidance.

General Effects

Antipsychotics. Chlorpromazine produces a *selective* effect in both discrete trial and continuous avoidance procedures. This effect has been demonstrated in rats, dogs and monkeys and occurs following a variety of other phenothiazine derivatives, reserpine (also see Chapter 5) and haloperidol. Figure 9-10 illustrates the effect of chlorpromazine on a discrete trial avoidance procedure. Rats were trained to turn a wheel in order to avoid or escape shock. A buzzer sounded for seven seconds prior to the scheduled occurrence of shock, and it remained on until the shock was presented or a response occurred. Chlorpromazine (4.0 mg/kg) decreased avoidance responding to 20% of control, while escape responding remained at 95–100% control. Smaller doses produced a similar effect, but avoidance responding was reduced less. For example, 2.5 mg/kg of

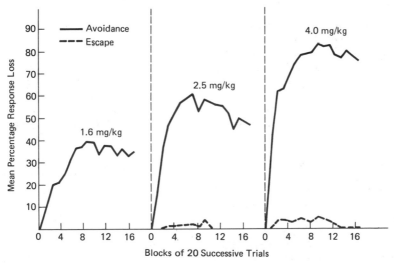

Fig. 9-10. Percentage of avoidance and escape responses blocked by three doses of chlorpromazine as a function of 20 successive trials. (From Verhave *et al.*, 1958.)

TABLE 9-3. Drug effects on behavior maintained by negative reinforcement

Schedule	Effect	Reference
PSYCHOMOTOR STIMULANTS (*d*-amphetamine, methamphetamine, cocaine, pipradrol, methylphenidate)		
Continuous avoidance	usually increases avoidance responding; however, decreases have been reported at very high doses that also produce decreases in overall response rate	Verhave (1958); Weissman (1959, 1963); Heise and Boff (1962); Stone (1964); Scheckel and Boff (1964); Pearl *et al.* (1968); Davis *et al.* (1973); Houser (1973)
ANTIPSYCHOTICS (amiperone, benperidol, chlorpromazine, chlorprothixene, clofluperol, cyclopromazine, droperidol, fluanisone, fluphenazine, haloperidol, moperone, perphenazine, pimozide, pipamperone, promazine, reserpine, spiramide, spirilene, spiroperidol, tetrabenazine, thioperazine, trifluoperazine, trifluperidol, triflupromazine, thioridazine)		
Discrete trial avoidance	decreases avoidance responding at doses that do not produce escape failure	Courvoisier *et al.* (1953); Cook and Weidley (1957); Smith *et al.* (1957); Verhave *et al.* (1958); John *et al.* (1958); Maffii (1959); Irwin *et al.* (1959); Herz (1960); Domino *et al.* (1963); Clark and Samuel (1969)
Continuous avoidance	decreases avoidance responding at doses that do not decrease overall response rates or produce escape failure	Boren (1961b); Clark and Steele (1963); Heise and Boff (1962); Cook and Kelleher (1962); Stone (1964); Scheckel and Boff (1964); Hanson *et al.* (1967, 1970); Niemegeers *et al.* (1969)
ANTIANXIETY AGENTS (barbital, pentobarbital, secobarbital, phenobarbital, hexobarbital, chlordiazepoxide, diazepam)		
Discrete trial avoidance	decreases avoidance responding only at doses that produce escape failure	Cook and Weidley (1957); Verhave *et al.* (1957, 1959); Randall *et al.* (1960); Domino *et al.* (1963); Clark and Samuel (1969)
Continuous avoidance	generally decreases avoidance responding at doses that do not decrease overall response rates nor produce escape failure	Randall *et al.* (1960); Heise and Boff (1962); Cook and Kelleher (1962); Bignami *et al.* (1971)
NARCOTIC ANALGESICS AND NARCOTIC ANTAGONISTS (morphine, codeine, pentazocine, naloxone, levallorphan, cyclazocine)		
Discrete trial avoidance	decreases avoidance responding at doses that do not produce escape failure	Cook and Weidley (1957); Maffii (1959); Verhave *et al.* (1959); Clark and Samuel (1969)
Continuous avoidance	usually decreases avoidance responding at doses that do not change overall response rates or produce escape failure; however, increases have been reported in rats	Heise and Boff (1962); Cook and Kelleher (1962); Holtzman and Jewett (1972a, b); Steinert *et al.* (1973); Holtzman (1974a, b, c, d)

Schedule	Effect	Reference
TRICYCLIC ANTIDEPRESSANTS (imipramine, amitriptyline, doxepin, butriptylin, nortriptyline)		
Continuous avoidance	either has no effect or decreases avoidance responding at doses that decrease response rate	Heise and Boff (1962); Cook and Kelleher (1963); Scheckel and Boff (1964); Owen and Rathbun (1966); Molinengo and Ricci-Gamalero (1972)
ETHANOL		
Discrete trial avoidance	decreases avoidance responding at doses that produce escape failure	Herz (1960)
Continuous avoidance	increases avoidance responding at low doses; decreases avoidance responding at doses that decrease overall response rate	Heise and Boff (1962); Reynolds and van Sommers (1960)
HALLUCINOGENS (LSD)		
Discrete trial avoidance	decreases avoidance responding at doses that do not produce escape failure	Cook and Weidley (1957)
Continuous avoidance	decreases avoidance responding at doses that do not decrease overall response rate; however, low doses have been reported to increase avoidance responding	Jarrard (1963); Wray (1972)
TETRAHYDROCANNABINOL (THC)		
Continuous avoidance	usually decreases avoidance responding	Scheckel *et al.* (1968); Barry and Kubena (1970)
CHOLINERGIC BLOCKERS (scopolamine, atropine, benactyzine)		
Continuous avoidance	usually decreases avoidance responding at doses that decrease overall response rate; however, increases in responding have been reported at low doses	Herrnstein (1958); Heise and Boff (1962); Scheckel and Boff (1964); Stone (1964)
CHOLINERGIC AGONISTS (nicotine)		
Continuous avoidance	increases avoidance responding at doses that increase overall response rate	Pradhan (1970)

chlorpromazine decreased avoidance responding to 40% of control; 1.6 mg/kg decreased it to 60% of control (Verhave *et al.*, 1958).

Chlorpromazine also alters avoidance responding (i.e., increases shock rate) in the continuous avoidance procedure, while overall response rates are unchanged (Boren, 1961b). The fact that shock rates increased while response rates remained unchanged can be attributed to the pattern of responding generated by the continuous avoidance procedure. On those occasions when the rat failed to avoid a shock following chlorpromazine, responding occurred at a very high rate immediately after the shock (called postshock bursts). When these postshock bursts were averaged in with lower response rates before shock presentation, overall response rates did not change. Boren (1961a) further examined postshock bursts with the following procedure: rats were trained to avoid shock on one lever and escape it on a second lever. He found that postshock bursts which followed the escape response occurred only on the escape lever, indicating that escape responses were distinct from avoidance responses which occurred on the other lever.

Narcotic Analgesics and Narcotic Antagonists. In general, the effects of morphine are similar to those of chlorpromazine. That is, in both discrete trial and continuous avoidance procedures, morphine has a selective effect on avoidance (see Table 9-3). Holtzman and his colleagues, however, reported that morphine increased avoidance responding in rats at low doses (0.3–3.0 mg/kg) and decreased it at higher doses (10 mg/kg) (Holtzman, 1974c,d). Similar effects were reported for a variety of drugs with narcotic antagonist activity, including pentazocine, cyclazocine and nalorphine (Holtzman and Jewett, 1972a,b; 1973; Holtzman, 1974b,c,d). Naloxone had no effect on avoidance responding in the rat when given alone (Holtzman, 1974a; Steinert *et al.*, 1973); however, naloxone antagonized both the rate-increasing and rate-decreasing effects of pentazocine, cyclazocine and nalorphine (Holtzman and Jewett, 1972a,b; 1973; Holtzman, 1974b,c) (see Fig. 9-11).

Antianxiety Agents. The effects of the barbiturates and benzodiazepines differ from those of chlorpromazine and morphine on discrete trial avoidance. Figure 9-12 illustrates the effect of three doses of secobarbital on both escape and avoidance responses in a discrete trial avoidance procedure. These effects contrast with the effects of chlorpromazine illustrated in Fig. 9-10, in which chlorpromazine was shown to decrease avoidance responding without affecting escape responding.

On continuous avoidance procedures, phenobarbital, hexobarbital, diazepam and chlordiazepoxide generally decrease avoidance responding at doses that do not decrease overall response rates or produce escape failure. While these effects have generally been confirmed, all data are not consistent. For example, the dose of phenobarbital that increased shock rate on a continuous shock avoid-

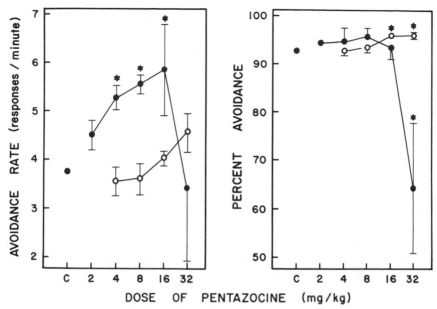

Fig. 9-11. Avoidance rate and percent avoidance as a function of dose of pentazocine when given alone (●———●) and when given with 8 mg/kg of naloxone (○———○) in rats. Each point in the dose-response curves represents the mean of one observation in each of four rats. The points at *C* represent the mean level of performance of the four rats in a total of 33 control sessions. The vertical lines represent ±S.E.M. Where vertical lines are not shown, the S.E.M. was less than the radius of the point. *, Significantly different from control; *P* < .05. (From Holtzman and Jewett, 1972a.)

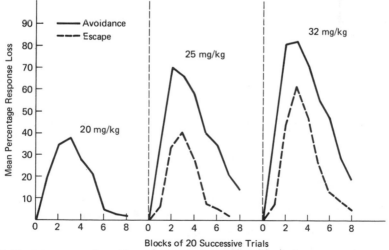

Fig. 9-12. Percentage of avoidance and escape responses blocked by three doses of seco-barbital as a function of 20 successive trials. (From Verhave *et al.*, 1958.)

ance procedure in squirrel monkeys also produced a failure to escape the shock and was accompanied by ataxia (Cook and Kelleher, 1962).

Therefore, the effects of the antianxiety agents on avoidance depend on the particular drug and avoidance procedure examined. On discrete trial avoidance, both barbiturates and benzodiazepines decrease avoidance responding only at doses that also block escape responding. On continuous avoidance, the benzodiazepines and some barbiturates have been reported to decrease avoidance at doses which do not produce escape failure (Table 9-2).

Table 9-3 presents a summary of the effects of a variety of other drugs on avoidance responding. The effects of the psychomotor stimulants, the tricyclic antidepressents, ethanol, LSD, THC and cholinergic agents on avoidance have been examined less frequently than those of the drugs discussed above, and reports are often variable. Chlorpromazine-like effects (i.e., decreases in avoidance at doses that do not affect overall response rate or produce escape failure) have been reported for LSD. Decreases in avoidance only at doses which also decrease overall response rate or produce escape failure are usually reported for the tricyclic antidepressants and ethanol. Both nicotine and amphetamine have been reported to increase avoidance.

While these studies have shown that different drugs affect avoidance responding differentially, and that these effects may depend on the particular avoidance procedure employed, it is always important to recall that any generalization about a drug effect must be qualified by the dose of the drug, the experimental subject and the particular conditions of the experiment. Moreover, we saw earlier in this chapter that rate of responding is an important determinant of drug effects on behavior maintained by positive reinforcement. Therefore, it is interesting to examine the relationship between rate of responding and a drug's effect on behavior maintained by negative reinforcement.

Rate-Dependency

The question of whether a drug affects avoidance responding by virtue of its effect on overall rate of responding is answered in part in the discrete trial avoidance procedure by the fact that one response—the avoidance response—is decreased, while another response—the escape response—is not affected. The question is complicated however, in the continuous avoidance procedure since the pattern of responding as well as the rate of responding determines the number of shocks received. Recall that the overall rate of responding in a continuous avoidance procedure does not always correlate with the number of shocks received. Since each response postpones shock for a specified interval, and since the timing of the interval starts immediately after the response, a few evenly spaced responses will postpone shock longer than a burst of responses. Therefore, it is important to look at both pre-drug shock rate and pre-drug response rate in examining the possibility that drug-induced changes in avoidance responding depend upon pre-drug response rate.

Bignami *et al.* (1971) examined the relationship between pre-drug response rates and shock rates and the effects of phenobarbital, chlordiazepoxide and diazepam on a continuous avoidance procedure. They found that the pre-drug shock rate rather than pre-drug response rate determined the effect of the drugs. Chlordiazepoxide, phenobarbital and diazepam produced decreases in shock rate in rats with high pre-drug shock rates, whereas increases were seen in rats with low pre-drug shock rates. When these drugs decreased shock rate, response rates did not necessarily increase, since the drugs tended to produce a more evenly spaced pattern of responding. (See also Weissman, 1963.)

Other Variables

A number of variables have been shown to interact with drug effects on avoidance. In Chapter 1, the acquisition and maintenance of avoidance responding was shown to depend on such factors as the shock level used, the nature of the

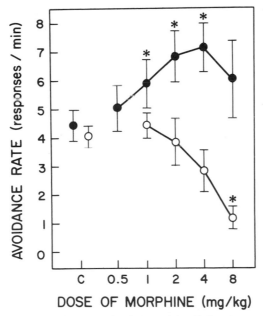

Fig. 9-13. Avoidance rate under two shock intensities (1.3 mA, ●————● and 0.8 mA, ○————○) as a function of dose of morphine in rats. Each point represents the mean of one observation in each of five rats. Vertical lines represent ±1 S.E.M. The control values (*C*) for each group are represented by the isolated points at the left. *, Significantly different from control; *P* < 0.05. (From Holtzman and Jewett, 1972c.)

preshock stimulus (buzzer, light, tone) and the interval between shocks. These factors, and others, may modify drug effects as well.

One important variable which has been shown to interact with drug effects on discrete trial avoidance performance is the time between the onset of the preshock stimulus and the shock. For example, Low et al. (1966) trained rats to avoid shock in a shuttle box. They used three different intervals between the preshock stimulus and the shock (5, 10 or 15 sec). Chlorpromazine did not decrease avoidance responding with the 5- or 10-sec interval, but did with the 15-sec interval.

Holtzman and Jewett (1972c) found that the effects of morphine on a continuous avoidance schedule in rats depended on shock intensity. While control rates of responding did not differ when an 0.8-mA or a 1.3-mA shock was used, morphine (0.5-8.0 mg/kg) increased response rate in rats at the high shock intensity, while it either had no effect or decreased responding at the low shock intensity (see Fig. 9-13).

Other factors that have been shown to interact with drug effects in both discrete trial and continuous avoidance procedures are rate of acquisition (Latz et al., 1969), species (Clark and Samuel, 1969), strain (Fuller, 1966), age (Doty and Doty, 1966) and the nature of the preshock stimulus (John et al., 1958; Cook and Catania, 1964).

PROCEDURES THAT DECREASE RESPONSE RATE

Under many conditions response rate is decreased when an event such as electric shock is presented following a response. The barbiturates and benzodiazepines generally produce increases in responding suppressed by shock presentation. In this respect they differ from the antipsychotics, psychomotor stimulants, narcotics and a variety of other drugs that normally do not restore behavior suppressed by shock. For example, diazepam has been reported to increase punished responding in rats. In a punishment procedure responding is usually maintained by a schedule of positive reinforcement, and shock is presented contingent on a response. Figure 9-14 illustrates the response pattern of one rat in a punishment procedure before and after diazepam. Note that response rates were high when responding was simply followed by food presentation alone. When every tenth response was followed by food and shock, responding was suppressed. Responding suppressed during the punishment component was increased following diazepam.

Table 9-4 presents the effects of a variety of drugs on two procedures generally used to decrease response rate, i.e., punishment and conditioned suppression. Recall from Chapter 1 that conditioned suppression is established by presenting a stimulus followed by an unavoidable shock. The effects of the barbiturates and benzodiazepines, antipsychotics, psychomotor stimulants and narcotics will

TABLE 9-4. Drug effects on behavior maintained by procedures that decrease response rate

Schedule	Effect	Reference
PSYCHOMOTOR STIMULANTS (*d*-, *dl*-amphetamine, cocaine)		
Punishment	usually does not increase responding suppressed by punishment; however, small increases have been reported under special conditions	Geller and Seifter (1960); Kelleher and Morse (1964); Hendry and Van Toller (1964); Hanson *et al.* (1967); Morrison (1969); Foree *et al.* (1973); McMillan (1973a); Miczek (1973b)
Conditioned suppression	does not increase responding suppressed by noncontingent shock	Brady (1956a, b); Lauener (1963); Hill *et al.* (1967); Tenen (1967); Miczek (1973a)
ANTIPSYCHOTICS (chlorpromazine, trifluoperazine, reserpine, tetrabenazine)		
Punishment	usually does not increase responding suppressed by punishment; however, increases have been reported when punished responding occurs at a very low rate	Geller and Seifter (1960); Grossman (1961); Geller *et al.* (1963); Morse (1964); Cook and Catania (1964); Kelleher and Morse (1964); Hanson *et al.* (1967); McMillan (1973a, b); Stitzer (1974)
Conditioned suppression	usually does not increase responding suppressed by noncontingent shock; however, increases have been reported under special conditions	Brady (1956a, b); Yamahiro *et al.* (1961); Kinnard *et al.* (1962); Lauener (1963); Tenen (1967); Hill *et al.* (1967)
ANTIANXIETY AGENTS (pentobarbital, phenobarbital, amobarbital, barbital, chlordiazepoxide, diazepam)		
Punishment	increases responding suppressed by punishment.	Geller and Seifter (1960); Geller *et al.* (1962); Morse (1964); Kelleher and Morse (1964); Cook and Catania (1964); Hanson *et al.* (1967); Morrison (1969); Wuttke and Kelleher (1970); McMillan (1973a); Cook and Davidson (1973); Miczek (1973b); McMillan and Leander (1975)
Conditioned suppression	increases responding suppressed by noncontingent shock	Lauener (1963); Tenen (1967); Hill *et al.* (1967); Scobie and Garske (1970); Miczek (1973a)
NARCOTIC ANALGESICS (morphine, methadone, meperidine)		
Punishment	usually decreases responding suppressed by punishment; however, increases have been reported	Geller *et al.* (1963); Kelleher and Morse (1964); Holtzman and Villarreal (1973); McMillan (1973a); Cook and Davidson (1973); Stitzer (1974)

Schedule	Effect	Reference
Conditioned suppression	either increases responding suppressed by noncontingent shock or has no effect	Lauener (1963); Hill *et al.* (1957, 1966, 1967)
TRICYCLIC ANTIDEPRESSANTS (imipramine)		
Punishment	either decreases further responding suppressed by punishment or has no effect	Morse (1964); Wuttke and Kelleher (1970); McMillan (1973a); Cook and Davidson (1973)
ETHANOL		
Punishment	variable effects	Hendry and Van Toller (1964); Cook and Davidson (1973); McMillan and Leander (1975)
Conditioned suppression	no effect	Lauener (1963)
HALLUCINOGENS (LSD, mescaline)		
Punishment	does not increase responding suppressed by punishment	Appel (1971); McMillan (1973a)
Conditioned suppression	increases responding suppressed by noncontingent shock under special conditions	Hill *et al.* (1967)
TETRAHYDROCANNABINOLS (Δ^8-THC; Δ^9-THC)		
Punishment	decreases further responding suppressed by punishment	McMillan (1973a)
CHOLINERGIC BLOCKERS (scopolamine)		
Punishment	either decreases further responding suppressed by punishment or has no effect	Hanson *et al.* (1970); Miczek (1973b)
Conditioned suppression	no effect	Miczek (1973a)
CHOLINERGIC AGONISTS (nicotine)		
Punishment	usually does not increase responding suppressed by punishment	Morrison (1969)

be discussed in detail. Variables important in determining drug effects on behavior suppressed by shock presentation will also be examined. These include pre-drug response rate, shock intensity and shock frequency.

General Effects

Antianxiety Agents. The barbiturates and the benzodiazepines generally increase responding suppressed by punishment. Moreover, it has been shown

RAT CONFLICT – PUNISHMENT

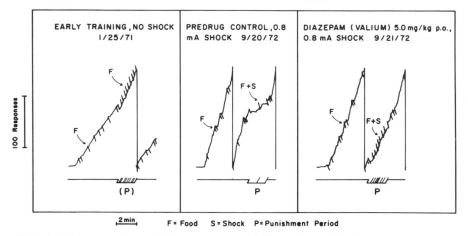

Fig. 9-14. Segments of cumulative response records illustrating: (1) high rates of responding when responding was maintained on a VI 30-sec schedule of food presentation; (2) suppressed responding during periods when every tenth response was followed by shock (P); and (3) increases in responding in P following diazepam. (From Cook and Sepinwall, 1975.)

that while these drugs usually increase responding suppressed by shock, they either do not change or decrease responding maintained by positive reinforcement.   For example, Geller *et al.* (1962) reported that chlordiazepoxide increased responding in the following schedule: Rats were maintained on a VI 2-min schedule of food presentation.   At certain times a tone was presented during which every response was followed by both food and shock.   While chlordiazepoxide (7.5–15.0 mg/kg) increased responding during the tone (i.e., when responding was punished), lower doses (7.5 mg/kg) did not affect variable interval rates and high doses (15–30 mg/kg) decreased variable interval rates.

Cook and Davidson (1973) report similar effects with several benzodiazepines and some barbiturates.   Figure 9-15 illustrates the effects of chlordiazepoxide on a procedure in which responding was maintained on a VI schedule of food presentation in one component of a multiple schedule.   In the other component, every tenth response was followed by food and shock.

Similar effects have been reported in rats, squirrel monkeys and pigeons (see Table 9-4).   Moreover, pentobarbital increased responding suppressed either by response-contingent shock or by time out from food presentation (McMillan, 1967).   These drugs also increased responding suppressed by a stimulus paired with an unavoidable shock in the conditioned suppression procedure, while responding maintained by positive reinforcement was not altered.

Antipsychotics.   In general, the antipsychotics do not increase responding that has been suppressed by punishment in pigeons, rats or squirrel monkeys (see

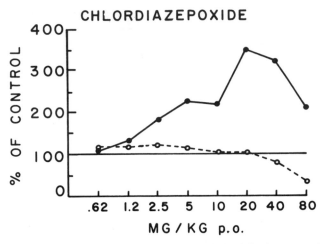

Fig. 9-15. Percent of control responding on a VI schedule of food presentation (o----o) and during a punishment component in which every tenth response was followed by food and shock (●————●) as a function of several oral doses of chlordiazepoxide. The solid horizontal line represents control level. At least 10 rats were examined at each dose except the 80 mg/kg-dose, at which 7 rats were examined. (From Cook and Sepinwall, 1975.)

Table 9-4).   There are reports, however, that chlorpromazine does increase punished responding occurring at a very low rate (McMillan, 1973a; Grossman, 1961; Dinsmoor and Lyon, 1961).   McMillan examined punished responding in pigeons on an FI schedule of food presentation in which every response was also followed by shock.   While overall rates of punished responding were not increased, the low rates of punished responding that occurred early in the FI were increased by chlorpromazine.

The antipsychotics are usually reported to have no effect on responding in the conditioned suppression paradigm (see Table 9-4); however, occasional increases have been reported (Appel, 1963; Brady, 1956a,b).   Brady (1956a,b) reported an increase with reserpine in the following procedure: Monkeys and rats were maintained on a VI 1-min schedule of juice or water presentation. A clicking noise was presented at regular intervals for a period of time (3-min in rats; 5-min in monkeys).   One-third to one-half of the times the clicker was presented, it terminated with a shock.   Daily doses of reserpine (0.2 mg/kg) increased response rates which had been suppressed during the clicker presentation, while rates during the nonclicker periods were decreased.   When responses that occurred during the clicker presentation were punished with shock, reserpine did not increase punished responding.   On the other hand, Yamahiro et al. (1961) reported no effect with reserpine (0.2 mg/kg–0.6 mg/kg daily) on a conditioned suppression paradigm in which a 4-min tone always terminated with shock.   It should be noted that in Brady's procedure, shock did not always follow the preshock stimulus, whereas in the Yamahiro *et al.* study, shock always followed the preshock stimulus. Moreover, intermittent shock presentation produced less suppression than when shock always followed the preshock stimulus. This difference in degree of response suppression may account for the different effects.

Psychomotor Stimulants. While amphetamine generally has no rate-increasing effect on responding followed by shock (see Table 9-4), in a few instances low doses of amphetamine have been reported to increase responding suppressed by shock. For example, low doses (0.1–1.0 mg/kg) of *d*-amphetamine increased punished responding in rats when responding was maintained on a VI 3-min schedule of food presentation in which every twelfth response was followed by shock. Shock intensities were adjusted so that the rate of punished responding was 35–65% of the rate before punishment (Miczek, 1973b). Similarly, McMillan (1973a) reported that in pigeons *d*-amphetamine (0.3–3.0 mg/kg) increased very low rates of punsihed responding that occurred early in an FI 5-min schedule. High rates of punished responding that occurred later in the FI were decreased. Moreover, McKearney and Barrett (1975) report that *d*-amphetamine increased punished responding in squirrel monkeys when periods of punished responding were alternated with shock avoidance periods.

Narcotic Analgesics. Increases in responding suppressed by punishment are usually not reported following morphine in rats (0.25–7.5 mg/kg), pigeons (0.3–10.0 mg/kg) or rhesus monkeys (0.5–4.0 mg/kg). Indeed, Holtzman and Villarreal (1973) report that in rhesus monkeys morphine further decreased responding suppressed by punishment; however, occasional increases in punished responding have been reported with morphine (see McMillan, 1973a; Stitzer, 1974; Cook and Davidson, 1973). The effects of morphine on the conditioned suppression procedure are not consistent, in that both increases (Hill *et al.*, 1967) or no effect (Lauener, 1963) have been reported.

Table 9-4 presents a summary of the effects of several drugs in punishment and conditioned suppression procedures with representative references. Briefly, responding suppressed by punishment or conditioned suppression procedures usually is not increased by imipramine, ethanol, mescaline, LSD, THC, scopolamine or nicotine.

As with all the procedures we have discussed, there are several variables that influence responding in punishment and conditioned suppression procedures and which determine how drugs affect behavior maintained by these procedures. For example, drug effects on punished responding have been related to pre-drug response rate, shock intensity and shock frequency. These variables are discussed below.

Rate-dependency

Since punished responding usually occurs at a low rate, the increase in responding following administration of a drug such as chlordiazepoxide may be merely an instance of a general tendency of these agents to increase low response rates, rather than a specific interaction between these drugs and punished responding. For example, when the effects of chlordiazepoxide, diazepam and nitrazepam were compared on equal rates of punished and unpunished responding in pigeons, it was shown that these drugs increased low rates equally under both conditions (Wuttke and Kelleher, 1970). On the other hand, Cook and Sepinwall (1975) found that chlordiazepoxide and diazepam did not increase equal rates of punished and unpunished responding to the same extent in squirrel monkeys. The following concurrent schedule was used: On one lever responding was maintained by a VI 1.5-min schedule of food presentation and a VR 24 schedule of footshock presentation. On another lever responding was main-

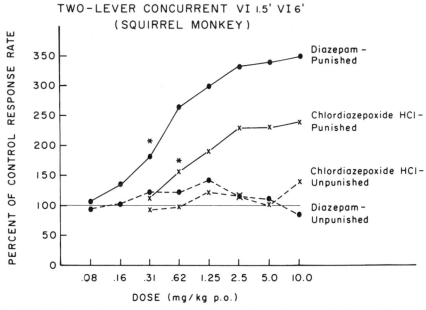

Fig. 9-16. Percent of control response rate on punished and unpunished responding in the squirrel monkey as a function of dose of diazepam or chlordiazepoxide. Unpunished responding was maintained on a VI 6-min schedule of food presentation, and punished responding was maintained on a VI 1.5-min schedule of food presentation and a VR 24 schedule of shock presentation. Shock level was adjusted (1.3–1.6 mA, 0.5 sec) so the two rates were roughly equal in control sessions. Solid horizontal line represents control performance. Each point represents the mean value for four monkeys. (From Cook and Sepinwall, 1975.)

tained by a VI 6-min schedule of food presentation. The rates of responding on the punished and unpunished levers were about equal. Chlordiazepoxide and diazepam increased punished responding more than unpunished responding (see Fig. 9-16). (See also Cook and Catania, 1964.)

Similarly, McMillan (1973a) reported that diazepam and chlordiazepoxide increased low rates of punished responding more than equally low rates of unpunished responding. McMillan used a multiple schedule. In one component responding was maintained by an FI 5-min schedule of food presentation, and in the other component responding was maintained by an FI 5-min schedule of food presentation in which all responses were also followed by shock (punished). While chlordiazepoxide and diazepam increased low rates of responding in both punished and unpunished components, punished responding was increased more than unpunished responding. Pentobarbital also increased low rates of punished responding more than equally low rates of unpunished responding. On the other hand, chlorpromazine and d-amphetamine increased low rates of unpunished responding more than equally low rates of punished responding. Therefore, while evidence is not always consistent, it appears that increases in punished responding following administration of the barbiturates or benzodiazepines cannot be attributed only to general rate-increasing effects.

Shock Intensity

Another important variable which determines a drug's effect on punished responding is shock intensity. For example, McMillan (1973b) found that diazepam and pentobarbital showed little tendency to increase overall rates of punished responding when shock intensity was low (2.5 mA); however, punished responding was increased when shock intensity was higher (4.3 mA and 5.2 mA).

It is important to note that the 2.5-mA shock barely suppressed responding, while the 4.3- and 5.2-mA shocks both decreased responding to near zero rates, suggesting that these effects may depend on the rate of responding maintained by various shock intensities rather than on the shock intensity itself. Nevertheless, responding was increased more following diazepam when the shock intensity was 4.3 mA than when it was 5.2 mA, even though both shock intensities suppressed responding equally, indicating that shock intensity and response rates are both important determinants of a drug effect (see Fig. 9-17).

Moreover, chlorpromazine, which normally does not increase responding suppressed by shock, will increase overall rates of responding suppressed by intense shock (3.4–5.2 mA), but only at a very high dose (30 mg/kg in pigeons) (McMillan, 1973b). On the other hand, morphine, which usually does not increase responding suppressed by shock, will increase punished responding when responding is moderately suppressed (74%) (Stitzer, 1974).

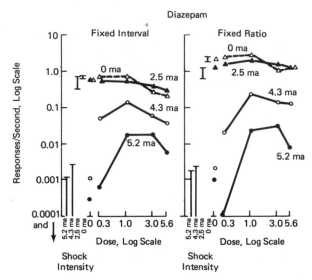

Fig. 9-17. Rate of responding under a multiple FI 5-min FR 30 schedule of food presentation in which all responses also produced electric shock at three different intensities (2.5 mA, 4.3 mA and 5.2 mA) as a function of dose of diazepam. The brackets represent the range of control rates observed during 12 sessions when injections were not given. The points at 0 on the abscissa show the effects of the injection vehicle. The shock intensity in milliamperes is shown beside each dose effect curve. Each point is the mean of a single observation in each of three birds. (From McMillan, 1973b.)

Other Variables

In some punishment procedures every response is followed by shock, while in others shock is only presented intermittently. Drug effects have also been shown to depend on the frequency of shock presentation (Foree *et al.*, 1973; Stitzer, 1974). Similarly, in a conditioned suppression procedure reserpine only increased rates when the noncontingent shock occurred one-third to one-half of the times that the preshock stimulus was presented (Brady, 1956a,b), while the same dose of reserpine did not increase responding when shock followed every presentation of the preshock stimulus (Yamahiro *et al.*, 1961).

Drug effects have also been related to the nature of the stimulus that precedes the shock in the conditioned suppression procedure (Hill *et al.*, 1967) and the nature of the unavoidable stimulus (i.e., food vs. shock) (Miczek, 1973a), as well as the schedule of reinforcement maintaining responding in punishment procedures (Foree *et al.*, 1973; McKearney and Barrett, 1975). (See McMillan, 1975, for a review of variables important in determining a drug effect on punished responding.)

Therefore, the effects of drugs on responding suppressed by shock depend on a variety of factors, including dose, intensity and schedule of presentation of the shock and pre-drug response rate. While some drugs increase responding in punishment and conditioned suppression paradigms, this effect depends on the degree to which responding is suppressed. Moreover, drugs that do not usually increase responding suppressed by shock will produce an increase under certain conditions, pointing again to the dependence of drug effects on experimental parameters.

COMPARISON OF DRUG EFFECTS ON BEHAVIOR MAINTAINED BY POSITIVE OR NEGATIVE REINFORCEMENT

Drugs have different effects on responding maintained by different procedures. For example, while chlorpromazine has a selective effect on avoidance responding in that it decreases avoidance responding without affecting escape responding, it generally does not affect responding in punishment or conditioned suppression procedures. On the other hand, the barbiturates and benzodiazepines generally increase responding suppressed by shock but have variable effects on avoidance responding that depend on the procedure and the particular drug examined. In addition, many drugs have been reported to have effects on avoidance responding that are different from their effects on responding maintained by food presentation (Weissman, 1959; Cook and Catania, 1964; Cook and Kelleher, 1962). In view of these differential effects it would be interesting to make a direct comparison of drug effects on behavior maintained by positive or negative reinforcement. Since drug effects depend on pre-drug rates and patterns of responding, it is important to make such a comparison under conditions in which equivalent response rates and patterns are generated by schedules of positive and negative reinforcement. For example, Kelleher and Morse (1964) trained monkeys to respond on a schedule of negative reinforcement or a schedule of positive reinforcement in which comparable rates and patterns of responding were maintained. Three food-deprived monkeys were trained on a multiple fixed-interval, fixed-ratio schedule of positive reinforcement. In the presence of a red light, responding was maintained on an FR 30 schedule of food presentation. In the presence of a white light, responding was maintained on an FI 10-min schedule of food presentation. Another group of three monkeys were trained on a multiple FI FR schedule of reinforcement; however, in the presence of a red light, shocks occurred at 30-sec intervals. Thirty responses (FR 30) terminated the light and produced a stimulus during which no shocks were delivered. In the presence of a white light, shocks occurred at 1-sec intervals starting after 10 min; the first response after 10-min terminated the white stimulus light and produced the shock-free stimulus. Table 9-5 outlines this procedure. Rates and patterns of responding were the same in both groups of monkeys regardless of the nature of the stimuli that maintained responding. The

TABLE 9-5. Design of a schedule of positive and negative reinforcement that generates equal response patterns.

Positive reinforcement		Negative reinforcement	
Red light		*Red light* (shock every 30-sec)	
30 responses - - - - - - - - - food (FR 30) presentation		30 responses - - - - - - stimulus during which (FR 30) no shocks occur	
White light		*White light* (shock every 1-sec)	
1st response after 10-min - - - - - - - - - food (FI 10-min) presentation		1st response after 10 min - - - - - - stimulus during which (FI 10-min) no shocks occur	

effects of chlorpromazine and *d*-amphetamine were shown to depend on the schedule of reinforcement maintaining the behavior rather than on the nature of the reinforcer (see Fig. 9-18). *d*-Amphetamine increased FI rates except at the highest dose, and decreased FR response rates. Chlorpromazine decreased rates of responding under both the FR and FI schedules. These effects were the same in the monkeys whose behavior was maintained by termination of a stimulus correlated with shock as those obtained in monkeys whose behavior was maintained by food presentation.

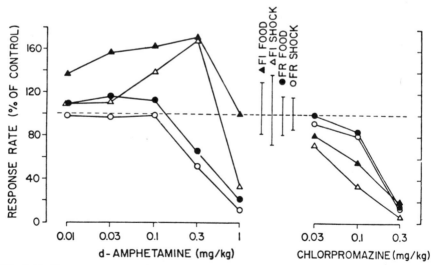

Fig. 9-18. Response rate under multiple FI FR schedules of food presentation and stimulus-shock termination in squirrel monkeys as a function of dose of *d*-amphetamine or chlorpromazine. Each point represents two or more observations in three monkeys under each multiple schedule. Vertical lines signify the range of control (non-drug) observations. Note the similarity of the pairs of dose-effect curves for FI and for FR components regardless of the type of reinforcing event. (From Kelleher and Morse, 1964.)

Cook and Catania (1964) examined a situation in which responding was either maintained on an FI 10-min schedule of food presentation or on an FI 10-min schedule of shock termination (shock pulsed continuously throughout the FI interval and the first response after 10-min terminated the shock). Rates and patterns of responding were similar under FI food presentation and under FI shock termination. Chlorpromazine and imipramine decreased responding maintained by both shock termination or food presentation, while amphetamine, meprobamate and chlordiazepoxide increased rates under both schedules. Figure 9-19 illustrates the effects of one dose of chlorpromazine, imipramine,

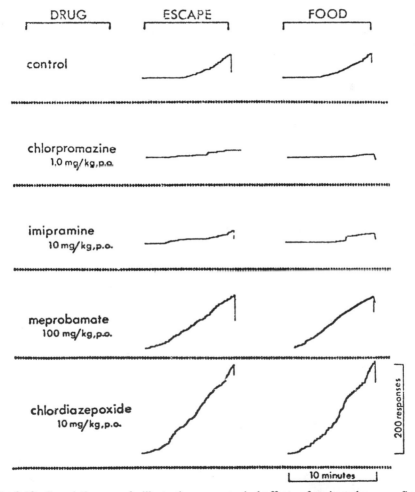

Fig. 9-19. Cumulative records illustrating some typical effects of various drugs on fixed-interval responding maintained by a schedule of negative reinforcement (escape) or positive reinforcement in squirrel monkeys. (From Cook and Catania, 1964.)

meprobamate, and chlordiazepoxide on the pattern of FI responding maintained by food or shock.

Another procedure that has been used to examine drug effects on responding maintained by different events is the response-dependent shock paradigm. In Chapter 1 we noted that while the presentation of electric shock following a response ordinarily results in response suppression, under some conditions response-dependent electric shock can maintain responding. Moreover, responding under these conditions is characteristic of responding maintained by food presentation. McKearney (1974) compared the effects of d-amphetamine, morphine and chlorprozamine on responding under comparable FI schedules of food presentation and shock presentation. d-Amphetamine increased responding under the FI schedule of food presentation and the FI schedule of

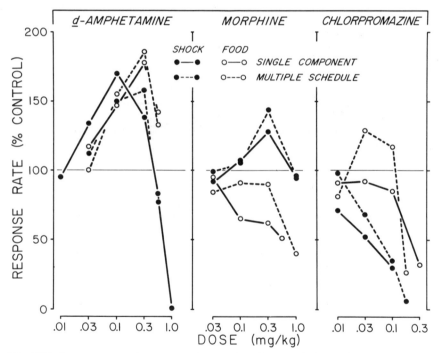

Fig. 9-20. Response rate (as percent of control) under FI schedules of shock presentation and food presentation and under a multiple schedule of shock presentation and food presentation as a function of dose of d-amphetamine, morphine or chlorpromazine in squirrel monkeys. Points are means of the average rates of responding (expressed as percent of control) at a given dose for each subject. Note the qualitatively similar effects of d-amphetamine under all schedules, but the different effects of morphine depending on whether responding was maintained by food or shock presentation. (From McKearney, 1974.)

shock presentation.   In general, chlorpromazine decreased responding under both schedules, but the magnitude of decrease at a given dose was usually greater under the FI schedule of shock presentation.   On the other hand, morphine increased responding under the FI schedule of shock presentation but at the same doses it decreased responding under the FI schedule of food presentation.   The effects of d-amphetamine, chlorpromazine and morphine are presented in Fig. 9-20.

Thus it appears that if the rates and patterns of responding are equal in schedules maintained by food and shock, many drugs affect behavior maintained by food and shock similarly, pointing to the importance of rate and pattern of responding in determining a drug effect.   Whether the results of these studies will hold under different shock values, deprivation conditions, schedules of reinforcement, and different drugs remains to be investigated.

ADDITIONAL CONSIDERATIONS

In this chapter the importance of behavioral determinants of a drug effect has been emphasized.   While it has been noted repeatedly that the dose of a drug is a fundamental determinant of drug effect, some additional pharmacological variables deserve attention.   Moreover, drug effects have sometimes been shown to depend on the species examined. These variables are discussed below.

Time Course

In studies presented in this chapter, neither the time nor the route of drug administration was discussed.   Moreover, the length of the experimental session was usually not specified.   Since drugs vary in onset and duration of action, description of a drug effect may vary depending on when the effect was observed and the route of administration (see Chapter 2).   In many instances, drug effects are described in terms of changes in overall response rate during an experimental session.   If an experimental session is long (e.g., four hours) a drug might have effects early in the session that are different from effects occurring later in the session.   For example, nicotine produces an initial decrease in rate of responding that is usually followed by an increase in response rate (Morrison, 1967, 1968).   Similar effects have been reported for LSD (Appel and Freedman, 1965; Appel, 1971).

In addition, the onset and duration of a drug effect depends on the dose examined.   Clark and Steele (1966) examined the effects of d-amphetamine on a multiple FR FI extinction schedule over a four-hour period.   The effects of amphetamine depended on the schedule, the dose and the time since drug administration.   For example, while 0.5 mg/kg (im) increased FI rates during the first hour of the session, larger doses (1.0–2.0 mg/kg) did not increase FI rates until the second hour. Chlorpromazine has been shown to have similar time-dependent effects (Clark, 1969).

Tolerance

In the work discussed in this chapter, drugs were usually administered once or twice a week. When drugs are administered repeatedly (every day or several times a day), a progressive diminution in the magnitude of the drug effect is often observed. This is referred to as tolerance. For example, a single dose of Δ^9-tetrahydrocannabinol, which decreased rate of responding on FI schedules of reinforcement following one injection, had no effect if the same dose was given at daily intervals (McMillan et al., 1970a). Similar effects have been reported with a variety of other drugs, including methamphetamine, amphetamine, morphine and methadone (Fischman and Schuster, 1974; Schuster et al., 1966; McMillan and Morse, 1967; Holtzman and Villarreal, 1973; Heifetz and McMillan, 1971; Holtzman, 1974d).

The degree to which tolerance occurs depends on the behavior examined. Heifetz and McMillan (1971) have shown that while the effects of both morphine and methadone on a multiple FR FI schedule of food presentation were reduced following daily injections, tolerance was less complete under the fixed ratio component than under the fixed interval component. Moreover, while tolerance occurred to morphine- and methadone-induced decreases in responding on the FI component of the multiple schedule, tolerance did not occur to increases in response rate produced by low doses of these drugs.

The importance of behavioral variables in the development of tolerance has also been demonstrated with amphetamine. Schuster et al. (1966) examined the effects of chronic administration of d-amphetamine in rats maintained on a multiple DRL 30-sec FI 30-sec schedule of food presentation and on a shock avoidance schedule. The effects of one dose of 1.0 mg/kg d-amphetamine in rats were compared to the effects of daily injections of the same dose of d-amphetamine. A single dose of d-amphetamine generally increased rates of responding on both components of the multiple schedule (DRL and FI) and on the shock avoidance schedule. Following repeated administration of d-amphetamine, tolerance occurred to the increases in responding on the DRL component but not to the increases in responding on the FI component or the shock avoidance schedule. Schuster et al. suggested that tolerance develops only when a drug interferes with reinforcement frequency. While an increase in response rate on a DRL schedule reduces reinforcement frequency, an increase in response rate on an FI schedule or a shock avoidance schedule does not, suggesting that schedules of reinforcement are important determinants in the occurrence of tolerance.

Campbell and Seiden (1973) investigated further the behavioral determinants of tolerance in the following situation: Two groups of rats were maintained on a

DRL schedule of food presentation. Both groups were given daily doses of *d*-amphetamine for several weeks. In one group, *d*-amphetamine was administered 20 min before daily experimental sessions so that performance took place in the presence of the drug. In the second group, *d*-amphetamine was administered 20 min after the experimental session so that performance did not take place in the presence of the drug. Tolerance developed in the group that received *d*-amphetamine before the experimental session. In this group a 1.5-mg/kg dose of *d*-amphetamine initially increased response rate. Following repeated daily injections of the same dose of *d*-amphetamine, responding gradually returned to control levels. In the second group, no changes occurred as a result of repeated administration of *d*-amphetamine. Following development of tolerance in the group receiving amphetamine before the experimental session, the groups were switched. That is, animals that had received amphetamine before the experimental session now received it after the session and vice versa. The animals were run under these conditions for an additional 12 days. When rats that had previously received amphetamine before the session and had become tolerant to its effects were given amphetamine following the session, responding remained at pre-drug levels. When rats that had been receiving *d*-amphetamine after the session were given amphetamine before the session, amphetamine produced an increase in response rate, indicating that these rats had not developed tolerance to the drug when it was given after the experimental session. This finding suggests that the development of tolerance depends on the relationship between the time of injection and the time at which the behavior was performed and not just on the repeated administration of the drug. Therefore, drug tolerance involves factors related to the behavior examined and the time of drug administration.

Species

In order to investigate a drug effect across species, it is important to establish comparable patterns of responding in the different species to be examined. While very little work has been done in the area of comparative behavioral pharmacology, in a few instances similar rates and patterns of responding have been established with different species so that comparisons of a drug effect could be made between species. For example, *d*-amphetamine has been examined on a multiple FR 30 FI 5-min schedule of food presentation in pigeons (McMillan, 1969) and squirrel monkeys (McMillan, 1968b). In rats, *d*-amphetamine has been examined on a multiple FR 25 FI 4-min schedule (Clark and Steele, 1966). In each case, response rates and patterns were similar and *d*-amphetamine increased responding maintained by the FI schedule of food presentation and decreased responding on the FR schedule in a relatively similar dose range.

On the other hand, the effects of chlorpromazine vary depending on the species examined. Chlorpromazine usually decreases overall response rates on FI schedules of food presentation in rats (Boren, 1961b; Clark, 1969), squirrel monkeys (Kelleher and Morse, 1964; Cook and Kelleher, 1962; Hanson *et al.*, 1967; McKearney, 1974) and pigeons (Dews, 1958a; Bignami and Gatti, 1969; McMillan, 1971; Leander, 1975), while it increases response rates in chimpanzees (Byrd, 1974). Similarly, Byrd (1975) has shown that morphine produces effects on schedule-controlled behavior in the chimpanzee that are different from effects in other primates. Byrd maintained responding in chimpanzees and baboons on a multiple FI 10-min FR 30 schedule of food presentation. Response rates and patterns were similar in both species. Morphine (0.3–3.0 mg/kg) increased rates of responding in the FR and FI components in the chimpanzee, but in the baboon it decreased responding in the FR component and either had no effect or decreased FI responding at high doses (3.0–10.0 mg/kg). Decreases in responding on FR schedules are usually reported for squirrel monkeys and rhesus monkeys following morphine in a similar dose range (0.1–3.0 mg/kg) (Goldberg and Morse, 1974; Woods and Schuster, 1971; Woods, 1969; McMillan and Morse, 1967). Therefore, morphine appears to have effects in the chimpanzee qualitatively different from its effects in other nonhuman primates.

SUMMARY

In this chapter we have examined the effects of drugs on behavior maintained by positive reinforcement, negative reinforcement and responding in punishment and conditioned suppression procedures. We have seen that drug effects upon responding maintained by different schedules of reinforcement depend on a variety of factors, including the rate of responding engendered by the schedule of reinforcement and the dose of the drug.

In procedures that employ positive schedules of reinforcement, it has been shown that most drugs increase rates of responding on schedules which generate low pre-drug rates of responding and decrease rates of responding on schedules which generate high pre-drug rates of responding, at least in some dose range. While rate of responding was shown to be an important determinant of a drug effect, the importance of other variables such as discriminative and punishing stimuli was also emphasized.

In avoidance procedures, it was shown that some drugs decrease responding maintained by the postponement of shock without producing ataxia or failure to escape a shock, while other drugs decreased avoidance responding only at doses that decreased overall rates of responding or produced failure to escape. The importance of procedural variables in this effect was also discussed.

The barbiturates and the benzodiazepines usually increase responding in punishment and conditioned suppression procedures, while most other drugs do not increase responding suppressed by shock. It was noted, however, that whether a drug increased punished responding depended on factors such as shock intensity, frequency and degree of response suppression.

Direct comparisons of identical patterns and rates of responding maintained by schedules of positive and negative reinforcement showed that several drugs produced the same effects on behavior maintained by shock or food when the rates and patterns of responding were equal, supporting the notion that the behavioral variables are important determinants of a drug effect.

REFERENCES

Altman, J. L. and J. B. Appel. 1975. LSD and fixed-interval responding in the rat. *Pharmacol. Biochem. Behav.* **3**: 151–155.

Appel, J. B. 1963. Drugs, shock intensity, and the CER. *Psychopharmacologia* **4**: 148–153.

Appel, J. B. 1971. Effects of LSD on time-based schedules of reinforcement. *Psychopharmacologia* **21**: 174–186.

Appel, J. B. and D. X. Freedman. 1965. The relative potencies of psychotomimetic drugs. *Life Sci.* **4**: 2181–2186.

Barrett, J. E. 1974. Conjunctive schedules of reinforcement I: Rate-dependent effects of pentobarbital and *d*-amphetamine. *J. Exp. Anal. Behav.* **22**: 561–573.

Barry, H. III and R. K. Kubena. 1970. Effects of Δ^1-tetrahydrocannabinol on avoidance by rats and monkeys. *Proc. 78th Ann. Conv. APA* 805–806.

Bignami, G. and G. L. Gatti. 1969. Analysis of drug effects on multiple fixed ratio 33-fixed interval 5-min in pigeons. *Psychopharmacologia* **15**: 310–332.

Bignami, G., L. deAcetis and G. L. Gatti. 1971. Facilitation and impairment of avoidance responding by phenobarbital sodium, chloridazepoxide and diazepam—the role of performance base lines. *J. Pharmacol. Exp. Ther.* **176**: 725–732.

Boren, J. J. 1961a. Isolation of post-shock responding in a free operant avoidance procedure. *Psychol. Rep.* **9**: 265–266.

Boren, J. J. 1961b. Some effects of adiphenine, benactyzene, and chlorpromazine upon several operant behaviors. *Psychopharmacologia* **2**: 416–424.

Boren, J. J. and A. P. Navarro. 1959. The action of atropine, benactyzine and scopolamine upon fixed-interval and fixed-ratio behavior. *J. Exp. Anal. Behav.* **2**: 107–115.

Brady, J. V. 1956a. A comparative approach to the evaluation of drug effects upon affective behavior. *Ann. N.Y. Acad. Sci.* **64**: 632–643.

Brady, J. V. 1956b. Assessment of drug effects on emotional behavior. *Science* **123**: 1033–1034.

Branch, M. N. 1974. Behavior as a stimulus: Joint effects of *d*-amphetamine and pentobarbital. *J. Pharmacol. Exp. Ther.* **189**: 33–41.

Branch, M. N. 1975. Effects of chlorpromazine and *d*-amphetamine on observing responses during a fixed-interval schedule. *Psychopharmacologia* **42**: 87–93.

Branch, M. N. and L. R. Gollub. 1974. A detailed analysis of the effects of *d*-amphetamine on behavior under fixed-interval schedules. *J. Exp. Anal. Behav.* **21**: 519–539.

Brown, R. M. and L. S. Seiden. 1975. Interresponse time changes as a function of water deprivation and amphetamine. *J. Pharmacol. Exp. Ther.* **193**: 701–712.

Byrd, L. D. 1973. Effects of *d*-amphetamine on schedule-controlled key pressing and drinking in the chimpanzee. *J. Pharmacol. Exp. Ther.* **185**: 633–641.

Byrd, L. D. 1974. Modification of the effects of chlorpromazine on behavior in the chimpanzee. *J. Pharmacol. Exp. Ther.* **189**: 24–32.

Byrd, L. D. 1975. Contrasting effects of morphine on schedule-controlled behavior in the chimpanzee and baboon. *J. Pharmacol. Exp. Ther.* **193**: 861–869.

Campbell, J. C. and L. S. Seiden. 1973. Performance influence on the development of tolerance to amphetamine. *Pharmacol. Biochem. Behav.* **1**: 703–708.

Carey, R. J. and R. P. Kritkausky. 1972. Absence of a response-rate-dependent effect of *d*-amphetamine on a DRL schedule when reinforcement is signalled. *Psychon. Sci.* **26**: 285–286.

Clark, F. C. 1969. Effects of chlorpromazine on behavior maintained by a multiple schedule of reinforcement. *J. Pharmacol. Exp. Ther.* **166**: 179–188.

Clark, F. C. and B. J. Steele. 1963. Some observations on the interaction of chlorpromazine and free operant avoidance bursts. *Psychopharmacologia* **4**: 221–231.

Clark, F. C. and B. J. Steele. 1966. Effects of *d*-amphetamine on performance under a multiple schedule in the rat. *Psychopharmacologia* **9**: 157–169.

Clark, R. and G. K. Samuel. 1969. Drug effects on a discrete conditioned avoidance response in dogs, rhesus monkeys and rats. *Psychopharmacologia* **14**: 106–114.

Conrad, D. G., T. F. Elsmore and F. J. Sodetz. 1972. Δ^9-Tetrahydrocannabinol: Dose-related effects on timing behavior in chimpanzee. *Science* **175**: 547–550.

Cook, L. and A. C. Catania. 1964. Effects of drugs on avoidance and escape behavior. *Fed. Proc.* **23**: 818–835.

Cook, L. and A. B. Davidson. 1973. Effects of behaviorally active drugs in a conflict-punishment procedure in rats. *In* S. Garattini, E. Mussini and L. O. Randall (eds.), *The Benzodiazepines*. Raven Press, New York.

Cook, L. and R. T. Kelleher. 1962. Drug effects on the behavior of animals. *Ann. N.Y. Acad. Sci.* **96**: 315–335.

Cook, L. and R. T. Kelleher. 1963. Effects of drugs on behavior. *Ann. Rev. Pharmacol.* **3**: 205–222.

Cook, L. and J. Sepinwall. 1975. Reinforcement schedules and extrapolations to humans from animals in behavioral pharmacology. *Fed. Proc.* **34**: 1889–1897.

Cook, L. and E. Weidley. 1957. Behavioral effects of some psychopharmacological agents. *Ann. N.Y. Acad. Sci.* **66**: 740–752.

Courvoisier, S., J. Fournel, R. Ducrot, M. Kolsky and P. Koetschet. 1953. Propriétés pharmacodynamiques du chlorhydrate de chloro-3 (diméthyl-amino-3'-propyl)-10 phénothiazine (4.560 R. P.). *Arch. Int. Pharmacodyn.* **92**: 305–361.

Davis, T. R. A., C. J. Kensler and P. B. Dews. 1973. Comparison of behavioral effects of nicotine, *d*-amphetamine, caffeine, and dimethylheptyl-tetrahydrocannabinol in squirrel monkeys. *Psychopharmacologia* **32**: 51–65.

Dews, P. B. 1955. Studies on behavior. I. Differential sensitivity to pentobarbital of pecking performance in pigeons depending on the schedule of reward. *J. Pharmacol. Exp. Ther.* **113**: 393–401.

Dews, P. B. 1958a. Effects of chlorpromazine and promazine on performance on a mixed schedule of reinforcement. *J. Exp. Anal. Behav.* **1**: 73–82.

Dews, P. B. 1958b. Studies on Behavior. IV. Stimulant actions of methamphetamine. *J. Pharmacol. Exp. Ther.* **122**: 137–147.

Dews, P. B. 1962. A behavioral output enhancing effect of imipramine in pigeons. *Int. J. Neuropharmacol.* **1**: 265–272.

Dews, P. B. 1964. A behavioral effect of amobarbital. *Naunyn Schmiedebergs Arch. Exp. Path. Pharmakol.* **248**: 296–307.

Dews, P. B. 1971. Commentary *in* J. A. Harvey (ed.), *Behavioral Analysis of Drug Action*. Scott Foresman & Co., Glenview, Illinois, pp. 22–25.

Dinsmoor, J. A. and D. O. Lyon. 1961. The selective action of chlorpromazine in behavior suppressed by punishment. *Psychopharmacologia* **2**: 456–460.

Domino, E. F., A. J. Karoly and E. L. Walker. 1963. Effects of various drugs on a conditioned avoidance response in dogs resistant to extinction. *J. Pharmacol. Exp. Ther.* **141**: 92–99.

Doty, B. A. and L. A. Doty. 1966. Facilitative effects of amphetamine on avoidance conditioning in relation to age and problem difficulty. *Psychopharmacologia* 9: 234–241.

Dykstra, L. A., D. E. McMillan and L. S. Harris. 1974. Antagonism of morphine by long acting narcotic antagonists. *Psychopharmacologia* 39: 151–162.

Dykstra, L. A., D. E. McMillan and L. S. Harris. 1975. Effects of Δ^9-THC and a water soluble ester of Δ^9-THC on schedule-controlled behavior. *Pharmacol. Biochem. Behav.* 3: 29–32.

Ferraro, D. P., D. M. Grilly and W. C. Lynch. 1971. Effects of marijuana extract on the operant behavior of chimpanzees. *Psychopharmacologia* 22: 333–351.

Fischman, M. W. and C. R. Schuster. 1974. Tolerance development to chronic methamphetamine intoxication in the rhesus monkey. *Pharmacol. Biochem. Behav.* 2: 503–508.

Foree, D. D., F. H. Moretz and D. E. McMillan. 1973. Drugs and punished responding II: *d*-amphetamine-induced increases in punished responding. *J. Exp. Anal. Behav.* 20: 291–300.

Frankenheim, J. M. 1974. Effects of repeated doses of *l*-Δ^8-trans-tetrahydrocannabinol on schedule-controlled temporally-spaced responding of rats. *Psychopharmacologia* 38: 125–144.

Frankenheim, J. M., D. E. McMillan and L. S. Harris. 1971. Effects of *l*-Δ^9 and *l*-Δ^8-trans-tetrahydrocannabinol and cannabinol on schedule-controlled behavior of pigeons and rats. *J. Pharmacol. Exp. Ther.* 178: 241–252.

Fry, W., R. T. Kelleher and L. Cook. 1960. A mathematical index of performance on fixed-interval schedules of reinforcement. *J. Exp. Anal. Behav.* 3: 193–199.

Fuller, J. L. 1966. Variation in effects of chlorpromazine in three strains of mice. *Psychopharmacologia* 8: 408–414.

Geller, I. and J. Seifter. 1960. The effects of meprobamate, barbiturates, *d*-amphetamine and promazine on experimentally induced conflict in the rat. *Psychopharmacologia* 1: 482–492.

Geller, I., I. Bachman and J. Seifter. 1963. Effects of reserpine and morphine on behavior suppressed by punishment. *Life Sci.* 2: 226–231.

Geller, I., J. T. Kulak and J. Seifter. 1962. The effects of chlordiazepoxide and chlorpromazine on a punishment discrimination. *Psychopharmacologia* 3: 374–385.

Goldberg, S. R. and W. H. Morse. 1974. Some behavioral effects of morphine, naloxone and nalorphine alone and in combination, compared in the squirrel monkey and the pigeon. *Fed. Proc.* 33: 550.

Grisham, M. G. and D. P. Ferraro. 1972. Biphasic effects of Δ^9-tetrahydrocannabinol on variable interval schedule performance in rats. *Psychopharmacologia* 27: 163–169.

Grossman, S. P. 1961. Effects of chlorpromazine and perphenazine on bar-pressing performance in an approach-avoidance conflict. *J. Comp. Physiol. Psychol.* 54: 517–521.

Hanson, H. M., C. A. Stone and J. J. Witoslawski. 1970. Antagonism of the antiavoidance effects of various agents by anticholinergic drugs. *J. Pharmacol. Exp. Ther.* 173: 117–124.

Hanson, H. M., J. J. Witoslawski and E. H. Campbell. 1967. Drug effects in squirrel monkeys trained on a multiple schedule with a punishment contingency. *J. Exp. Anal. Behav.* 10: 565–569.

Hearst, E. and J. R. Vane. 1967. Some effects of *d*-amphetamine on the behavior of pigeons under intermittent reinforcement. *Psychopharmacologia* 12: 58–67.

Heifetz, S. A. and D. E. McMillan. 1971. Development of behavioral tolerance to morphine and methadone using the schedule-controlled behavior of the pigeon. *Psychopharmacologia* 19: 40–52.

Heise, G. A. and E. Boff. 1962. Continuous avoidance as a base-line for measuring behavioral effects of drugs. *Psychopharmacologia* 3: 264–282.

Hendry, D. P. and C. Van Toller. 1964. Fixed-ratio punishment with continuous reinforcement. *J. Exp. Anal. Behav.* 7: 293–300.

Herrnstein, R. J. 1958. Effects of scopolamine on a multiple schedule. *J. Exp. Anal. Behav.* 1: 351–358.

Herz, A. 1960. Drugs and conditioned avoidance behavior. *Int. Rev. Neurobiol.* 2: 229–277.

Hill, H. E., E. C. Bell and A. Wikler. 1967. Reduction of conditioned suppression: actions of morphine compared with those of amphetamine, pentobarbital, nalorphine, cocaine, LSD-25 and chlorpromazine. *Arch. Int. Pharmacodyn.* 165: 212–226.

Hill, H. E., R. E. Belleville, F. T. Pescor and A. Wikler. 1966. Comparative effects of methadone, meperidine and morphine on conditioned suppression. *Arch. Int. Pharmacodyn.* 163: 341–352.

Hill, H. E., F. T. Pescor, R. E. Belleville and A. Wikler. 1957. Use of differential bar-pressing rates of rats for screening analgesic drugs. I. Techniques and effects of morphine. *J. Pharmacol. Exp. Ther.* 120: 388–397.

Hines, G., A. E. Lee and W. T. Miller. 1970. Effect of atropine dose level on the suppression of water-reinforced VI responding. *Psychon. Sci.* 20: 37–38.

Hines, G., W. T. Miller and A. E. Lee. 1969. The effects of atropine on food-reinforced vs. water-reinforced VI responding. *Psychon. Sci.* 17: 33–34.

Holloway, F. A. and D. R. Vardiman. 1971. Dose-response effects of ethanol on appetitive behaviors. *Psychon. Sci.* 24: 218–220.

Holtzman, S. G. 1974a. Behavioral effects of separate and combined administration of naloxone and *d*-amphetamine. *J. Pharmacol. Exp. Ther.* 189: 51–60.

Holtzman, S. G. 1974b. Effects of nalorphine on avoidance behavior and locomotor activity in the rat. *Arch. Int. Pharmacodyn.* 212: 199–204.

Holtzman, S. G. 1974c. Narcotic antagonists as stimulants of behavior in the rat: Specific and nonspecific effects. *In* M. C. Braude, L. S. Harris, E. L. May, J. P. Smith and J. E. Villarreal (eds.), *Narcotic Antagonists. Advances in Biochemical Psychopharmacology* 8: 371–382, Raven Press, New York.

Holtzman, S. G. 1974d. Tolerance to the stimulant effects of morphine and pentazocine on avoidance responding in the rat. *Psychopharmacologia* 39: 23–37.

Holtzman, S. G. and R. E. Jewett. 1972a. Some actions of pentazocine on behavior and brain monoamines in the rat. *J. Pharmacol. Exp. Therap.* 181: 346–356.

Holtzman, S. G. and R. E. Jewett. 1972b. Stimulation of behavior in the rat by cyclazocine. *Proc. V Int. Cong. Pharmacol.* Bethesda, Maryland, p. 105.

Holtzman, S. G. and R. E. Jewett. 1972c. Shock intensity as a determinant of the behavioral effects of morphine in the rat. *Life Sci.* 11: 1085–1091.

Holtzman, S. G. and R. E. Jewett. 1973. Stimulation of behavior in the rat by cyclazocine: Effects of naloxone. *J. Pharmacol. Exp. Ther.* 187: 380–390.

Holtzman, S. G. and J. E. Villarreal. 1973. Operant behavior in the morphine-dependent rhesus monkey. *J. Pharmacol. Exp. Ther.* 184: 528–541.

Houser, V. P. 1973. Modulation of avoidance behavior in squirrel monkeys after chronic administration and withdrawal of *d*-amphetamine or α-methyl-*p*-tyrosine. *Psychopharmacologia* 28: 213–234.

Hunt, H. F. 1957. Some effects of meprobamate on conditioned fear and emotional behavior. *Ann. N.Y. Acad. Sci.* 67: 712–722.

Irwin, S., M. Slabok, P. L. Debiase and W. M. Govier. 1959. Perphenazine (trilafon), a new potent tranquilizer and antiemetic: I. Behavior profile, acute toxicity and behavioral mode of action. *Arch. Int. Pharmacodyn.* 118: 358–374.

Jarrard, L. E. 1963. Effect of D-lysergic acid diethylamide on operant behavior in the rat. *Psychopharmacologia* 5: 39–46.

John, E. R., B. M. Wenzel and R. D. Tschirgi. 1958. Differential effects of reserpine on conditioned responses in cats. *Science* 127: 25–26.

Kelleher, R. T. and W. H. Morse. 1964. Escape behavior and punished behavior. *Fed. Proc.* **23**: 808–817.

Kelleher, R. T. and W. H. Morse. 1968. Determinants of the specificity of behavioral effects of drugs. *Ergebn. Physiol. Biol. Chem. Exp. Pharmakol.* **60**: 1–56.

Kelleher, R. T., W. Fry, J. Deegan and L. Cook. 1961. Effects of meprobamate on operant behavior in rats. *J. Pharmacol. Exp. Ther.* **133**: 271–280.

Kinnard, W. J., M. D. G. Aceto and J. P. Buckley. 1962. The effects of certain psychotropic agents on the conditioned emotional response behavior pattern of the albino rat. *Psychopharmacologia* **3**: 227–230.

Kornetsky, C. 1965. A comparison of the effects of desipramine and imipramine on two schedules of reinforcement. *Int. J. Neuropharmacol.* **4**: 13–16.

Kosersky, D. S., D. E. McMillan and L. S. Harris. 1974. Δ^9-tetrahydrocannabinol and 11-hydroxy-Δ^9-tetrahydrocannabinol: Behavioral effects and tolerance development. *J. Pharmacol. Exp. Ther.* **189**: 61–65.

Laties, V. G. 1972. The modification of drug effects on behavior by external discriminative stimuli. *J. Pharmacol. Exp. Ther.* **183**: 1–13.

Laties, V. G. 1975. The role of discriminative stimuli in modulating drug action. *Fed. Proc.* **34**: 1880–1888.

Laties, V. G. and B. Weiss. 1962. Effects of alcohol on timing behavior. *J. Comp. Physiol. Psychol.* **55**: 85–91.

Laties, V. G. and B. Weiss. 1966. Influence of drugs on behavior controlled by internal and external stimuli. *J. Pharmacol. Exp. Ther.* **152**: 388–396.

Latz, A., G. T. Bain and C. Kornetsky. 1969. Attenuated effect of chlorpromazine on conditioned avoidance as a function of rapid acquisition. *Psychopharmacologia* **14**: 23–32.

Lauener, H. 1963. Conditioned suppression in rats and the effect of pharmacological agents thereon. *Psychopharmacologia* **4**: 311–325.

Leander, J. D. 1975. Rate-dependent effects of drugs. II. Effects of some major tranquilizers on multiple fixed-ratio, fixed-interval schedule performance. *J. Pharmacol. Exp. Ther.* **193**: 689–700.

Leander, J. D. and D. E. McMillan. 1974. Rate-dependent effects of drugs. I. Comparison of *d*-amphetamine, pentobarbital and chlorpromazine on multiple and mixed schedules. *J. Pharmacol. Exp. Ther.* **188**: 726–739.

Leander, J. D., D. E. McMillan and F. W. Ellis. 1974. Ethanol and isopropanol: Comparison of behavioral effects. *Pharmacologist* **16**, Abstract.

Low, L. A., M. Eliasson and C. Kornetsky. 1966. Effect of chlorpromazine on avoidance acquisition as a function of CS-US interval length. *Psychopharmacologia* **10**: 148–154.

MacPhail, R. C. 1971. Rate-dependent effects of amphetamine are also schedule dependent. *Proc. 79th Ann. Conv. APA*, 755–756.

MacPhail, R. C. and L. R. Gollub. 1975. Separating the effects of response rate and reinforcement frequency in the rate-dependent effects of amphetamine and scopolamine on the schedule-controlled performances of rats and pigeons. *J. Pharmacol. Exp. Ther.* **194**: 332–342.

Maffii, G. 1959. The secondary conditioned response of rats and the effects of some psychopharmacological agents. *J. Pharm. Pharmacol.* **11**: 129–139.

Manning, F. G. 1973. Acute tolerance to the effects of delta-9-tetrahydrocannabinol on spaced responding by monkeys. *Pharmacol. Biochem. Behav.* **1**: 665–671.

Marr, M. J. 1970. Effects of chlorpromazine in the pigeon under a second-order schedule of food presentation. *J. Exp. Anal. Behav.* **13**: 291–299.

McKearney, J. W. 1968. The relative effects of *d*-amphetamine, imipramine and harmaline on tetrabenazine suppression of schedule-controlled behavior in the rat. *J. Pharmacol. Exp. Ther.* **159**: 429–440.

McKearney, J. W. 1970. Rate-dependent effects of drugs: Modification by discriminative stimuli of the effects of amobarbital on schedule-controlled behavior. *J. Exp. Anal. Behav.* **14:** 167–175.

McKearney, J. W. 1972. Schedule-dependent effects: effects of drugs, and maintenance of responding with response-produced electric shocks. *In* R. M. Gilbert and J. D. Keehn (eds.), *Schedule Effects: Drugs, Drinking and Aggression.* University of Toronto Press, pp. 3–25.

McKearney, J. W. 1974. Effects of *d*-amphetamine, morphine and chlorpromazine on responding under fixed-interval schedules of food presentation or electric shock presentation. *J. Pharmacol. Exp. Ther.* **190:** 141–153.

McKearney, J. W. and J. E. Barrett. 1975. Punished Behavior: Increases in responding after *d*-amphetamine. *Psychopharmacologia* **41:** 23–26.

McKim, W. A. 1973. The effect of scopolamine on fixed-interval behaviour in the rat. A rate-dependency effect. *Psychopharmacologia* **32:** 255–264.

McKim, W. A. 1974. The effects of scopolamine and physostigmine on fixed-interval behaviour in the rat. *Psychopharmacologia* **39:** 237–244.

McMillan, D. E. 1967. A comparison of the punishing effects of response-produced shock and response-produced time out. *J. Exp. Anal. Behav.* **10:** 439–449.

McMillan, D. E. 1968a. The effect of sympathomimetic amines on schedule-controlled behavior in the pigeon. *J. Pharmacol. Exp. Ther.* **160:** 315–325.

McMillan, D. E. 1968b. Some interactions between sympathomimetic amines and amine-depleting agents on the schedule-controlled behavior of the pigeon and the squirrel monkey. *J. Pharmacol. Exp. Ther.* **163:** 172–187.

McMillan, D. E. 1969. Effects of *d*-amphetamine on performance under several parameters of multiple fixed-ratio, fixed-interval schedules. *J. Pharmacol. Exp. Ther.* **167:** 26–33.

McMillan, D. E. 1971. Interactions between naloxone and chlorpromazine on behavior under schedule control. *Psychopharmacologia* **19:** 128–133.

McMillan, D. E. 1973a. Drugs and punished responding I: Rate dependent effects under multiple schedules. *J. Exp. Anal. Behav.* **19:** 133–145.

McMillan, D. E. 1973b. Drugs and punished responding III. Punishment intensity as a determinant of drug effect. *Psychopharmacologia* **30:** 61–74.

McMillan, D. E. 1975. Determinants of drug effects on punished responding. *Fed. Proc.* **34:** 1870–1879.

McMillan, D. E. and R. J. Campbell. 1970. Effects of *d*-amphetamine and chlordiazepoxide on spaced responding in pigeons. *J. Exp. Anal. Behav.* **14:** 177–184.

McMillan, D. E. and L. S. Harris. 1972. Behavioral and morphine-antagonist effects of the optical isomers of pentazocine and cyclazocine. *J. Pharmacol. Exp. Ther.* **180:** 569–589.

McMillan, D. E. and J. D. Leander. 1975. Drugs and punished responding V. Effects of drugs on responding suppressed by response-dependent and response-independent electric shock. *Arch. Int. Pharmacodyn. Ther.* **213:** 22–27.

McMillan, D. E. and W. H. Morse. 1967. Some effects of morphine and morphine antagonists on schedule controlled behavior. *J. Pharmacol. Exp. Ther.* **157:** 175–184.

McMillan, D. E., L. S. Harris, J. M. Frankenheim and J. S. Kennedy. 1970a. *l*-Δ^9-trans-tetrahydrocannabinol in pigeons: Tolerance to the behavioral effects. *Science* **169:** 501–503.

McMillan, D. E., P. S. Wolf and R. A. Carchman. 1970b. Antagonism of the behavioral effects of morphine and methadone by narcotic antagonists in the pigeon. *J. Pharmacol. Exp. Ther.* **175:** 443–458.

Miczek, K. A. 1973a. Effects of scopolamine, amphetamine and benzodiazepines on conditioned suppression. *Pharmacol. Biochem. Behav.* **1:** 401–411.

Miczek, K. A. 1973b. Effects of scopolamine, amphetamine and chlordiazepoxide on punishment. *Psychopharmacologia* 28: 373–389.

Miller, L. L. and W. G. Drew. 1974. Cannabis: Review of behavioral effects in animals. *Psychol. Bull.* 81: 401–417.

Miller, R. E., J. V. Murphy and I. A. Mirsky. 1957. The effect of chlorpromazine on fear-motivated behavior in rats. *J. Pharmacol. Exp. Ther.* 120: 379–387.

Molinengo, L. and S. Ricci-Gamalero. 1972. The action of imipramine, amitriptyline, doxepin and butriptyline in an operant conditioning schedule. *Psychopharmacologia* 24: 247–257.

Morrison, C. F. 1967. Effects of nicotine on operant behaviour of rats. *Int. J. Neuropharmacol.* 6: 229–240.

Morrison, C. F. 1968. A comparison of the effects of nicotine and amphetamine on DRL performance in the rat. *Psychopharmacologia* 12: 176–180.

Morrison, C. F. 1969. The effects of nicotine on punished behaviour. *Psychopharmacologia* 14: 221–232.

Morse, W. H. 1962. Use of operant conditioning techniques for evaluating the effects of barbiturates on behavior. *The First Hahnemann Symposium on Psychosomatic Medicine.* Lea and Febiger, New York.

Morse, W. H. 1964. Effect of amobarbital and chlorpromazine on punished behavior in the pigeon. *Psychopharmacologia* 6: 286–294.

Niemegeers, C. J. E., F. J. Verbruggen and P. A. J. Janssen. 1969. The influence of various neuroleptic drugs on shock avoidance responding in rats. I. nondiscriminated Sidman avoidance procedure. *Psychopharmacologia* 16: 161–174.

Owen, J. E., Jr. 1960. The influence of *dl-, d-*, and *l*-amphetamine and *d*-methamphetamine on a fixed-ratio schedule. *J. Exp. Anal. Behav.* 3: 293–310.

Owen, J. E., Jr. and R. C. Rathbun. 1966. Sustained changes of a avoidance behavior after chronic nortriptyline administration. *Psychopharmacologia* 9: 137–145.

Paasonen, M. K. and P. B. Dews. 1958. Effects of raunescine and isoraunescine on behaviour and on the 5-hydroxytryptamine and noradrenaline contents of brain. *Brit. J. Pharmacol. and Chemotherapy.* 13: 84–88.

Pearl, J., M. D. Aceto and J. J. Fitzgerald. 1968. Stimulant drugs and temporary increases in avoidance responding. *J. Comp. Physiol. Psychol.* 65: 50–54.

Pradhan, S. N. 1970. Effects of nicotine on several schedules of behavior in rats. *Arch. Int. Pharmacodyn.* 183: 127–138.

Pradhan, S. N. and S. N. Dutta. 1970. Comparative effects of nicotine and amphetamine on timing behavior in rats. *Neuropharmacology* 9: 9–16.

Randall, L. O., W. Schallek, G. A. Heise, E. F. Keith and R. E. Bagdon. 1960. The psychosedative properties of methaminodiazepoxide. *J. Pharmacol. Exp. Ther.* 129: 163–171.

Reynolds, G. S. and P. van Sommers. 1960. Effects of ethyl alcohol on avoidance behavior. *Science* 132: 42–43.

Richelle, M., B. Xhenseval, O. Fontaine and L. Thone. 1962. Action of chlordiazepoxide on two types of temporal conditioning in rats. *Int. J. Neuropharmacol.* 1: 381–391.

Rutledge, C. O. and R. T. Kelleher. 1965. Interactions between the effects of methamphetamine and pentobarbital on operant behavior in the pigeon. *Psychopharmacologia* 7: 400–408.

Sanger, D. J. and D. E. Blackman. 1975a. The effects of tranquillizing drugs on timing behaviour in rats. *Psychopharmacologia* 44: 153–156.

Sanger, D. J. and D. E. Blackman. 1975b. Rate-dependent effects of drugs on the variable-interval behavior of rats. *J. Pharmacol. Exp. Ther.* 194: 343–350.

Sanger, D. J., M. Key and D. E. Blackman. 1974. Differential effects of chlordiazepoxide and d-amphetamine on responding maintained by a DRL schedule of reinforcement. *Psychopharmacologia* **38:** 159–171.

Scheckel, C. L. and E. Boff. 1964. Behavioral effects of interacting imipramine and other drugs with d-amphetamine, cocaine, and tetrabenazine. *Psychopharmacologia* **5:** 198–208.

Scheckel, C. L., E. Boff, P. Dahlen and T. Smart. 1968. Behavioral effects in monkeys of two biologically active marijuana constituents. *Science* **160:** 1467–1469.

Schuster, C. R., W. S. Dockens and J. H. Woods. 1966. Behavioral variables affecting the development of amphetamine tolerance. *Psychopharmacologia* **9:** 170–182.

Scobie, S. R. and G. Garske. 1970. Chlordiazepoxide and conditioned suppression. *Psychopharmacologia* **16:** 272–280.

Sidman, M. 1955. Technique for assessing the effects of drugs on timing behavior. *Science* **122:** 925.

Skinner, B. F. and W. T. Heron. 1937. Effects of caffeine and benzedrine upon conditioning and extinction. *Psychol. Rec.* **1:** 340–346.

Smith, C. B. 1964. Effects of d-amphetamine upon operant behavior of pigeons: enhancement by reserpine. *J. Pharmacol. Exp. Ther.* **146:** 167–174.

Smith, R. P., A. I. Wagman, W. Wagman, C. C. Pfeiffer and A. J. Riopelle. 1957. Effects of some tranquilizing and depressant drugs on conditioned avoidance behavior in monkeys. *J. Pharmacol. Exp. Ther.* **119:** 317–323.

Steinert, H. R., S. G. Holtzman and R. E. Jewett. 1973. Some agonistic actions of the morphine antagonist levallorphan on behavior and brain monoamines in the rat. *Psychopharmacologia* **31:** 35–48.

Stitzer, M. 1974. Comparison of morphine and chlorpromazine effects on moderately and severely suppressed punished responding in the pigeon. *J. Pharmacol. Exp. Ther.* **191:** 172–178.

Stitzer, M., J. Morrison and E. F. Domino. 1970. Effects of nicotine in fixed-interval behavior and their modification by cholinergic antagonists. *J. Pharmacol. Exp. Ther.* **171:** 166–177.

Stone, G. C. 1964. Effects of drugs on nondiscriminated avoidance behavior. I. Individual differences in dose-response relationships. *Psychopharmacologia* **6:** 245–255.

Tenen, S. S. 1967. Recovery time as a measure of CER strength: Effects of benzodiazepines, amobarbital, chlorpromazine and amphetamine. *Psychopharmacologia* **12:** 1–17.

Thompson, D. M. and P. B. Corr. 1974. Behavioral parameters of drug action: signalled and response-independent reinforcement. *J. Exp. Anal. Behav.* **21:** 151–158.

Thompson, T., J. Trombley, D. Luke and D. Lott. 1970. Effects of morphine on behavior maintained by four simple food-reinforcement schedules. *Psychopharmacologia* **17:** 182–192.

Tilson, H. A. and S. B. Sparber. 1973. Similarities and differences between mescaline, lysergic acid diethlamide-25 (LSD) and d-amphetamine on various components of fixed interval responding in the rat. *J. Pharmacol. Exp. Ther.* **184:** 376–384.

Verhave, T. 1958. The effect of methamphetamine on operant level and avoidance behavior. *J. Exp. Anal. Behav.* **1:** 207–219.

Verhave, T., J. E. Owen, Jr. and E. B. Robbins. 1957. Effects of secobarbital and pentobarbital on escape and avoidance behavior. *Psychol. Rep.* **3:** 421–428.

Verhave, T., J. E. Owen, Jr. and E. B. Robbins. 1958. Effects of chlorpromazine and secobarbital on avoidance and escape behavior. *Arch. Int. Pharmacodyn.* **116:** 45–53.

Verhave, T., J. E. Owen, Jr. and E. B. Robbins. 1959. The effect of morphine sulfate on avoidance and escape behavior. *J. Pharmacol. Exp. Ther.* **125:** 248–251.

Wagman, W. D. and G. C. Maxey. 1969. The effects of scopolamine hydrobromide and methyl scopolamine hydrobromide upon the discrimination of interoceptive and exteroceptive stimuli. *Psychopharmacologia* **15:** 280–288.

Waller, M. B. 1961. Effects of chronically administered chlorpromazine on multiple-schedule performance. *J. Exp. Anal. Behav.* **4**: 351–359.
Waller, M. B. and W. H. Morse. 1963. Effects of pentobarbital on fixed-ratio reinforcement. *J. Exp. Anal. Behav.* **6**: 125–130.
Waller, M. B. and P. F. Waller. 1962. Effects of chlorpromazine on appetitive and aversive components of a multiple schedule. *J. Exp. Anal. Behav.* **5**: 259–264.
Wayner, M. J., I. Greenberg, S. Fraley and S. Fisher. 1973. Effects of Δ^9-tetrahydrocannabinol and ethyl alcohol on adjunctive behavior and the lateral hypothalamus. *Physiol. Behav.* **10**: 109–132.
Wedeking, P. W. 1968. Stimulating effects of chlordiazepoxide in rats on a food reinforced FR schedule. *Psychon. Sci.* **12**: 31–32.
Wedeking, P. W. 1974. Schedule-dependent differences among anti-anxiety drugs. *Pharmacol. Biochem. Behav.* **2**: 465–472.
Weiss, B. and C. T. Gott. 1972. A microanalysis of drug effects on fixed-ratio performance in pigeons. *J. Pharmacol. Exp. Ther.* **180**: 189–202.
Weiss, B. and V. G. Laties. 1963. Effects of amphetamine, chlorpromazine and pentobarbital on behavioral thermo-regulation. *J. Pharmacol. Exp. Ther.* **140**: 1–7.
Weiss, B. and V. G. Laties. 1964. Drug effects on the temporal patterning of behavior. *Fed. Proc.* **23**: 801–807.
Weissman, A., 1959. Differential drug effects upon a three-ply multiple schedule of reinforcement. *J. Exp. Anal. Behav.* **2**: 271–287.
Weissman, A. 1963. Correlation between baseline nondiscriminated avoidance behavior in rats and amphetamine-induced stimulation. *Psychopharmacologia* **4**: 294–297.
Willis, R. D. and L. M. Windland. 1968. Effects of repeated administrations of atropine on two multiple schedules. *Psychon. Sci.* **13**: 139–140.
Woods, J. H. 1969. Effects of morphine, methadone, and codeine on schedule-controlled behavior in the pigeon and rhesus monkey. *Fed. Proc.* **28**: 511.
Woods, J. H. and C. R. Schuster. 1971. Opiates as reinforcing stimuli. *In* T. Thompson and R. Pickens (eds.), *Stimulus Properties of Drugs.* Appleton-Century-Crofts, New York, pp. 163–175.
Wray, S. R. 1972. A correlative evaluation of cyclazocine, LSD and naloxone on continuous discriminated avoidance in rats. *Psychopharmacologia* **26**: 29–43.
Wuttke, W. and R. T. Kelleher. 1970. Effects of some benzodiazepines on punished and unpunished behavior in the pigeon. *J. Pharmacol. Exp. Ther.* **172**: 397–405.
Yamahiro, R. S., E. C. Bell and E. Hill. 1961. The effects of reserpine on a strongly conditioned emotional response. *Psychopharmacologia* **2**: 197–202.

10
Drug Effects on Discrimination

The integration and execution of every behavior an organism engages in requires discrimination in one or more of the primary sensory modalities. Therefore, a drug might be expected to alter behavior by virtue of its effects on discrimination. For example, there is a large body of literature concerned with reports of perceptual abnormalities and distortions following the administration of drugs such as mescaline and LSD (Hoffer and Osmond, 1967). Moreover, the narcotic analgesics are used clinically because they are thought to decrease sensitivity to painful stimuli (Goodman and Gilman, 1970). In light of these reports, one might inquire about the way in which these effects can be measured in experimental situations.

The experimenter confronts a number of methodological problems in investigating drug effects on discrimination. Therefore, while this chapter will examine various methods used to examine drug-induced changes in discrimination, methodological difficulties will be emphasized. Since this area has not received much attention, sufficient data are not available to make generalizations about drug effects on discrimination. Illustrative drug studies will be described in order to point out the strengths and weaknesses of the various procedures. Drug studies are not meant to be exhaustive.

Changes in discrimination can only be examined by measuring a change in behavior that is assumed to index a change in discrimination. Attempts to determine a drug's effect on discrimination therefore involve the measurement of behavior in the presence of discriminative stimuli. Alterations in discrimination are inferred from these behavioral measures. For example, in order to determine how a drug might alter afferent input to the visual system, the organism's behavior in response to the input is measured. If a drug alters the behavior in some way, it might be inferred that the drug effect was mediated by an alteration in discrimination. It is difficult, however, to separate the effects of drugs on discriminatory processes from their effects on the behavior used to measure these effects.

The various procedures that have been used to examine drug-induced changes in discrimination can be divided into two general groups. In one group, rates and patterns of responding are used as indicators of discrimination. In the other group, discrete responses are examined. Traditional rate measures are time-based schedules of reinforcement, multiple schedules and stimulus generalization procedures. Discrete trial procedures include matching-to-sample and signal detection procedures. Threshold measures may use rate measures or discrete trials. Each of these procedures will be discussed. Their strengths and weaknesses will be noted, and experiments that have used these procedures will be presented. We will see that there are many problems inherent in using rate of responding to measure discrimination. Some of these problems can be minimized by using discrete trial procedures.

RATE MEASURES

In this section, procedures will be discussed in which differential rates and patterns of responding are used as a measure of discrimination.

Time-based Schedules

In time-based schedules of reinforcement such as an FI or a DRL, the animal's behavior changes as a function of the passage of time. (See Chapter 1 for a thorough description of these schedules.) Under the DRL schedule, responses are reinforced only if a specified period of time without a response has occurred (e.g., in a DRL 20-sec schedule, only a response that follows the preceding response by more than 20-sec is reinforced). The time between responses is called an interresponse time (IRT) (see Chapter 1). Typical DRL 20-sec performance consists of a large percentage of IRTs of 20 sec or more, although there are usually also several very short IRTs (1–2 sec). Drug-induced alterations in IRT distributions have often been interpreted as an effect on temporal discrimination.

Responding under FI schedules has also been shown to change as a function of the passage of time. In the FI schedule, reinforcement is produced by the first response after a specified interval has elapsed. After extended training, responding follows a temporal pattern in which pausing usually occurs at the beginning of the interval, followed by an acceleration in rate towards the end of the interval (Skinner, 1938).

Both DRL and FI response patterns have been shown to change following drug administration (see Chapter 9, Table 9-1). For example, amphetamine has been reported to increase the number of short IRTs on a DRL 20-sec schedule, leading to a reduction in reinforcement frequency (Sidman, 1955). Amphetamine has also been shown to alter FI response patterns as measured by a change in quarter life (see Chapter 1, p. 16) (Stitzer *et al.*, 1970).

It is difficult however, to determine whether a drug alters DRL or FI performance as a result of changes in temporal discrimination. For example, the changes in DRL and FI performance produced by amphetamine may not be due to disruption of temporal discrimination, but rather may reflect the drug's rate-dependent effects (see Chapter 9). Amphetamine has been shown to reduce long IRTs and increase short IRTs on both time-based and *non*-time-based schedules of reinforcement (Segal, 1962; Dews and Morse, 1961). Moreover, many drugs increase low rates of responding early in the FI interval and decrease high rates occurring later in the interval, thereby flattening the response pattern in the FI and decreasing the quarter life. While these effects indicate a change in the temporal pattern of responding, they do not necessarily indicate that a drug has altered discriminative function.

Multiple Schedules

The multiple schedule (see Chapter 1) has also been used to examine drug effects on discrimination, but in general it suffers from problems similar to those of the time-based schedules. Each component of the multiple schedule is associated with a different discriminative stimulus, and a different rate and pattern of responding occurs in the presence of each discriminative stimulus. These different rates and patterns are used as a measure of discrimination. We have seen, however, that drug effects are often rate-dependent; therefore, it is difficult to separate a drug's effect on response rate from its effects on discrimination when rate of responding is the measure of discrimination. For example, in a multiple DRL 10-sec VR 30 schedule of reinforcement, low rates of responding occur in the presence of the DRL stimulus and high rates occur in the presence of the VR stimulus. Let us suppose that the DRL 10-sec component produces responding at the rate of 0.1 response per second and the VR component produces responding at the rate of 2.0 responses per second. Now suppose amphetamine is administered and responding increases to 1.0 response per second in the DRL component and decreases to 1.0 response per second in the VR component. It might be said that the animal's ability to discriminate between the two discriminative stimuli had been altered by the drug, and therefore the organism was unable to determine which schedule of reinforcement was in effect. Alternatively, the drug effect may be accounted for by the drug's characteristic rate-dependent effects on the two different schedule-controlled patterns of responding, *without* affecting the discrimination. If amphetamine normally increases response rate on DRL schedules and normally decreases response rate on VR schedules, then the performance changes seen after the drug in a multiple schedule would not necessarily be indicative of a loss of discrimination. Therefore, the multiple schedule is not a convenient way to measure drug effects on discrimination.

Stimulus Generalization Procedures

The generalization procedure is considered to be a useful tool for analyzing the sensitivity of normal and/or drug treated animals to changes in their external environment. In studies involving stimulus generalization, the subject is initially trained either to respond in the presence of one discriminative stimulus or to respond differentially in the presence of two or more stimuli. A generalization test is then given during extinction; the discriminative stimulus is varied along one of its dimensions (frequency, intensity), and the animal's response rate in the presence of each variation of the stimulus is recorded. For example, during discrimination training, an animal's responses are followed by reinforcement only in the presence of a 1000-Hz tone. During generalization testing, several tones of different frequencies (600, 800, 1200, 1400 Hz) are presented to the animal, and responding is measured during each. When response rates are plotted as a function of each stimulus value, they produce a function describing a generalization gradient. The extent to which an animal's behavior is controlled by variations in the stimulus is related to the slope of the gradient obtained. A flat gradient, showing equal rates of responding in the presence of all test stimuli, indicates little discrimination, whereas a steep gradient, showing maximal responding to the training stimulus and little responding to the test stimuli, indicates that the animal discriminated the training stimulus easily (see Fig. 10-1). The effect of a drug on generalization can be determined by measuring the amount of generalization under drugged and nondrugged conditions.

While generalization procedures have been used to measure drug effects (Hanson and Guttman, 1961; Hearst, 1964; Lyons et al., 1973a,b), these procedures are also confounded by using rate of responding as a measure of discrimination. For example, Dykstra and Appel (1970, 1972) found that the alterations in a generalization test produced by LSD were attributable to drug-induced changes in rate of responding. This work points out the importance of eliminating the confounding effect of changes in response rate from measures of generalization, and demonstrates that whether or not a drug affects ability to discriminate depends on the measure used to examine discrimination.

THRESHOLD MEASURES

Another method for determining whether a drug alters discrimination is an adaptation of techniques developed in the human psychophysical laboratory

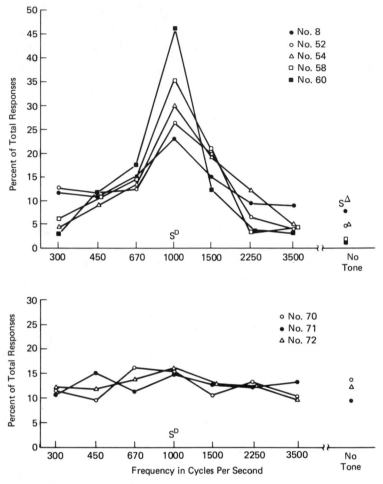

Fig. 10-1. Individual generalization gradients of tonal frequency obtained from pigeons. Upper figure shows a peaked generalization gradient with maximal responding at the training stimulus, less responding in presence of other test stimuli. Lower figure shows approximately equal responding in presence of each stimulus, producing a flat gradient. (From Jenkins and Harrison, 1960.)

to measure threshold levels for auditory stimuli (Békésy, 1947). Blough used the following threshold technique to examine the effects of LSD on a visual discrimination in the pigeon. In brief, pigeons were trained to view a stimulus and to peck one key when the stimulus was visible and another key when the stimulus was not visible. A peck on the "stimulus visible" key operated a control circuit that decreased the stimulus intensity, whereas a peck on the "stimulus not visible" key produced an increase in stimulus intensity. The exact schedule for this procedure is described in detail elsewhere (Blough, 1958). Changes in stimulus intensity produced by the animal's responses were recorded and indicated the animal's threshold over time (see Fig. 10-2). Blough (1957a) found that pigeons produced reliable and consistent thresholds under control conditions. When LSD was given (0.1 mg/kg), a rise was seen in threshold, which remained elevated for several hours before returning to control levels.

Threshold measures have also been used to study the effects of drugs that are thought to alter pain sensitivity. The procedure is similar to the threshold technique used by Blough (1958) to study vision. In general, small increments

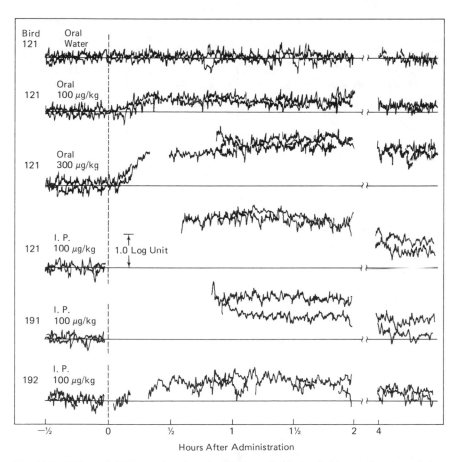

Fig. 10-2. Effect of LDS on the pigeon's absolute visual threshold as a function of time after drug administration. Vertical shifts in the curves represent changes in the brightness of a "just visible" stimulus patch. LSD was given in two oral doses (100 and 300 μg/kg) and one intraperitoneal dose (100 μg/kg). (From Blough, 1957a.)

in some stimulus (usually a shock) are automatically programmed to occur at a specified interval, and decrements in the stimulus intensity follow an appropriate response by the subject. The level at which the subject maintains the shock is said to reflect its tolerance of the shock stimulus. The titration technique has been shown to be a valuable way to examine the analgesic effectiveness of various drugs (Fields and Glusman, 1969; Weiss and Laties, 1961, 1964; Weitzman and Ross, 1962; Scheckel *et al.*, 1968; Pert and Yaksh, 1975; Malis *et al.*, 1975). Weiss and Laties (1958, 1961) used the titration procedure to examine the effects of morphine, aspirin and sodium salicylate in rats. Administration of morphine, sodium salicylate and aspirin produced a rise in the median shock level. Figure 10-3 presents this effect for aspirin.

Weiss and Laties (1964) also examined this schedule with rhesus monkeys. Increases in median shock level were observed following morphine and cyclazocine (a benzomorphan narcotic antagonist), but *not* with the narcotic antagonist nalorphine, which has been shown to be an effective clinical analgesic. Work by Dykstra and McMillan (1974) showed that pentazocine, propoxyphene and morphine increased median shock levels under a titration schedule in squirrel

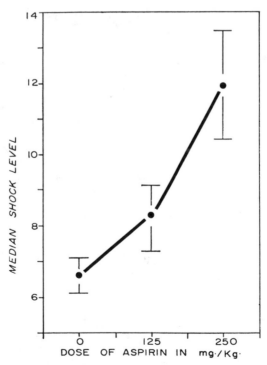

Fig. 10-3. Median shock levels following vehicle alone and 125 and 250 mg/kg aspirin delivered via stomach tube. Data are the mean of 10 animals. Brackets represent standard errors. (From Weiss and Laties, 1961.)

monkeys.   No changes were seen with chlorpromazine, nalorphine or naloxone.

While techniques such as titration are promising and should be developed further, they suffer from the same difficulty as do all methods which are based on the assumption that a sensory threshold must exist which is independent of presumably nonsensory variables such as response rate or other parameters of the experimental situation.   For example, in the work of Weiss and Laties (1959, 1961, 1963) it was found that the level at which rats maintained a shock depended on how rapidly the shock level was increased.   When the time interval between shock intensity increments was short, the animals tolerated a higher shock level.   A similar relationship was seen between the number of responses required to produce a decrease in shock level and the level at which the animal maintained the shock.   The effects of morphine and sodium salicylate were examined under the titration schedule with an interval between shock increments of 2 sec or 10 sec (i–i interval).   It was found that the drug effect depended on the schedule of shock presentation (see Fig. 10-4).   When the i–i interval was short (2 sec), the median shock level was maintained at higher intensities and it was increased more following both morphine and sodium salicylate than when the i–i interval was 10 sec.

Thus, once again we find that the effects of drugs on presumed indexes of discriminability are confounded by effects that may be independent of purely sensory variables.

DISCRETE TRIAL PROCEDURES

One way to minimize the confounding effects of variations in response rate on measures of discrimination is to use discrete trial procedures.   Since most drugs have been reported to produce marked variation in response rate (see Chapter 9), a discrete trial procedure in which a single response is made in the presence of each stimulus might be more appropriate for studying discrimination than procedures in which rate is a variable.

Discrete trial discrimination tasks are similar to free operant discriminations such as the multiple schedule in that in both cases an animal is trained by differential reinforcement to respond in a certain way in the presence of one stimulus (or class of stimuli) and in another way in the presence of another stimulus (Keller and Schoenfeld, 1950).   The organism is said to discriminate between the two stimuli to the extent that its behavior in the presence of one stimulus is different from its behavior in the presence of another stimulus (Gilbert and Sutherland, 1969).   In the case of a discrete trial procedure, differential behavior may be right or left lever presses, right or left turns in a maze or responding in the presence of one stimulus but not responding in the presence of another stimulus.   The measure of responding is a probability rather than a rate.

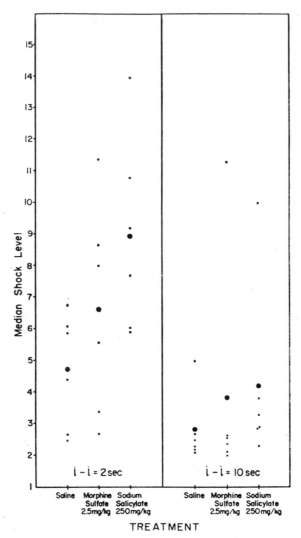

Fig. 10-4. Median shock levels with saline, 2.5 mg/kg morphine sulfate and 250 mg/kg sodium salicylate at i-i = 10 sec and i-i = 2 sec. The large dots show the means of the medians. The individual subjects are shown by the small dots. (From Weiss and Laties, 1961.)

Successive Discriminations

Among the most common discrete trial procedures are those which use a *successive* discrimination. In a successive discrimination, one response is correct following the presentation of one stimulus, and a different response is correct following the presentation of some other stimulus. Only one stimulus is presented on each trial. These procedures have been used to study drug effects (McFarlain, 1973; Heise and Lilie, 1970; Stubbs and Thomas, 1974; Elsmore, 1972b; Heise, 1975). For example, Elsmore (1972b) used a two-lever discrimination task to examine the effects of THC on temporal discrimination. He trained chimps to discriminate between two durations of a visual stimulus. Following presentation of a 100-sec visual stimulus, a left response was correct; following presentation of a visual stimulus for less than 100-sec, a right response was correct. Elsmore found that THC (1.0–16 mg/kg) reduced the number of discrimination trials initiated by the chimps and also reduced discrimination accuracy in a dose-related manner. Similarly, Stubbs and Thomas (1974) reported that d-amphetamine (0.23–2.5 mg/kg) decreased the accuracy with which pigeons discriminated between a visual stimulus that was presented either for 1–5 sec or for 6–10 sec.

Matching to Sample

Another discrete trial procedure is the matching-to-sample task. It is of special interest because it provides a technique for examining complex discriminations. In the matching-to-sample procedure, a sample stimulus and two or more comparison stimuli are used. The sample stimulus is usually presented first, and then removed following a response. Then two or more comparison stimuli are presented simultaneously, and the subject's task is to indicate by a response which of the comparison stimuli matches the previously presented sample stimulus (see Fig. 10-5).

As with the successive discrimination task described above, matching-to-sample procedures have been used for the study of drug effects (Blough, 1957b; Berryman et al., 1962; Pragay et al., 1969). Various modifications can be made in this basic procedure. For example, one can manipulate the time between presentation of the sample and comparison stimuli in order to study the effect of delay on discrimination. Glick and Jarvik (1969a,b) have shown that amphetamine decreases the accuracy of delayed matching tasks. Similarly THC and ethanol have been reported to disrupt delayed matching tasks (Scheckel et al., 1968; Ferraro and Grilly, 1974; Mello, 1971).

Complex discriminations can also be investigated by requiring the subject to match classes of stimuli; for example, if the standard stimulus is a triangle, the subject may be required to make a match with other forms having the characteristics of a triangle. Siegel (1969) trained animals on a visual discrimination task which required conditional responding along the dimensions of form and color. A sample stimulus was first presented to the animal on a center key. This stimulus pattern was either a white triangle, another form or a color. When the white triangle was presented, responses on the center key were correct;

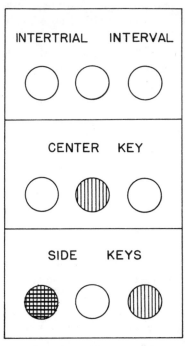

MATCHING - TO - SAMPLE

INTERTRIAL   INTERVAL

CENTER   KEY

SIDE   KEYS

Fig. 10-5. Schematic representation of matching-to-sample procedure. During the intertrial interval all keys are dark. A trial is started by illuminating the center key with one of the three hues. As soon as the bird pecks the center key, it is turned off and both side keys are illuminated, one with a hue matching that on the center key, the other with one of the two nonmatching hues. The two side keys remain illuminated until the bird pecks either of the side keys. When the side key response is made, all the key lights are turned off. If this response was to the side key of matching hue, food is presented for 3 sec; if it was to the nonmatching side key, the chamber lights are turned off, and the bird is left in total darkness for 3 sec. The intertrial interval follows either the reinforcement or the blackout.

if a color appeared on the center key, right key responses were correct; if a form appeared on the center key, left key responses were correct. LSD and cannabis increased responding on the color dimension. In other words, following drug administration pigeons reported color changes when no color changes were occurring on the center key, suggesting to Siegel that the animals were experiencing color hallucinations.

Discrete trial studies such as these provide a promising direction for research with drugs on discrimination. The results obtained to date are sketchy, however. Each experiment has used different drugs or dose ranges, different stimulus modalities or different tasks. For example, it has been reported that LSD may either increase (Becker et al., 1967), decrease (Fuster, 1959; Sharpe et al., 1967; Siegel, 1969) or have no effect (Berryman et al., 1962) on the accuracy of discrimination problems. Each of these studies, however, differs from the others in some important way, in terms of either the stimuli examined, the drug doses, the species or the routes of drug administration.

More important, however, is the fact that although discrete trial procedures avoid the difficulties inherent in the use of response rate to measure drug effects on discrimination, they do not solve the basic problem that a drug's effect on the measure used to evaluate performance cannot be separated from its effect on ability to discriminate. For example, d-amphetamine is known to increase response perseveration or stereotypy (see Chapter 6). If, in a discrete trial discrimination, accuracy (percent correct responding) decreases, this could be caused either by a drug-induced reduction in ability to discriminate or by a drug-induced increase in the probability that the animal will continue to do on trial $t + 1$ whatever he happened to be doing on trial t.

For example, Stubbs and Thomas (1974) trained pigeons on a two-key choice procedure that involved discriminating visual stimuli of varying durations. One response was reinforced following stimuli of short durations, and another response was reinforced following stimuli of longer durations. They reported that d-amphetamine decreased discrimination accuracy in this task. They also reported, however, that pigeons tended to respond on the same key as the dose level of d-amphetamine increased. Therefore, accuracy decreased because the pigeon tended to emit one class of responses (e.g., left responses) regardless of the stimuli presented.

It is unlikely that any procedure can eliminate this difficulty, even though many attempts have been made to separate the effects of response perseveration from measures of accuracy. For example, blank trials (i.e., trials in which no stimulus or an irrelevant stimulus is presented) may be introduced from time to time, and tendency to respond or not to respond (or to respond right or left) may be determined when no sensory discrimination is possible. Perhaps the most systematic effort to separate accuracy or sensitivity measures from perseveration or bias has been the application of signal detection theory.

Signal Detection

The theory of signal detection (SDT) provides a way to separate the ability to detect a stimulus from factors that affect response bias. The model has been applied successfully in human and animal psychophysics (Blough, 1967; Boneau and Cole, 1967; Hack, 1963; Nevin, 1964, 1970; Terman, 1970; Irwin and Terman, 1970; Clopton, 1972; Elsmore, 1972a; Hodos and Bonbright, 1972; Terman and Terman, 1973) and has also recently been extended to the study of drug action in animals (Dykstra and Appel, 1974; Warburton and Brown, 1971, 1972; Brown and Warburton, 1971) and in man (Schneider and Carpenter, 1969; Chapman *et al.*, 1973; Rappaport *et al.*, 1971, 1972; Chapman and Feather, 1973). While both elementary (McNicol, 1972) and more detailed explications of signal detection theory (Green and Swets, 1966) are available, it might be well to review some of the basic assumptions of this model before proceeding further.

In a signal detection procedure, the subject's task is to detect whether a stimulus (or signal) has been presented in background noise during a discrete trial period. In reporting whether or not a signal has been presented on a specific trial, at least two factors might affect the subject's decision to respond "Yes, it has been presented" or "No, it has not"; these two factors are (1) the subject's ability to detect the stimulus, i.e., his sensitivity, and (2) the subject's overall tendency to respond, i.e., his bias. Sensitivity is usually a function of the physical characteristics of the stimuli, while bias is usually a function of the consequences that follow the detection response. For example, if the subject is reinforced with a dime for responding yes to a signal that has actually been presented, but is penalized one dollar for responding yes when a signal has not been presented, the subject will probably only respond yes to clearly audible signals. On the other hand, if the relative reinforcing value of a yes or no response is reversed so that the subject now earns a dollar for responding yes in the presence of a signal but is only fined a dime for a yes response when the signal is absent, he will probably respond yes even when he is not sure the signal has been presented. The observer's sensitivity has not changed from one set of contingencies to the other, but his bias or tendency to respond yes has changed.

In order to separate the measure of sensitivity from the measure of bias, the relative frequencies of a subject's responses are examined over several detection trials. When a signal-noise discrimination is made, four possible stimulus-response combinations can occur. These combinations are shown below.

RESPONSE

		Signal	Noise
STIMULUS	Signal	HIT	MISS
	Noise	FALSE ALARM	CORRECT REJECTION

If the subject reports a signal on a trial when in fact a signal has been presented, a *hit* occurs. Reporting a signal on a trial when no signal has been presented is a *false alarm*. Reporting noise when in fact no signal has been presented is a *correct rejection*, and failing to report a signal when a signal has been presented is a *miss*. For purposes of determining sensitivity and bias, noise and signal stimuli are presented, and the number of times the subject makes a hit and a false alarm are recorded. Therefore hit rate equals number of hits/number of trials on which a signal is presented, and false alarm rate equals number of false alarms/number of trials on which a signal is not presented. Only hit and false alarm rates are needed since P (Miss) $= 1 - P$ (Hit), and P (Correct Rejection) $= 1 - P$ (False Alarm). Usually hit and false alarm rates are determined under several different experimental conditions in which the consequences of making various responses are manipulated. For example, in one condition hits and false alarms might be reinforced equally, and in another condition the relative reinforcing value might be greater for a hit than for a correct rejection. Then the P (Hit) is plotted as a function of P (False Alarm), and a receiver operating characteristic or relative operating characteristic (ROC) curve is obtained. The ROC curve is an analytical technique used in signal detection analysis to isolate response bias from sensitivity. A sensitivity and a bias measure can be obtained from each point on the ROC curve. The area under the curve is used as a measure of sensitivity, and bias is measured by the position of each point on a curve relative to the negative diagonal. (See Hodos, 1970; Pollack and Norman, 1964; Grier, 1971; Green and Swots, 1966, for details of the measuring procedure.)

The following study (Dykstra and Appel, 1974) describes one way in which a signal detection procedure can be designed. Rats were trained on a two-lever, discrete trial, auditory discrimination task involving two stimuli—a high (5000-Hz) or a low (2000-Hz) tone. A response on the left lever in the presence of the 2000-Hz tone was arbitrarily designated a hit, and a response on the right lever in the presence of the other tone (5000 Hz) was arbitrarily designated a correct rejection. The two complementary responses—a left response in the presence of a 5000-Hz tone and a right response in the presence of the 2000-Hz tone—were designated as false alarm and miss, respectively. For example, with a 2000–5000-Hz discrimination, the following situation was in effect:

	Left response	Right response
2000 Hz	Hit	Miss
5000 Hz	False alarm	Correct rejection

The experiment was designed so that differential consequences could be attached to each response. Reinforcement followed every tenth hit and tenth correct rejection (10, 10), tabulated independently. False alarms and misses were always followed by a time-out of 4 sec.

After stable baseline levels of accuracy were obtained with this symmetrical reinforcement schedule in which probabilities of reinforcement on each lever were identical and bias was minimal, LSD was given ip in doses of 0.04, 0.08 and 0.16 mg/kg immediately before certain sessions. The relative reinforcing value of a hit and a correct rejection was then altered by changing the number of correct responses required for reinforcement. Therefore, instead of there being equal reinforcement for both a hit and a correct rejection, the probability of the rat's being reinforced for a hit was greater than for a correct rejection. Milk reinforcement occurred every tenth hit and every second correct rejection (10, 2); later these values were reversed (2, 10). The same dosages of LSD were then readministered. The stimulus parameters were then changed by varying the distance between the stimuli to be discriminated (e.g., 3000–4000 Hz and 3800–3300 Hz), and new data were obtained for control and drug days at each of the reinforcement contingencies already outlined (10, 10; 10, 2; 2, 10).

The data obtained from the three stimulus conditions (2000 vs. 5000, 3000 vs. 4000, and 3300 vs. 3800 Hz) under each of the three reinforcement conditions (10, 10; 10, 2; 2, 10) were then plotted as receiver operator characteristic curves (ROC curves). The ROC curve was obtained in the following way: under a fixed stimulus condition, e.g., tones of 2000 and 5000 Hz, a left response in the presence of the 2000-Hz tone $[P$ (Hit)$]$ was plotted as a function of the probability of left response in the presence of the 5000-Hz tone $[P$ (False Alarm)$]$. These probabilities were obtained under each reinforcement condition; each point on the curve then represents the subject's performance in a given reinforcement condition. A similar curve was generated for each stimulus condition. Points generated from the same stimulus condition fell along the same curve; under different stimulus conditions points fell along a different curve.

Figure 10-6 shows actual ROC curves generated from the performance of one rat on three different discriminations (A = 2000 vs. 5000 Hz; B = 3000 vs. 4000 Hz; C = 3300 vs. 3800 Hz). Sensitivity was a direct function of the degree of separation of the tones (i.e., task difficulty); it was greatest during the 2000 vs. 5000 Hz discrimination and least during the 3300 vs. 3800 Hz discrimination (Fig. 10-6). The relative frequency of reinforced trials for left or right responses (2, 10; 10, 10; 10, 2) affected the animal's bias systematically but did not alter sensitivity (Fig. 10-6).

The question of interest is whether LSD affected sensitivity or bias, or both. Suppose the drug is given under the symmetrical 10, 10 contingency with a discrimination of 3000–4000 Hz. With reference to the ROC curve of Fig. 10-6, at least two things might occur, i.e., the point P (Hit) as a function of P (FA) obtained following drug can (1) move along curve B, relative to where it had been following saline—an effect on bias; or (2) it can jump to another

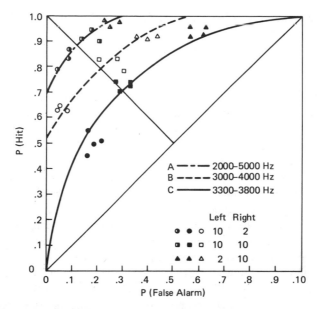

Fig. 10-6. Three receiver operator characteristic (ROC) curves for the performance of one rat on three frequency discriminations. Points were obtained by plotting the probability of making a hit (i.e., responding on the left lever in the presence of a low tone) as a function of the probability of making a false alarm (i.e., responding on the left lever in the presence of a high tone). Points represent at least three determinations at each discrimination for three reinforcement conditions. In one reinforcement condition, every tenth correct response on the left lever and every second correct response on the right lever were reinforced. In the second condition every tenth correct response on the left lever and every tenth correct response on the right lever were reinforced. The third condition was the opposite of the first condition: every second correct response on the left lever and every tenth correct response on the right lever were reinforced. Conditioned reinforcement followed all correct responses. The curves were fitted to these points by inspection. (From Dykstra and Appel, 1974.)

curve—an effect on sensitivity. In fact, no dose or dose regimen of LSD had any effect on sensitivity. However, the drug did alter bias, i.e., produced movement along the ROC curve. These changes were significant at doses greater than 0.04 mg/kg.

The results of this analysis suggest that the effects of LSD might be due more to drug-induced changes in decision to respond (or, more accurately, to respond more often on one lever than on another) than to changes in ability to detect differences in frequency of auditory stimuli. The drug acts as if it mimics the effect of variables such as frequency of reinforcement that alter bias.

Dykstra and Appel (1974) report identical results in a discrimination involving temporal stimuli. Rats were required to discriminate between tones with a duration of 1.25 or 2.25 sec. At doses greater than 0.04 mg/kg, LSD altered response preference (bias) but had no effect on ability to detect differences in duration of auditory stimuli.

SENSORY VARIABLES

We have emphasized numerous methodological variables that affect the measurement of drug effects on sensory function. While it can be concluded that more consistent methodology is needed before generalizations can be drawn about a drug's effect on discrimination, it should also be noted that in order to make an extensive investigation of a drug's effect on discrimination, sensory variables such as the difficulty of the discrimination and the physical properties of the stimuli must also be considered, as well as the familiar variables of dose, species and route of drug administration.

For example, it has been shown that a drug's effect may be determined by the difficulty of the discrimination. LSD alters complex discriminations but not more simple discriminations (Polidora, 1963; Sharpe et al., 1967). Similarly, secobarbital has been shown to produce greater impairment of more difficult tasks than of simpler tasks (Pragay et al., 1969). It has also been shown that a dose of a drug that has little or no effect on stimulus control exerted by a single stimulus disrupts complex conditional discriminations involving at least three stimuli (Dews, 1955). Dews trained pigeons to respond on an S^D, S^Δ discrimination. In the simple discrimination pecking was reinforced in the presence of a red light and not reinforced in the presence of a blue light. This discrimination was not disrupted by pentobarbital, methamphetamine or scopolamine. In the complex discrimination pecking was reinforced according to a conditional discrimination. Pentobarbital and methamphetamine disrupted this more complex (conditional) discrimination in a dose-dependent fashion.

Variability in a drug's effect also may be due to the stimulus modality examined. Blough (1957b) reported that 0.1–0.3 mg/kg of LSD given orally to pigeons had an enhancing effect on a complex visual discrimination based on brightness, but Berryman et al. (1962) found no change after LSD (0.05 mg/kg) when pigeons performed a similar discrimination with hue. Therefore, drug effects on discrimination behavior depend on numerous variables, each of which must be specified in order to describe a drug effect accurately.

SUMMARY

This chapter has reviewed some of the data and problems associated with assessing a drug's effect on discrimination. We have seen that it is difficult to isolate discrimination as a discrete process, since "stimulus control of behavior involves simultaneous consideration of the stimuli governing and behavior governed" (Dews, 1970, p. 398).   Sufficient data are not available to make generalizations about drug effects on sensory function.   Investigations of drug effects on sensory function await a consistent methodology so that effects can be examined over a broad range of drug doses, in several species and taking into account such variables as the physical characteristics of the stimuli discriminated, and the consequences maintaining the behavior examined.

REFERENCES

Becker, D. I., J. B. Appel and D. X. Freedman. 1967.   Some effects of lysergic acid diethylamide on visual discrimination in pigeons. *Psychopharmacologia* 11: 354–364.

Békésy, G. V. 1947. A new audiometer. *Acta Oto-Laryng.* 35: 411–422.

Berryman, R., M. E. Jarvik and J. A. Nevin. 1962.   Effects of pentobarbital, lysergic acid diethylamide and chlorpromazine on matching behavior in the pigeon. *Psychopharmacologia* 3: 60–65.

Blough, D. S. 1957a.   Effect of lysergic acid diethylamide on absolute visual threshold of the pigeon. *Science* 126: 304–305.

Blough, D. S. 1957b.   Effects of drugs on visually controlled behavior in pigeons. *In* S. Garattini and V. Ghetti (eds.), *Psychotropic Drugs.* Amsterdam, Elsevier, pp. 110–118.

Blough, D. S. 1958.   A method for obtaining psychophysical thresholds from the pigeon. *J. Exp. Anal. Behav.* 1: 31–43.

Blough, D. S. 1967.   Stimulus generalization as signal detection in pigeons. *Science* 158: 940–941.

Boneau, C. A. and J. L. Cole. 1967.   Decision theory, the pigeon, and the psychophysical function. *Psych. Rev.* 74: 123–135.

Brown, K. and D. M. Warburton. 1971.   Attenuation of stimulus sensitivity by scopolamine. *Psychon. Sci.* 22: 297–298.

Chapman, C. R. and B. W. Feather. 1973.   Effects of diazepam on human pain tolerance and pain sensitivity. *Psychosom. Med.* 35: 330–340.

Chapman, C. R., T. M. Murphy and S. H. Butler. 1973.   Analgesic strength of 33 percent nitrous oxide: A signal detection theory evaluation. *Science* 179: 1246–1248.

Clopton, B. M. 1972.   Detection of increments in noise intensity by monkeys. *J. Exp. Anal. Behav.* 17: 473–481.

Dews, P. B. 1955.   Studies on Behavior. II. The effects of pentobarbital, methamphetamine, and scopolamine on performances in pigeons involving discriminations. *J. Pharmacol. Exp. Ther.* 115: 380–389.

Dews, P. B. 1970.   Drugs in psychology. A commentary on Travis Thompson and Charles R. Schuster's *Behavioral Pharmacology. J. Exp. Anal. Behav.* 13: 395–406.

Dews, P. B. and W. H. Morse. 1961.   Behavioral pharmacology. *Ann. Rev. Pharmacol.* 1: 145–174.

Dykstra, L. A. and J. B. Appel. 1970.   Effects of LSD on auditory generalization. *Psychon. Sci.* 21: 272–274.

Dykstra, L. A. and J. B. Appel. 1972.   Lysergic acid diethylamide and stimulus generalization: Rate-dependent effects. *Science* 177: 720–722.

Dykstra, L. A. and J. B. Appel. 1974.   Effects of LSD on auditory perception: A signal detection analysis. *Psychopharmacologia* 34: 289–307.

Dykstra, L. A. and D. E. McMillan. 1974.   Shock-intensity adjustment by squirrel monkeys under a titration procedure following administration of morphine, nalorphine, pentazocine, propoxyphene, Δ^8-tetrahydrocannabinol (Δ^8-THC) or chlorpromazine. *Fed. Proc.* **33**: 516.

Elsmore, T. F. 1972a. Duration discrimination: effects of probability of stimulus presentation. *J. Exp. Anal. Behav.* **18**: 465–469.

Elsmore, T. F. 1972b. Effects of delta-9-tetrahydrocannabinol on temporal and auditory discrimination performances of monkeys. *Psychopharmacologia* **26**: 62–72.

Ferraro, D. P. and D. M. Grilly. 1974. Effects of chronic exposure to Δ^9-tetrahydrocannabinol on delayed matching-to-sample in chimpanzees. *Psychopharmacologia* **37**: 127–138.

Fields, L. and M. Glusman. 1969. Titration of aversive thresholds in cats: escape and avoidance components. *J. Comp. Physiol. Psychol.* **68**: 334–337.

Fuster, J. M. 1959. Lysergic acid and its effects on visual discrimination in monkeys. *J. Nerv. Ment. Dis.* **129**: 252–256.

Gilbert, R. M. and N. S. Sutherland (eds.). 1969. *Animal Discrimination Learning.* Academic Press, New York.

Glick, S. D. and M. E. Jarvik. 1969a. Amphetamine, scopolamine and chlorpromazine interactions on delayed matching performance in monkeys. *Psychopharmacologia* **16**: 147–155.

Glick, S. D. and M. E. Jarvik. 1969b. Impairment by *d*-amphetamine of delayed matching performance in monkeys. *J. Pharmacol. Exp. Ther.* **169**: 1–6.

Goodman, L. S. and A. Gilman. 1970. *The Pharmacological Basis of Therapeutics.* Macmillan Pub. Co., Inc. New York.

Green, D. M. and J. A. Swets. 1966. *Signal Detection Theory and Psychophysics.* Wiley, New York.

Grier, J. B. 1971. Nonparametric indexes for sensitivity and bias: computing formulas. *Psychol. Bull.* **75**: 424–429.

Hack, H. 1963. Signal detection in the rat. *Science* **139**: 758–759.

Hanson, H. M. and N. Guttman. 1961. The use of a behavioral stimulant in the study of stimulus generalization. *J. Exp. Anal. Behav.* **4**: 209–212.

Hearst, E. 1964. Drug effects on stimulus generalization gradients in the monkey. *Psychopharmacologia* **6**: 57–70.

Heise, G. A. 1975. Discrete trial analysis of drug action. *Fed. Proc.* **34**: 1898–1903.

Heise, G. A. and N. L. Lilie. 1970. Effects of scopolamine, atropine, and *d*-amphetamine on internal and external control of responding on non-reinforced trials. *Psychopharmacologia* **18**: 38–49.

Hodos, W. 1970. Nonparametric index of response bias for use in detection and recognition experiments. *Psychol. Bull.* **74**: 351–354.

Hodos, W. and J. C. Bonbright, Jr. 1972. The detection of visual intensity differences by pigeons. *J. Exp. Anal. Behav.* **18**: 471–479.

Hoffer, A. and H. Osmond. 1967. *The Hallucinogens.* Academic Press, New York.

Irwin, R. J. and M. Terman. 1970. Detection of brief tones in noise by rats. *J. Exp. Anal. Behav.* **13**: 135–143.

Jenkins, H. M. and R. H. Harrison. 1960. Effect of discrimination training on auditory generalization. *J. Exp. Psychol.* **59**: 246–253.

Keller, F. S. and W. N. Schoenfeld. 1950. *Principles of Psychology.* Appleton-Century-Crofts, New York.

Lyons, J., W. D. Klipec and R. Eirick. 1973a. The effect of chlorpromazine on the peak shift in the albino rat. *Physiol. Psychol.* **1**: 165–168.

Lyons, J., W. D. Klipec and G. Steinsultz. 1973b. The effect of chlorpromazine on discrimination performance and the peak shift. *Physiol. Psychol.* **1**: 121–124.

Malis, J. L., M. E. Rosenthale and M. I. Gluckman. 1975. Animal pharmacology of Wy-16, 225, a new analgesic agent. *J. Pharmacol. Exp. Ther.* **194**: 488–498.

McFarlain, R. A. 1973. Para-chlorophenylalanine: Its effects on auditory discrimination. *Psychopharmacologia* **29**: 263–270.

McNicol, D. 1972. *A Primer of Signal Detection Theory.* George Allen and Unwin, Ltd. London.

Mello, N. K. 1971. Alcohol effects on delayed matching to sample performance by rhesus monkey. *Physiol. Behav.* **7**: 77–101.

Nevin, J. A. 1964. A method for the determination of psychophysical functions in the rat. *J. Exp. Anal. Behav.* **7**: 169.

Nevin, J. A. 1970. On differential stimulation and differential reinforcement. *In* W. C. Stebbin (ed.), *Animal Psychophysics: The Design and Conduct of Sensory Experiments.* Appleton-Century-Crofts, New York, pp. 401–423.

Pert, A. and T. Yaksh. 1975. Localization of the antinociceptive action of morphine in primate brain. *Pharmacol. Biochem. Behav.* **3**: 133–138.

Polidora, V. J. 1963. A sequential response method of studying complex behavior in animals and its application to the measurement of drug effects. *J. Exp. Anal. Behav.* **6**: 271–277.

Pollack, I. and D. A. Norman. 1964. A non-parametric analysis of recognition experiments. *Psychon. Sci.* **1**: 125–126.

Pragay, E. B., A. F. Mirsky and J. M. Abplanalp. 1969. The effects of chlorpromazine and secobarbital on matching from sample and discrimination tasks in monkeys. *Psychopharmacologia* **16**: 128–138.

Rappaport, M., H. K. Hopkins and K. Hall. 1972. Auditory signal detection in paranoid and nonparanoid schizophrenics. *Arch. Gen. Psychiat.* **27**: 747–752.

Rappaport, M., J. Silverman, H. K. Hopkins and K. Hall. 1971. Phenothiazine effects on auditory signal detection in paranoid and nonparanoid schizophrenics. *Science* **174**: 723–725.

Scheckel, C. L., E. Boff, P. Dahlen and T. Smart. 1968. Behavioral effects in monkeys of racemates of two biologically active marijuana constituents. *Science* **160**: 1467–1469.

Schneider, E. W. and J. A. Carpenter. 1969. The influence of ethanol on auditory signal detection. *Quart. J. Stud. Alcohol* **30**: 357–370.

Segal, E. F. 1962. Effects of *dl*-amphetamine under concurrent VI DRL reinforcement. *J. Exp. Anal. Behav.* **5**: 105–112.

Sharpe, L. G., L. S. Otis and R. J. Schusterman. 1967. Disruption of size discrimination in squirrel monkeys (*saimiri sciureus*) by LSD-25. *Psychon. Sci.* **7**: 103–104.

Sidman, M. 1955. Technique for assessing the effects of drugs on timing behavior. *Science* **122**: 925.

Siegel, R. K. 1969. Effects of cannabis sativa and lysergic acid diethylamide on a visual discrimination task in pigeons. *Psychopharmacologia* **15**: 1–8.

Skinner, B. F. 1938. *The Behavior of Organisms.* Appleton-Century-Crofts, New York.

Stitzer, M., J. Morrison and E. F. Domino. 1970. Effects of nicotine on fixed-interval behavior and their modification by cholinergic antagonists. *J. Pharmacol. Exp. Ther.* **171**: 166–177.

Stubbs, D. A. and J. R. Thomas. 1974. Discrimination of stimulus duration and *d*-amphetamine in pigeons: A psychophysical analysis. *Psychopharmacologia* **36**: 313–322.

Terman, M. 1970. Discrimination of auditory intensities by rats. *J. Exp. Anal. Behav.* **13**: 145–160.

Terman, M. and J. S. Terman. 1973. Latency differentiation of hits and false alarms in an operant-psychophysical test. *J. Exp. Anal. Behav.* **20:** 439–445.

Warburton, D. M. and K. Brown. 1971. Attenuation of stimulus sensitivity induced by scopolamine. *Nature* **230:** 126–127.

Warburton, D. M. and K. Brown. 1972. The facilitation of discrimination performance by physostigmine sulphate. *Psychopharmacologia* **27:** 275–284.

Weiss, B. and V. G. Laties. 1958. Fractional escape and avoidance on a titration schedule. *Science* **128:** 1575–1576.

Weiss, B. and V. G. Laties. 1959. Titration behavior on various fractional escape programs. *J. Exp. Anal. Behav.* **2:** 227–248.

Weiss, B. and V. G. Laties. 1961. Changes in pain tolerance and other behavior produced by salicylates. *J. Pharmacol. Exp. Ther.* **131:** 120–129.

Weiss, B. and V. G. Laties. 1963. Characteristics of aversive thresholds measured by a titration schedule. *J. Exp. Anal. Behav.* **6:** 563–572.

Weiss, B. and V. G. Laties. 1964. Analgesic effects in monkeys of morphine, nalorphine, and a benzomorphan narcotic antagonist. *J. Pharmacol. Exp. Ther.* **143:** 169–173.

Weitzman, E. D. and G. S. Ross. 1962. A behavioral method for the study of pain perception in the monkey. The effects of some pharmacological agents. *Neurology* **12:** 264–272.

11
Drugs as Reinforcers

The fundamental principle of behavior analysis which was outlined in Chapter 1 was that the frequency and pattern of operant behavior is controlled by the events that follow it, i.e., consequences or reinforcers. In this chapter the ability of drugs to act as reinforcers will be examined. The acquisition and maintenance of drug-reinforced responding will be described, as well as the pattern of res-ponding generated when different drugs and different doses of a drug serve as reinforcers and also when they are presented on various schedules. Finally, the applications of this research to human drug abuse will be discussed along with models for predicting a particular drug's abuse potential.

In order to study drugs as reinforcers, it is necessary to develop a technique whereby drug delivery is contingent on the behavior of the organism, i.e., the drug should be self-administered. Ideally, the method should permit identifi-cation and subsequent manipulation of the variables that control the acquisition and maintenance of drug administration. The method used most often to ex-amine drugs as reinforcers involves delivery of the drug via the intravenous route. Oral methods are also used, but special inducements are often necessary to estab-lish administration with oral methods because many drugs have a bitter or sour taste. In addition, there is a delayed onset of pharmacological action when a drug is delivered by the oral route. Intragastric (Ellis and Pick, 1970; Yanagita and Takahashi, 1973; Götestam, 1973) and inhalational (Goldstein and Pal, 1971) techniques for drug delivery have also been used, but are less common. The oral and intravenous methods and data derived from these techniques are discussed below. It might be noted that the drugs self-administered by animals are also self-administered by man (Jaffe, 1970; Eddy et al., 1965).

ORAL ADMINISTRATION

Several methods have been used to examine drug administration by the oral route, including procedures in which animals are simply given free access to a drug solution as well as procedures in which special inducements are used to obtain drug administration. Because many drugs have an unpleasant taste, investigations in which the drug is made freely available to the animal have met with limited success. Techniques in which drug consumption is induced by placing the drug in the animals' sole source of food or water do produce substantial amounts of drug intake; however, they do not demonstrate that the drug is serving as a reinforcer. Similar problems occur with other procedures for inducing drug intake. Nevertheless, some provide a better demonstration of drug reinforcement than others. While a variety of drugs have been examined with these procedures, the majority of the work has been with ethanol. In assessing the reinforcing properties of ethanol, it is important to consider the fact that ethanol provides caloric content. (See Mello, 1973, for a discussion of these problems and a review of some procedures used to examine ethanol consumption.)

Free Access

In 1940 Richter and Campbell reported that rats would drink more ethanol than water when given concurrent access to water and ethanol (1.8-6% w/v) in their home cages. While more recent work has confirmed the fact that animals will freely consume certain concentrations of ethanol, the amount consumed is generally not sufficient to produce intoxication or physical dependence. Moreover, ethanol consumption has been shown to depend on a variety of factors, including the ethanol concentration, the sex, age and species or strain of the experimental subject, as well as factors such as position habits, food and water deprivation, previous ethanol history and the availability of alternative food and liquid sources (see Lester, 1966; Myers and Veale, 1972).

Forced Consumption

In the forced consumption method a drug is added to the only liquid (or food) available to the animal, and the animal is forced to drink (or eat) the drug to obtain fluid (or food). Work with this method has shown that animals will consume a variety of drug solutions under these conditions, including d-amphetamine, cocaine, several barbiturates, morphine, methadone, meperidine, etonitazene, meprobamate, chlordiazepoxide, lysergic acid diethylamide, ethanol and caffeine (Wikler et al., 1963; Harris et al., 1968; Stolerman et al., 1971; Mendelson and Mello, 1971; Pieper et al., 1972; McMillan et al., 1974b, 1976; Samson and Falk, 1974a; Freund, 1969; Wahlström, 1974; Vitiello and Woods, 1975). When animals are presented with a subsequent choice between food or water and a drug solution, preferences for the drug are sometimes observed. For example, rats presented with a choice between morphine and water after one month of forced morphine drinking, preferred the morphine solution (Kumar and Stolerman, 1972; Thompson and Ostlund, 1965). In most cases preferences for drug are only observed in those cases where physical dependence on the drug has occurred, i.e., where severe physical symptoms develop when use of the drug is discontinued. (See Chapter 6, p. 202 for a discussion of physical dependence.)

Animals have been shown to consume sufficient quantities of various narcotics with this procedure to produce signs of physical dependence following (1) removal of the drug from the liquid solution and (2) administration of a narcotic antagonist such as nalorphine or naloxone (Risner and Khavari, 1973; McMillan et al., 1974b, 1976). (See Chapter 6, p. 202.) For example, McMillan et al., (1976) reported signs of dependence (wet shakes, weight loss, salivation, abnormal posture, diarrhea) following a naloxone injection in rats drinking morphine, meperidine, methadone or etonitazene, a very potent narcotic. In addition, forced consumption procedures have been shown to produce ethanol intake at a level sufficient to produce signs of withdrawal when ethanol is discontinued (Pieper et al., 1972; Freund, 1969). Therefore, forced consumption procedures have shown that animals will ingest considerable quantities of a drug when the drug is the sole liquid or food source available; however, since drug intake is so closely tied to food and water intake, it cannot be concluded that the drug is serving as a reinforcer in these procedures.

Schedule-induced Polydipsia

Another method for the oral administration of drugs makes use of a phenomenon that was described by Falk (1961). Falk observed that rats drank large quantities of water shortly after a food pellet was delivered on an FI schedule. This pattern of excessive drinking after food presentation has been called *schedule-induced polydipsia*. Since Falk's initial discovery, schedule-induced polydipsia has also been obtained with several other schedules of response-contingent reinforcement (Carlisle, 1971; Hymowitz, 1971; Segal and Holloway, 1963; Rosenblith, 1970; Segal and Bandt, 1966), as well as when food is given intermittently without a response requirement (Burks, 1970).

Recently, this method has been used to induce ingestion of a variety of drug solutions. For example, Falk et al. (1972) induced extensive ethanol intake in rats by simply substituting ethanol solutions for water in the schedule-induced polydipsia paradigm. Feeding periods were provided in which a pellet of food was delivered every two minutes, and ethanol was concurrently available in varying concentrations (1–6% v/v). Feeding periods occurred for an hour every four hours throughout the day (i.e., six one-hour feeding periods per day). Figure 11-1 shows the mean daily intake of ethanol as a function of the ethanol concentration.

The schedule-induced polydipsia procedure has been used extensively to examine ethanol consumption (Holman and Myers, 1968; Lester, 1961; Everett

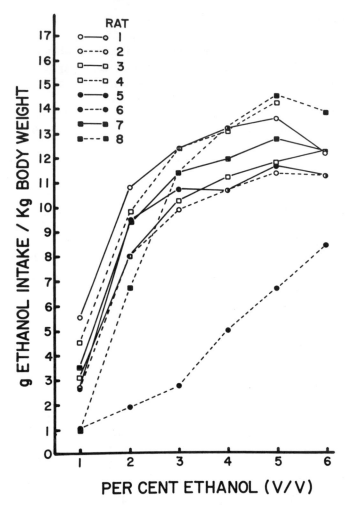

Fig. 11-1. Mean daily amounts of ethanol drunk by individual rats as a function of the available ethanol concentration. (From Falk *et al.*, 1972.)

and King, 1970; Freed *et al.*, 1970; Freed, 1974; Mello and Mendelson, 1971; Meisch and Thompson, 1971, 1972a, 1974b; Falk *et al.*, 1972; Ogata *et al.*, 1972; Gilbert, 1974; McMillan *et al.*, 1974a; Samson and Falk, 1974a,b). A number of conclusions can be drawn from these studies: (1) The frequency of ethanol consumption depends on the concentration of the solution. Although the frequency of ethanol consumption decreases with increasing concentrations, the total amount consumed increases with the concentration (Meisch and Thompson, 1972a). (2) When food reinforcement is discontinued, schedule-induced ethanol consumption persists, whereas schedule-induced water consumption often stops (Meisch and Thompson, 1971, 1974b; Freed et al., 1970; Gilbert, 1974). (3) Ethanol consumption may be sufficient to produce physical dependence (Falk et al., 1972; Samson and Falk, 1974a,b), especially when the periods of ethanol consumption occur several times throughout the day, although the occurrence of dependence has been questioned (Heintzelman et al., 1976).

Schedule-induced polydipsia is also an effective means of inducing rats to drink large daily doses of several narcotics (Leander et al., 1975; Leander and McMillan, 1973) and some barbiturates (Meisch, 1969; Kodluboy and Thompson, 1971). Therefore, schedule-induced polydipsia produces excessive drug consumption without forcing the animals to consume the drug in order to obtain food or water. It is questionable whether drug consumption produced by schedule-induced polydipsia is a demonstration of drug reinforcement; however, it does provide a procedure for examining variables related to excessive drug consumption.

Operant Responding

Food-deprived rats will press a lever when responding is followed by presentation of an ethanol solution (Mello and Mendelson, 1964; Meisch and Thompson, 1972b, 1973, 1974a; Anderson and Thompson, 1974). Responding can also be maintained in morphine-dependent rats by access to etonitazene, an extremely potent narcotic which does not have a bitter taste (Lewis et al., 1975).

Responding maintained by ethanol presentation occurs under a variety of conditions. For example, responding for ethanol can be maintained over a broad range of ethanol concentrations (2, 4, 8, 16 and 32% w/v) (Meisch and Thompson, 1972b). While the frequency of responding decreases as ethanol concentration increases, the total quantity of ethanol consumed increases as the ethanol concentration increases (Fig. 11-2a,b). Responding can also be maintained by ethanol presentation under schedules of intermittent drug presentation. Meisch and Thompson (1973) presented ethanol (8% w/v) on fixed ratio (FR) schedules of drug presentation (FR 1, 2, 4, 8, 16, 32, 64, 128 and 256). The pattern of responding was similar to fixed ratio responding maintained by other reinforcers. When the FR requirement increased, ethanol intake declined. Similarly, Anderson and Thompson (1974) maintained responding in rats when ethanol (8% w/v) was presented on various fixed interval schedules (FI 1-, 2-, 3-, and 4-min). The pattern of responding was typical of fixed interval responding for non-drug reinforcers.

While rats were food-deprived in these studies, responding followed by ethanol presentation has been obtained in food-satiated rats (Fig. 11-3) (Meisch and Thompson, 1973, 1974a) and when water is concurrently available (Meisch and

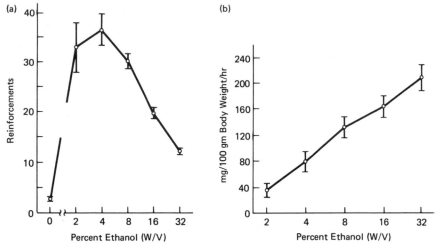

Fig. 11-2. Number of reinforcements (a) or total ethanol intake (b) as a function of ethanol concentration in rats pressing a lever for 4-sec presentations of ethanol. Each point is the mean of five 1-hr sessions from each of six rats. Brackets indicate the standard error of the mean. (From Meisch and Thompson, 1972b.)

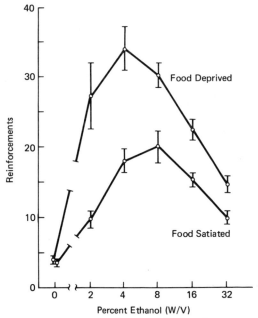

Fig. 11-3. Number of reinforcements as a function of ethanol concentration in rats pressing a lever for 4-sec presentations of ethanol. One group of rats was food-deprived, and one group was food-satiated. Each point is the mean of five 1-hr sessions from each of six rats. Brackets indicate the standard error of the mean. (From Meisch and Thompson, 1974a.)

Beardsley, 1975), indicating that the caloric or liquid value of ethanol is not the exclusive determinant of ethanol intake in these situations. Nevertheless, acquisition of responding for ethanol is usually established in food- and water-deprived animals. In summary, this work demonstrates that animals will consume large quantities of ethanol despite the fact that these solutions have an unpleasant taste and despite possible delays in onset of the pharmacological action of the drug by the oral route.

INTRAVENOUS ADMINISTRATION

Intravenous (iv) methods of drug administration have been used in rats (Weeks, 1962, 1964; Davis, 1966), rhesus monkeys (Yanagita et al., 1965; Wilson et al., 1971), squirrel monkeys (Stretch et al., 1971; Goldberg, 1973) and dogs (Jones and Prada, 1973). The fundamental aspect of the iv system is chronic implantation of an indwelling venous catheter which is connected to a motor-driven infusion pump. One end of the catheter is typically implanted into the external jugular or femoral vein, whereas the other end exits from the animal's back and passes through a protective metal coil which is attached to a wall of the experimental space and which allows the organism relatively unrestricted movement. Finally, connection is made to automatic programming equipment that controls delivery of the drug and the conditions under which the animal receives the drug. Delivery of the drug is almost always contingent on some response by the animal. Figure 11–4 shows the system used by Schuster and his associates at the University of Chicago. Work with the iv method of drug delivery has shown that a variety of drugs can serve as reinforcers under a variety of conditions.

Positive Reinforcement

In Chapter 1 a positive reinforcer was defined as any event which increased the probability of occurrence of the response it followed. Weeks (1962) found that a 10 mg/kg iv injection of morphine increased the rate of lever pressing in rats which were physically dependent on morphine. Moreover, Deneau et al. (1969) found that naive monkeys would self-administer a variety of drug solutions. They examined drug reinforcement with the following procedure: The monkeys' rate of responding was first determined when saline was delivered following each response. Most monkeys responded for saline at a low rate. This was referred to as the operant level of responding. The saline solution was then replaced by a drug solution, and subsequent changes in rate of response were compared to the operant level. If monkeys did not self-administer a drug within a specified period of time after substitution, injections were programmed automatically in an attempt to induce self-administration by priming the monkey with drug. Deneau et al. (1969) found that monkeys would self-administer morphine, codeine, co-

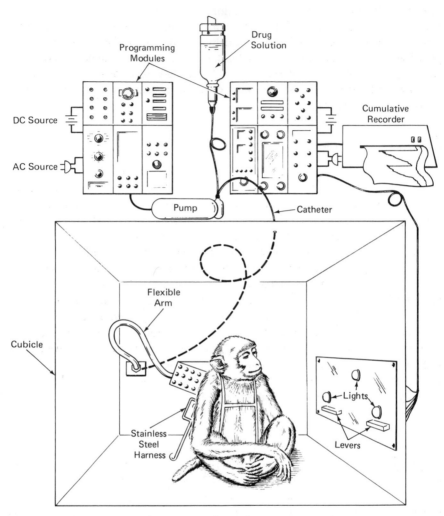

Fig. 11-4. System (used by Schuster at the University of Chicago) for automatic intravenous drug infusions with the rhesus monkey. The monkey is fitted with a steel harness connected to the wall of the cubicle by a metal coil. The catheter runs through the metal coil to an infusion pump. Drug availability is controlled by electrical programming equipment, and the relevant responses made by the monkeys are automatically recorded by this same equipment. (From Schuster and Johanson, 1974.)

caine, *d*-amphetamine, pentobarbital and sometimes ethanol. Caffeine was self-administered only by some monkeys and sometimes priming was required before administration was initiated. Nalorphine, mescaline and chlorpromazine were not self-administered, even after extensive priming periods. Subsequently, a variety of drugs have been tested with procedures very similar to those of

Deneau *et al*. Table 11-1 lists some drugs that have been self-administered by rats or monkeys, and Table 11-2 lists some drugs that have not been self-administered.

While rate of response has generally been used to determine whether a drug

TABLE 11-1. Some self-administered drugs

Drug	Reference
Psychomotor stimulants	
cocaine	Pickens (1968)
	Pickens and Thompson (1967, 1968)
	Yanagita *et al*. (1965, 1969)
	Deneau *et al*. (1969)
	Woods and Schuster (1968)
d-amphetamine	Pickens (1968)
	Pickens and Harris (1968)
	Pickens and Thompson (1967)
	Deneau *et al*. (1969)
	Yanagita *et al*. (1969)
	Hoffmeister *et al*. (1970)
	Balster and Schuster (1973a)
	Yokel and Pickens (1973, 1974)
l-amphetamine	Yokel and Pickens (1971, 1973, 1974)
	Balster and Schuster (1973a)
methamphetamine	Pickens (1968)
	Pickens *et al*. (1967)
	Deneau *et al*. (1969)
	Yanagita *et al*. (1970)
	Balster and Schuster (1973a)
phenmetrazine	Wilson *et al*. (1971)
	Yanagita *et al*. (1970)
methylphenidate	Wilson *et al*. (1971)
pipradrol	Wilson *et al*. (1971)
	Yanagita *et al*. (1970)
diethylproprion	Götestam and Andersson (1975)
Barbiturates and benzodiazepines	
chlordiazepoxide	Findley *et al*. (1972)
diazepam	Yanagita and Takahashi (1973)
amobarbital	Davis and Miller (1963)
	Davis *et al*. (1968)
	Woods and Schuster (1970)
hexobarbital	Davis *et al*. (1968)
pentobarbital	Schlichting *et al*. (1971)
	Woods and Schuster (1970)
	Goldberg *et al*. (1971b)
secobarbital	Findley *et al*. (1972)

TABLE 11-1. (*Continued*)

Drug	Reference
Narcotics	
morphine	Weeks (1962, 1964)
	Weeks and Collins (1964)
	Balster *et al.* (1971)
	Deneau *et al.* (1969)
	Hoffmeister and Schlichting (1972)
	Thompson and Schuster (1964)
	Woods and Schuster (1968)
	Yanagita *et al.* (1970)
meperidine	Yanagita *et al.* (1970)
codeine	Balster *et al.* (1971)
	Hoffmeister and Schlichting (1972)
	Schlichting *et al.* (1971)
propoxyphene	Balster *et al.* (1971)
	Hoffmeister and Schlichting (1972)
	Talley and Rosenblum (1972)
pentazocine	Hoffmeister and Schlichting (1972)
apomorphine	Baxter *et al.* (1974)
Others	
ethanol	Deneau *et al.* (1969)
	Winger and Woods (1973)
phencyclidine	Balster *et al.* (1973)
nicotine	Deneau and Inoki (1967)

TABLE 11-2. Some drugs that are *not* self-administered

Drug	Reference
Acetylsalicylic acid	Hoffmeister and Wuttke (1973b, 1975)
Caffeine	Yanagita *et al.* (1969)
	Deneau *et al.* (1969)
Chlorphentermine	Yanagita *et al.* (1969)
Fenfluramine	Woods and Tessel (1974)
Magnesium pemoline	Wilson *et al.* (1969)
Mescaline	Deneau *et al.* (1969)
Tetrahydrocannabinol	Harris *et al.* (1974)
Thiopental	Davis *et al.* (1968)
Chlorpromazine	Hoffmeister *et al.* (1970)
	Deneau *et al.* (1969)

can serve as a reinforcer, this measure should be used cautiously as an indicator of a drug's reinforcing properties, since drugs may have effects on rate of response that are independent of their ability to act as reinforcers. For example, very high doses of a variety of drugs produce nonspecific decreases in response rate. Alternative procedures for measuring drug reinforcement will be discussed in the section on abuse potential.

Negative Reinforcement

The drugs listed in Table 11-1 are positive reinforcers in that they increase the probability of the response they follow at least at some doses. Some drugs (e.g., cyclazocine, nalorphine, lysergic acid diethylamide) can serve as negative reinforcers in that they will maintain responding which avoids or terminates their presentation in drug naive monkeys (Hoffmeister and Wuttke, 1973a; Hoffmeister, 1975). Moreover, drugs have also been shown to act as negative reinforcers in morphine-dependent animals (Goldberg *et al.*, 1971a; Downs and Woods, 1975). For example, Goldberg *et al.*, made monkeys physically dependent on morphine and then tested them on a discrete trial avoidance schedule. In the avoidance procedure a 10-sec nalorphine injection was scheduled to occur every 30-sec, and a response postponed the nalorphine injection. Animals responded at high rates to avoid injections of nalorphine and naloxone, but not of saline.

Conditioned Reinforcement

Stimuli that accompany reinforcement can become conditioned reinforcers (see Chapter 1). Crowder *et al.* (1972) found that lever pressing in rats could be maintained by saline infusions if a buzzer that had previously been paired with morphine delivery was presented along with the saline infusion. Moreover, when morphine administration is accompanied by a light flash, the light flash will maintain responding when the opportunity to administer morphine is withdrawn (Thompson and Schuster, 1964; Schuster and Woods, 1968). Stimuli associated with delivery of the narcotic antagonist nalorphine can acquire conditioned negative reinforcing properties. For example, morphine-dependent monkeys will press a lever when the response terminates a stimulus previously paired with delivery of nalorphine (Goldberg *et al.*, 1971a).

Rates and Patterns of Responding Maintained by Drug Reinforcement

While a variety of drugs have been shown to be self-administered, the temporal pattern of administration varies considerably between drugs. The rate and pattern of drug administration depends on several variables, including the total amount of time each day the drug is available, the dose per infusion (unit dose) and the schedule of reinforcement.

Unlimited Access.   Deneau *et al.* (1969) investigated intake patterns for several drugs under conditions in which rhesus monkeys had unlimited access to the drug. They reported marked differences in intake patterns for the narcotics and the psychomotor stimulants under these conditions. Morphine intake increased daily for 20 to 30 days until it reached a stable level (50–100 mg/kg/day), with intake levels being higher during the day than at night (see Fig. 11-5). Codeine and pentobarbital produced a similar pattern. Cocaine, on the other hand, produced an erratic intake pattern without a long acquisition period. Co-

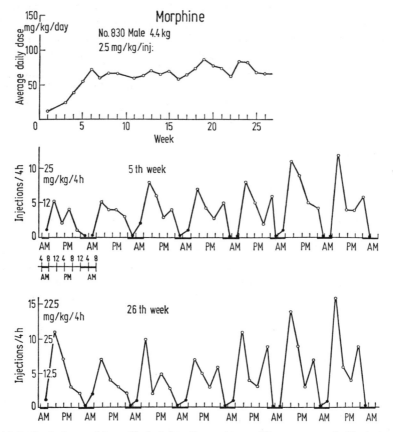

Fig. 11-5. Typical morphine self-administration pattern. The upper graph illustrates the fairly constant dosage level attained after a six-week period of rapid incrementation. The lower graphs illustrate the day-to-day consistency of morphine self-administration. (From Deneau *et al.*, 1969.)

caine intake consisted of rapid but erratic increases in drug intake with periods of high intake alternating with periods of abstinence. Cocaine was usually administered around the clock until exhaustion occurred, followed by one to five days of abstinence. Indeed, Deneau *et al.* (1969) found that when cocaine was offered without restriction, monkeys would administer cocaine until convulsions and death occurred, usually within 30 days. Figure 11-6 illustrates the erratic course of cocaine self-administration. A similar pattern was seen with *d*-amphetamine.

An erratic pattern of amphetamine intake has also been reported in the rat (Pickens and Thompson, 1971; Pickens *et al.*, 1967; Pickens and Harris, 1968). Rats administering *d*-amphetamine are highly excitable; they neither eat nor sleep and often exhibit highly stereotyped movements. Patterns similar to those of the rat and monkey have also been seen with intravenous stimulant administration in man.   For example, Kramer *et al.* (1967) reported that individuals administering intravenous methamphetamine typically inject methamphetamine about every two hours around the clock for periods of three to six days, during which time the individual remains awake continuously, eats little food, and engages in stereotyped behavior (see Chapter 6, p. 174).

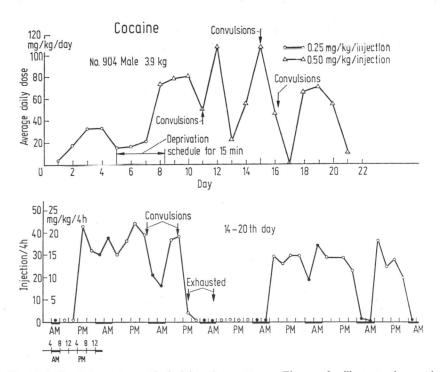

Fig. 11-6. Typical cocaine self-administration pattern.   The graphs illustrate the erratic course of cocaine self-administration. (From Deneau *et al.*, 1969.)

Limited Access. Limited access to the psychomotor stimulants produces a regular pattern of intake unlike the sporadic pattern seen when availability is unlimited (Pickens and Thompson, 1971; Balster and Schuster, 1973a). With morphine, however, limiting access to only one hour every five hours may or may not lower daily intake to a level below that taken when unlimited access is provided (Schuster and Johanson, 1974).

Extinction. When the opportunity to administer a psychomotor stimulant is withdrawn (i.e., extinction), a long burst of responses occurs at a very high rate followed by a gradual decrease in response rate. When the opportunity to administer a narcotic is withdrawn, responding continues at a low rate for weeks and even months (Thompson and Pickens, 1970).

Unit Dose. Total daily intake of narcotics can be modified by decreasing or increasing the unit dose, i.e., the amount of drug delivered per infusion (Woods and Schuster, 1968; Weeks and Collins, 1964; Schuster and Balster, 1973). As unit dosage increases, daily intake also increases, although rate of responding decreases (see Fig. 11-7). Similar effects have been shown with pentobarbital (Goldberg *et al.*, 1971b).

On the other hand, the total daily intake of the psychomotor stimulants (e.g., cocaine, methamphetamine, *d*-amphetamine) is only minimally determined by

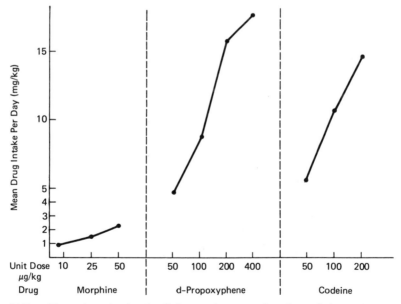

Fig. 11-7. Mean drug intake (mg/kg) per day as a function of dose of morphine, *d*-propoxyphene and codeine. (From Balster, personal communication.)

the unit dose. When unit dose is increased, rate of responding decreases proportionally, so that under limited access conditions, the amount of drug administered per day is fairly constant even though dosage may change (Wilson *et al.*, 1971; Pickens and Thompson, 1968; Pickens *et al.*, 1967; Pickens and Harris, 1968; Balster and Schuster, 1973a; Goldberg *et al.*, 1971b). Figure 11-8 shows this effect for methylphenidate. A 16-fold increase in dose produced little more than a twofold increase in intake. It has been suggested that daily intake of large unit doses of psychomotor stimulants is limited by the fact that large unit doses of these drugs produce behavioral disruption incompatible with high rates of responding (Wilson *et al.*, 1971). It is interesting to note that a similar disruption in responding occurs following administration of a high dose of cocaine in rats when responding is maintained by food presentation.

The relationship between rate of responding maintained by psychomotor stimulant administration and unit dose may only hold, however, when the drug is delivered following every response. Balster and Schuster (1973b) reported that rate of responding on an FI 9-min schedule of cocaine presentation in

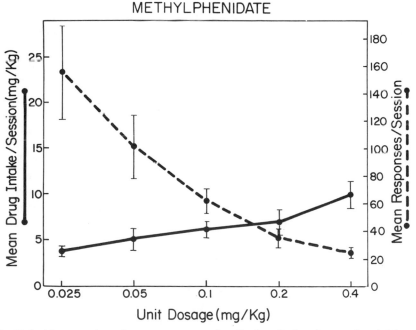

Fig. 11-8. Mean number of responses per session (broken line) and mean drug intake per session (solid line) as functions of unit dosage of methylphenidate hydrochloride. Each point represents the mean of data obtained from four subjects on days three through seven of exposure to each unit dosage. Vertical lines represent the range. (From Wilson *et al.*, 1971.)

monkeys increased as unit dose increased; however, others reported decreasing rates of responding in pigeons when responding was maintained by increasing doses of cocaine on an FI 200- or 400-sec schedule (Dougherty and Pickens, 1973). While these contradictory findings may reflect differences in species or FI values, it is important to note that Balster and Schuster added a 15-min time-out after each cocaine presentation, which might have eliminated drug-induced disruptions in responding, whereas Dougherty and Pickens did not have time-out periods. Moreover, Dougherty and Pickens reported that decreases in rate following large doses of cocaine were due primarily to long pauses at the beginning of the FI interval. In short, these data emphasize the importance of procedural variables in determining rates and patterns of drug-maintained responding. Therefore, generalizations about rate of responding and drug dose must be qualified by variables such as the schedule of reinforcement under which the drug is delivered.

Schedule Effects. Weeks (1962) examined morphine intake under several different FR schedules of reinforcement. When the FR requirement was increased from 1 to 5 responses per reinforcement, morphine intake decreased. When the FR requirement was further increased to an FR 10, however, the response rate doubled from its FR 5 level. Weeks and Collins (1964) also showed that higher FR requirements (e.g., 20, 32, 50) decreased the amount of morphine administered by rats. A similar effect was found with pentobarbital in rhesus monkeys (Goldberg *et al.*, 1971b). Total pentobarbital intake decreased as the FR requirement increased. On the other hand, total intake of the psychomotor stimulant cocaine did not decrease as the ratio requirement increased (Goldberg *et al.*, 1971b; Pickens, 1968; Pickens and Thompson, 1968). Figure 11-9 illustrates these differential effects for cocaine and pentobarbital, and Fig. 11-10 illustrates an effect similar to that of cocaine for *d*-amphetamine. Therefore, when psychomotor stimulants are delivered on an FR schedule of reinforcement, both rats and monkeys increase response rate as the ratio requirement increases, thereby keeping daily intake constant; whereas when morphine or pentobarbital is delivered on an FR schedule, response rate decreases, thereby decreasing daily intake levels.

Work with other schedules of drug reinforcement (e.g., fixed interval schedules, second order schedules) demonstrates that drug reinforcers generate response patterns characteristic of patterns generated by reinforcers such as food or water (Thompson and Schuster, 1964; Woods and Schuster, 1968; Goldberg, 1973; Dougherty and Pickens, 1973; Balster and Schuster, 1973b; Downs and Woods, 1974; Goldberg *et al.*, 1975).

While some generalizations can therefore be drawn about the rate and pattern of responding maintained by various drugs, these generalizations must always be qualified in terms of a number of procedural variables, including amount of time

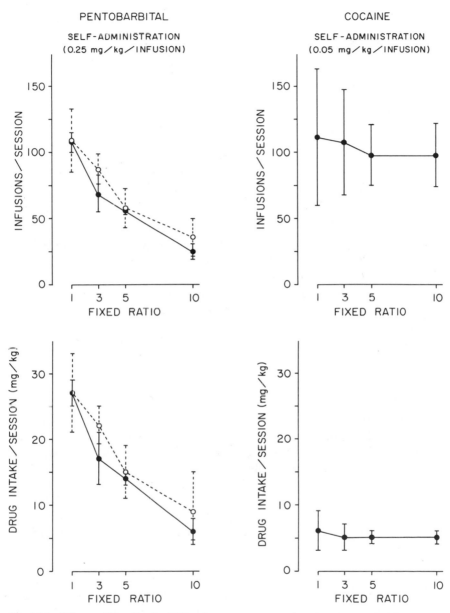

Fig. 11-9. Effects of fixed ratio (FR) value on response rate and total drug intake per session. In the top graphs the mean number of infusion/session for pentobarbital and cocaine is shown as a function of the FR value. In the bottom graphs the mean drug intake (mg/kg)/session for pentobarbital and cocaine is shown as a function of the FR value. (From Goldberg *et al.*, 1971b.)

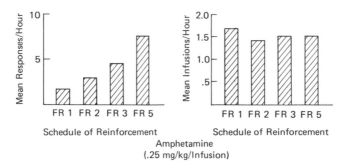

Fig. 11-10. Effects of fixed ratio (FR) value on response frequency and infusion frequency for *d*-amphetamine self-administration in one rat. In the left graph the mean number of responses/hour is shown as a function of the FR value. In the right graph the mean number of infusions/hour is shown as a function of the FR value. (From Pickens and Harris, 1968.)

the subject has access to the drug, the dose and parameters of the schedule of drug delivery. In addition to these variables, duration of the drug infusion has also been shown to be important (Balster and Schuster, 1973a). Moreover, rates and patterns of responding are not always constant throughout a session, even when parameters of dose and schedule remain the same. For example, high rates at the beginning of a session followed by decreases in response rate as the session progresses are often reported (Wilson *et al.*, 1971; Hoffmeister and Schlichting, 1972).

Other Variables Important in Drug Reinforcement

Although there is good indication from the above studies that certain drugs can be considered reinforcers in that they maintain responding followed by drug administration, there is still some question as to whether mere availability of a drug is a sufficient condition for administration.

Since morphine and morphine-like drugs (e.g., heroin, codeine) produce physical dependence as evidenced by severe withdrawal when the drug is discontinued, and since this withdrawal can be rapidly terminated by drug administration, it is possible that these drugs derive their reinforcing properties from their ability to alleviate withdrawal. In the earliest self-administration studies, animals were made physically dependent on morphine prior to being given an opportunity to administer the drug. Weeks (1962) first established physical dependence in rats by administering increasing (2.0–40.0 mg/kg) doses of morphine over a period of several days. Similarly, Thompson and Schuster (1964) made monkeys physically dependent on morphine before administration was established. Moreover, Deneau *et al.* (1969) occasionally found that it was necessary to prime monkeys with programmed injections of morphine before self-administration occurred.

It seems, however, that physical dependence is not a necessary antecedent condition for morphine administration to take place. Schuster and his associates maintain that morphine can be reinforcing in the absence of physical dependence (Schuster, 1970; Woods and Schuster, 1968; Schuster and Villarreal, 1968; Schuster and Thompson, 1969). Woods and Schuster (1970) report that monkeys will respond for doses of morphine as low as 0.01 mg/kg. This dose of morphine has not been reported to produce detectable signs of physical dependence. Moreover, it has been shown that animals will administer morphine when given the drug under conditions which will not produce physical dependence (three hours per day for a period not longer than six days) (Balster et al., 1971; Hoffmeister and Schlichting, 1972). We can conclude from this that "morphine is a positive reinforcer independently of its ability to terminate the withdrawal syndrome" (Schuster and Johanson, 1974, p. 7). The reinforcing efficacy of morphine is increased, however, if animals are physically dependent on it and undergoing withdrawal when the drug is available (Weeks and Collins, 1964; Thompson and Schuster, 1964; Woods and Schuster, 1968).

Since administration of psychomotor stimulants is often accompanied by highly excitable behavior (Pickens and Thompson, 1971; Deneau et al., 1969), one might question whether the high rates of responding maintained by stimulants are an indication of their reinforcing efficacy or are due simply to indirect stimulant effects of this class of drugs. Pickens (1968) investigated this question with the following experiment: A second lever was added to an experimental chamber so that one lever produced the drug, and the second lever had no consequence. If high rates of responding were due simply to generalized stimulant effects of the drug, then one would expect to see high rates of responding on both levers; however, little responding occurred on the non-drug lever. Secondly, when noncontingent drug injections were given at the same rate that drug was usually self-administered, no responding occurred. Responding resumed, however, when noncontingent injections were discontinued. Finally, if animals were paired and the experimental member of each pair was allowed to administer drug while the control (yoked) member was given a drug injection at the same time as its experimental partner, the response rate of the experimental animal was found to be significantly above that of the control animal. It can be concluded from these studies that high rates of stimulant administration cannot be attributed to a generalized motor stimulant effect.

DRUG INTERACTIONS

Drug intake patterns have been shown to be altered by pretreatment with other drugs.

Narcotics

Pharmacological variables which affect the administration pattern of narcotics are of particular interest because of their direct application to problems of drug abuse. Two types of pharmacological manipulations have been examined with narcotics. One involves substitution of another drug for morphine or heroin; a second involves blocking the effects of morphine or heroin with narcotic antagonists. We will discuss below the results of these manipulations, as well as their application to drug abuse treatment programs.

Drug Substitutions. Pretreatment with morphine or another narcotic will decrease the rate of responding for morphine. For example, when morphine, codeine or meperidine is continuously infused into rats administering 10 mg/kg of morphine, responding for morphine decreases (Weeks and Collins, 1964). Intake also decreases when etonitazene, a synthetic opiate-like drug, is added to their drinking water. Morphine and methadone pretreatment will also decrease morphine administration (Thompson, 1968; Thompson and Schuster, 1964). Since methadone is a long-acting drug and can be taken orally, it has been used extensively in outpatient clinics for treatment of drug abuse. The patient receives daily doses of methadone, and heroin administration is thereby eliminated, or at least reduced. Physical dependence upon methadone, however, continues (Dole and Nyswander, 1968).

Drug Antagonism. The narcotic antagonists block most of the effects of morphine and heroin (see Chapter 6, p. 202). A low dose of nalorphine or naloxone can elicit the withdrawal syndrome in morphine-dependent organisms. Since these antagonists elicit the withdrawal syndrome, it is not surprising that low doses of nalorphine and naloxone have been shown to increase morphine administration (Weeks and Collins, 1964; Thompson and Schuster, 1964; Goldberg *et al.*, 1969, 1971c, 1972). High doses of nalorphine however, will decrease morphine administration and produce withdrawal signs in morphine-dependent monkeys. Nalorphine pretreatment has no effect on cocaine administration (see Fig. 11-11).

Narcotic antagonists also block the development of tolerance to and dependence upon the narcotics (Woods, 1956; Martin, 1967). Because narcotic antagonists can block development of drug dependence, it has been suggested that narcotic antagonists might be useful in the prevention of relapse to narcotics (Martin *et al.*, 1966). Programs that use narcotic antagonists to treat drug abuse problems are organized around the following lines: Since narcotic antagonists do not maintain physical dependence, the individual first spends a period of time in inpatient care, during which he is withdrawn from morphine or heroin. After withdrawal, the antagonist is given periodically (usually daily) so that effects of future morphine or heroin drug-taking will be blocked. It is thought that if the effects of morphine or heroin are blocked, their positive reinforcing effects will be eliminated, and the drug-taking behavior will extinguish (Freedman, 1966; Martin and Gorodetzky, 1967).

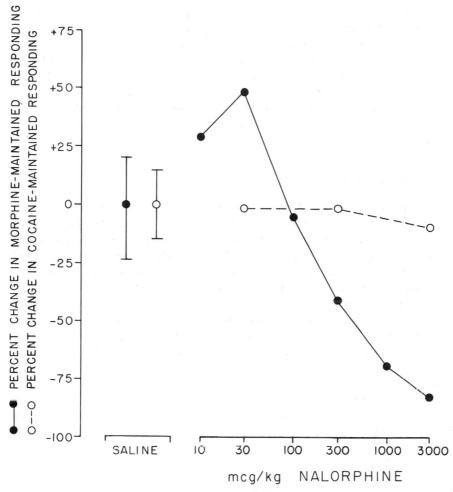

Fig. 11-11. Percent change in morphine- or cocaine-maintained responding as a function of nalorphine dose. The percent change in number of responses in a given session was calculated as follows:

$$\frac{\text{number of responses in} - \text{number of responses in mean}}{\text{pretreatment session}} \quad \text{of three control sessions}}{(\text{number of responses in mean of three previous control sessions})}$$

When the number of responses in the pretreatment session is equal to the number of responses in the control session, the percent change is zero. Each far-left point represents the average, and the brackets the range of saline pretreatment sessions. Closed circles: average of four sessions for each of four monkeys; open circles: average of six sessions, one for each of six monkeys. (From Goldberg et al., 1972.)

Unfortunately, the available narcotic antagonists have some disadvantages for long-term administration as prophylactics against relapse to narcotics. For example, both nalorphine (Lasagna and Beecher, 1954) and cyclazocine (Martin, 1967) produce a number of unpleasant side effects. Naloxone is limited by its short duration of antagonist activity (Jasinski *et al.*, 1967). Attention has recently shifted to naltrexone (EN-1639-A) and diprenorphine (M 5050), whose narcotic antagonist activities seem to be more potent and to have longer durations of action than those of naloxone (Hammond, 1971; Blumberg *et al.*, 1967; Martin *et al.*, 1973).

Psychomotor Stimulants

Much less work has been done on drug interactions with the psychomotor stimulants than with the narcotics. It has been shown, however, that satiation and substitution procedures are effective in decreasing intake levels. For example, administration of cocaine is decreased following administration of *d*-amphetamine (Wilson and Schuster, 1973b). Moreover, methamphetamine administration is decreased following methamphetamine pretreatment (Pickens *et al.*, 1968).

Most work on drug interactions among the psychomotor stimulants has been directed toward examining biochemical mechanisms which may underlie the reinforcing efficacy of these drugs, in particular mechanisms involved in regulating or limiting drug intake. As discussed above, when availability of the psychomotor stimulants is limited, a constant total amount of drug is usually administered each day. Furthermore, reductions in unit dose usually increase administration frequency such that the daily intake remains constant. In addition, when the psychomotor stimulants are administered on an FR schedule, response rate increases as the FR requirement increases, in such a way that daily intake remains constant.

The mechanisms underlying this stability have been examined by determining whether the reinforcing actions of psychomotor stimulants can be altered by treatment with other drugs. Specifically, attempts have been made to determine whether specific drugs can antagonize the reinforcing efficacy of these compounds. For example, if a drug interferes with the mechanism(s) whereby cocaine exerts its reinforcing effects, one might expect to see changes in the rate of cocaine administration. Recall (p. 372) that responding initially increases when the opportunity to administer a psychomotor stimulant is withdrawn. Therefore, if a drug prevents or decreases the ability of cocaine to act as a reinforcer, one might expect an increase in the rate of cocaine administration.

Administration of several psychomotor stimulants has been shown to increase following chlorpromazine and trifluoperazine (Wilson and Schuster, 1972; Wilson and Schuster, 1973b). Similarly, cocaine administration increases following alpha-methyltyrosine (AMT) in rhesus monkeys (Wilson and Schuster, 1974), and methamphetamine administration increases following AMT in rats (Pickens *et al.*, 1968). Moreover, Davis and Smith (1972) have shown that AMT blocks the development of *d*-amphetamine administration in rats.

On the basis of these results, it has been proposed that the reinforcing effects of the psychomotor stimulants are mediated through catecholaminergic systems. Alpha-methyltyrosine and chlorpromazine are thought to increase rates of psychomotor stimulant administration by preventing these drugs from acting as reinforcers. Blockade of the reinforcing effects of various psychomotor stimulants via catecholaminergic mechanisms is consistent with the presumed biochemical mechanism of action of chlorpromazine and alpha-methyltyrosine. Chlorpromazine is thought to produce receptor blockade in the catecholaminergic system and alpha-methyltyrosine is thought to inhibit synthesis of catecholamines (see Chapter 5, p. 123).

Further investigations of biochemical mechanisms underlying administration of psychomotor stimulants involve attempts to separate the action of dopamine (DA) and norepinephrine (NE) in psychomotor stimulant administration. Yokel and Wise (1975) have shown that *d*-amphetamine administration increases following pretreatment with pimozide, a dopamine blocking agent but not with phentolamine or *l*-propranolol, α or β noradrenergic blocking agents, respectively. Similarly, Wilson and Schuster (1974) report no change in self-administration of cocaine following pretreatment with the noradrenergic blocking agents, phentolamine and phenoxybenzamine. Cholinergic influences on cocaine administration have also been investigated (Wilson and Schuster, 1973a).

Similar investigations have been made of the reinforcing properties of morphine (Davis and Smith, 1972, 1975; Smith and Davis, 1973) and of intracranial self-stimulation (see Chapter 6, p. 184).

It must be recognized in interpreting these results that inferring biochemical mechanisms of drug action is difficult. Drugs have multiple effects, and while many are known to alter neurochemical transmission, drugs may have other important effects as well. Moreover, the rate at which an animal responds for a drug is also determined by multiple factors. For example, it has been suggested that psychomotor stimulant intake may be limited by nonspecific behavioral disrupting effects (see p. 373) such that large doses produce disruptions which are incompatible with high rates of responding. Therefore, chlorpromazine might increase cocaine intake by antagonizing these behavioral disrupting effects rather than by blocking the reinforcing efficacy of cocaine. For example, Wilson and Schuster (1975) have shown that when monkeys are maintained on an FR 10 schedule of food presentation, cocaine decreases responding. This decrement is partially blocked with chlorpromazine pretreatment, suggesting that chlorpromazine might nonspecifically antagonize the behavioral effects of cocaine.

Therefore, while this work makes some interesting suggestions about the biochemical mechanisms that may underlie the reinforcing efficacy of psychomotor stimulants, conclusions will have to await further data. Return to Chapters 4, 5 and 6 for a more thorough discussion of the problems involved in making correlations between a particular behavior and the biochemical mechanisms thought to underlie it.

ABUSE POTENTIAL

The intravenous method of drug administration is a valuable model for examining variables that maintain drug administration and for testing various drugs and procedures which might be used to treat drug abuse problems. Since there is a good correlation between a drug's ability to act as a positive reinforcer in infrahuman subjects and its abuse by man, these procedures are also being used to predict the abuse potential of new drugs.

Substitution Procedures

When testing the abuse potential of a new drug, one usually must investigate a wide range of drug doses. The process of running acquisition procedures for numerous doses of a drug is long and tedious. Yanagita *et al.* (1969) developed a procedure to get around this problem. They first train monkeys to administer some drug already shown to be reliably administered (e.g., morphine, cocaine). When the daily number of drug injections (called the baseline) is stable, the drug solution is replaced with saline, and administration of saline is continued until the daily number of saline injections stabilizes, presumably at a lower level than the baseline drug rate. This drug-saline procedure is repeated several times. Then a test drug is given instead of saline, and rate of responding maintained by the substituted drug is measured. If responding increases to a level above that observed under saline conditions, the substituted drug is considered a reinforcer. If responding does not increase to a level above the saline level, it is not considered a reinforcer. Yanagita *et al.* (1969, 1970) used the experimental compound SPA [(*l*)-1, 2-diphenyl-1-dimethylaminoethane], a psychomotor stimulant, as their baseline drug and then substituted several other drugs. The number of injections per day was high when monkeys were administering SPA and dropped considerably when the drug solution was replaced with saline. Yanagita *et al.* (1969, 1970) found that cocaine, *d*-amphetamine, methamphetamine, phenmetrazine and pipradrol were all reinforcing at certain unit dose levels for animals that had been administering SPA. They also showed that morphine and meperidine were reinforcers at low and intermediate doses in that they maintained responding above saline levels. Higher doses of these drugs did not maintain responding above saline levels (see Fig. 11-12). Monkeys only occasionally administered pentobarbital or chlordiazepoxide at a rate above that of saline (Fig. 11-12).

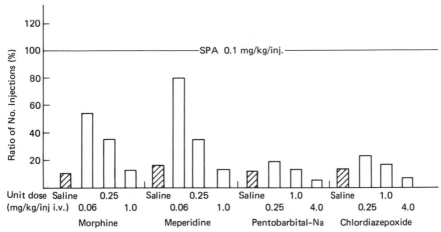

Fig. 11-12. Substitution tests with saline, morphine, meperidine, pentobarbital and chlordi-azepoxide in monkeys self-administering SPA (0.1 mg/kg/injections). The number of injec-tions of each of the test drugs is presented as a ratio of the number of injections of the baseline drug, SPA. The ratio is shown as a function of the dose of the test drugs. Each point is the mean of three monkeys. (From Yanagita et al., 1969.)

Chlorphentermine and caffeine were not administered above saline levels at any dose. Table 11-3 presents the results of several other studies that have used sub-stitution procedures to examine drug self-administration.

One variable which might be of particular importance in this type of study is the baseline drug used for comparison. A study by Schlichting et al. (1971) il-lustrates this point. In their study, three groups of three monkeys each re-sponded for drug on a fixed ratio schedule. Each group of monkeys received one of the following drugs: 0.05 mg/kg cocaine, 0.05 mg/kg codeine or 0.25 mg/kg pentobarbital. As in the Yanagita procedure, saline was then substituted for the drug and responding was measured. Then d-amphetamine was substi-tuted in a 0.05 mg/kg dose. Each group administered d-amphetamine above the saline levels, but at different rates. Higher rates of amphetamine administration were seen in the group of animals with a history of cocaine administration. Other studies have also suggested that animals experienced in administration of drugs of a certain class are more sensitive to the reinforcing effects of drugs of the same class. Hoffmeister and Schlichting (1972) found that animals with a history of codeine reinforcement administered opiates more often and at lower doses than animals with a history of cocaine reinforcement. Although the authors did not observe any indications of physical dependence, it is possible that codeine-trained animals might have developed physical dependence which might account for the higher rates of opiate administration in the codeine group over those of the cocaine group.

TABLE 11-3.   Studies demonstrating substitution across drugs

Baseline Drug	Substituted drugs administered above saline levels	Substituted drugs *not* administered above saline levels	Reference
SPA (*l*-1,2-diphenyl-1-dimethylaminoethane)	cocaine *d*-amphetamine	chlorphentermine caffeine	Yanagita *et al.* (1969)
SPA	phenmetrazine methamphetamine pipradrol morphine meperidine	pentobarbital chlordiazepoxide	Yanagita *et al.* (1970)
cocaine	codeine propoxyphene morphine		Schuster and Balster (1973)
cocaine	*d*-amphetamine morphine	imipramine chlorpromazine	Hoffmeister *et al.* (1970) Hoffmeister and Goldberg (1973)
codeine	pentazocine propiramfumarate dextropropoxyphene morphine codeine	nalorphine	Hoffmeister and Schlichting (1972)
cocaine	pentazocine propiramfumarate dextropropoxyphene morphine codeine	nalorphine	Hoffmeister and Schlichting (1972)
amphetamine	phenmetrazine diethylpropion	fenfluramine	Götestam and Andersson (1975)
cocaine	*d*-amphetamine *l*-amphetamine methamphetamine		Balster and Schuster (1973a)

These results indicate that the substitution procedure might be a good screening method for predicting the abuse liability of new drugs. Some problems remain, however. For example, Yanagita *et al.* (1970) did not find that pentobarbital, a known drug of abuse, was administered at rates above saline levels. Moreover, they found that higher doses of many drugs were not administered above saline levels. Schuster and Balster (1973) found that codeine was administered at a higher rate than propoxyphene and that propoxyphene was administered at a higher rate than morphine. If rate of administration is an indicator of reinforcing efficacy, then these results do not correlate with the abuse liability of these drugs in man (Jaffee, 1970).

There are problems with using the rate of drug administration as an indicator of its reinforcing properties. We discussed the problem of using rate as an indicator of a drug's reinforcing properties previously, but it is of sufficient importance to be reemphasized. Several drugs have general depressant effects that may interfere with frequency of administration. For example, in Hoffmeister and Schlichting's (1972) substitution study, animals administered pentazocine, propoxyphene and codeine at high rates, but usually only within very narrow dose ranges, whereas morphine was administered at more moderate rates, but over a very broad dose range. Therefore, the rate of administration may not be a good measure for evaluating the relative reinforcing properties of a given compound.

Preference Procedures

Preference procedures have been used to minimize problems in using response rate to examine reinforcement efficacy. A number of preference procedures have been developed (Johanson and Schuster, 1975; Iglauer and Woods, 1974; Findley et al. 1972). In all preference procedures, the subject is given a choice between two different drug conditions (e.g., two different doses of a drug, drug vs. saline, and so forth). The choice is made at a time when the drug's rate-modifying effects are minimal. For example, subjects can be tested 15 to 30 minutes after cocaine administration. At this time, immediate general suppressant actions of cocaine have dissipated (Nayak et al., 1975).

Johanson and Schuster (1975) designed a preference procedure in which two doses of a drug could be compared. In this procedure, monkeys made a choice between one of two drug solutions by responding on a lever associated with the preferred drug. The following procedure was used: Monkeys were first trained to administer some drug. Then they were presented with two sampling periods. During each sampling component, one of two different drug solutions could be administered. During administration of each of the two solutions, a stimulus light was on. For example, while the monkey self-administered one drug solution, a red light was on above the lever; while the monkey administered another drug or a different dose of the drug, a green light was on above the lever. Each different drug solution and light combination was sampled five times.

Thirty minutes after the preliminary sampling component, choice trials were begun. During choice trials, both stimulus lights were on (one color above each of the two levers). The two colors, one above each lever, were randomly changed for each trial. Therefore, if the monkey preferred drug A, and drug A had been administered only when the red light had been on over the lever, he should respond on whichever lever was illuminated with the red light; sometimes that would be the right lever and sometimes the left lever. To complete a choice trial, five responses had to be made on the same lever. Each choice trial was followed by a 15-minute time-out; then another choice trial occurred.

Johanson and Schuster (1975) made the following comparisons: Four doses of cocaine (0.05–1.5 mg/kg) and three doses of methylphenidate (0.075–0.7 mg/kg) were compared to saline. Low doses of cocaine were compared to higher doses of cocaine, and 0.75 mg/kg of methylphenidate was compared to higher doses of methylphenidate. Comparisons were also made between cocaine and methylphenidate. When monkeys were given a choice between either drug or saline, they showed a clear preference for drug. In addition, when given a choice between two solutions of various doses of cocaine or methylphenidate, they generally preferred the higher dose regardless of the drug. No preference was shown between equal doses of cocaine and methylphenidate. Moreover, Johanson and Schuster (1975) showed that rate of responding and drug dose were inversely related. For example, while monkeys consistently preferred higher doses of cocaine or methyphendiate during choice periods, rate of responding during sampling periods was markedly decreased by the higher doses of cocaine and methylphenidate. Thus, the preference procedure provides a measure of reinforcement minimally affected by drug-induced changes in response rate.

RELAPSE

The occurrence of relapse was and is still so common with all drug abuse treatment programs that much research has gone into trying to elucidate factors that contribute to it. Wikler (1965) has suggested that relapse to the narcotics has a lot to do with the dramatic withdrawal syndrome which follows cessation of drug taking in dependent subjects. Wikler suggested that the withdrawal syndrome could be classically conditioned to stimuli in the environment through repeated association of a specific environment with withdrawal. (See Chapter 1 for a discussion of classical conditioning.) Moreover, Wikler (1961) contends that treatment programs fail to extinguish the environmental stimuli associated with withdrawal. When patients are allowed to return to their home environment after treatment, these conditioned stimuli may precipitate withdrawal symptoms that have been relieved in the past by drug-taking behavior. Indeed, individuals no longer physically dependent upon heroin have described the recurrence of certain withdrawal symptoms upon returning to an environment in which they had engaged in drug-taking behavior. Wikler suggests that relapse is associated with the individual's history of having repeatedly reduced withdrawal distress by administering a drug. Wikler's two-factor theory, i.e., (1) conditioning of withdrawal phenomena to environmental situations and (2) previous reinforcement of drug-taking behavior through repeated reduction of withdrawal symptoms, has been demonstrated experimentally.

The first experimental observation of conditioned withdrawal was that of Irwin and Seevers (1952). They observed that nalorphine-induced withdrawal could be classically conditioned. Morphine-dependent monkeys that had undergone repeated nalorphine-induced withdrawal continued to show withdrawal-like symptoms, including increased salivation, vomiting, restlessness, tremors, etc., to both nalorphine and saline injections several months after having been withdrawn from morphine.

Wikler and Pescor (1967) also demonstrated the importance of conditioned withdrawal. They showed that conditioned withdrawal can be produced by returning rats to an environment previously associated with drug withdrawal. Rats showed an increase in the frequency of wet shakes (one of the symptoms of morphine withdrawal in rats) when they were returned to cages where they had experienced morphine abstinence. These occurred even after long drug-free periods (one to five months).

Goldberg and Schuster (1967) also demonstrated conditioning of morphine withdrawal. They produced these effects in the following way: Morphine-dependent monkeys responded on an FR 10 schedule of food presentation. When nalorphine was given to the dependent monkeys, FR responding was suppressed and physiological changes indicative of withdrawal occurred. Then a tone was presented along with the nalorphine injection. After several sessions in which the tone was paired with nalorphine, presentation of the tone alone suppressed responding and produced conditioned bradycardia, emesis and excessive salivation. Extinction, which consisted of daily pairings of the tone and saline, took 40 to 45 days (see Fig. 11-13).

Goldberg and Schuster (1970) extended their work to monkeys that had been withdrawn from morphine for several months. Monkeys were first made physically dependent on morphine. Withdrawal was produced in the morphine-dependent monkeys by nalorphine injections. A red light accompanied nalorphine injections. As with the tone, the light alone produced conditioned vomiting, salivation and response suppression. After this conditioning period, morphine injections were discontinued so that the animals underwent withdrawal. After 60 to 120 days, the animals were returned to the experimental situation and the red light was presented. Responding was still suppressed.

The increases in morphine administration which have been shown to follow injections of nalorphine in morphine-dependent monkeys (Thompson and Schuster, 1964) have also been shown to be conditionable (Goldberg et al., 1969). All these studies clearly demonstrate that stimuli associated with the nalorphine-induced withdrawal syndrome can produce dramatic conditioned effects which exist for a long time after the original conditioning.

We have seen that stimuli can obtain conditioned reinforcing effects by being paired with a drug reinforcer (see p. 369). Davis and Smith (1974) have shown that conditioned reinforcing stimuli may also be important in understanding relapse. They trained rats to bar press for an iv infusion of morphine paired with

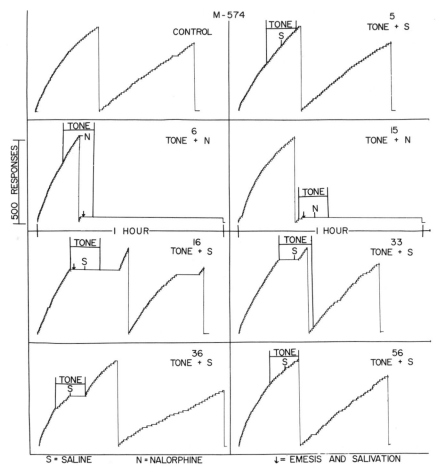

Fig. 11-13. Cumulative response records of selected sessions for one monkey, showing development and persistence of conditioned behavioral changes. Control: Session before CS (tone)–injection pairings. 5: Initial absence of response to tone paired with saline injections. 6: First acquisition session showing unconditioned effects of nalorphine (N) on food responding. 15: Tenth acquisition session showing conditioned responses to CS (tone). 16–56: Extinction sessions testing for persistence of the tone and saline injection as conditioned stimuli following cessation of chronic morphine treatment. Arrows indicate observation of emesis and excessive salivation. (From Goldberg and Schuster, 1967.)

a buzzer. Bar pressing was then extinguished, either by substituting saline for morphine or by administering naloxone. Extinction took place with or without the buzzer present. If the buzzer was present during extinction, bar pressing did not recover upon subsequent presentation of the buzzer. However, if the buzzer was *not* present during extinction, bar pressing did recover upon subsequent presentation. This study again points to the importance of eliminating both the pharmacological effects of a drug reinforcer and the stimuli that have become associated either with (1) the drug reinforcer or (2) withdrawal.

SUMMARY

In summary we can conclude that work with both oral and intravenous drug administration has been very successful in elucidating some of the variables that influence drug administration. It has been shown that, for many drugs, mere availability of the drug is sufficient to produce self-administration. The rate and pattern of administration depend on the drug, the drug dose, its availability and the schedule of reinforcement. This model has also been used to examine drug interactions and the abuse liability of various drugs.

REFERENCES

Anderson, W. W. and T. Thompson. 1974. Ethanol self-administration in water satiated rats. *Pharmacol. Biochem. Behav.* **2**: 447–454.

Balster, R. L. and C. R. Schuster. 1973a. A comparison of *d*-amphetamine, *l*-amphetamine and methamphetamine self-administration in rhesus monkeys. *Pharmacol. Biochem. Behav.* **1**: 67–71.

Balster, R. L. and C. R. Schuster. 1973b. Fixed-interval schedule of cocaine reinforcement: effect of dose and infusion duration. *J. Exp. Anal. Behav.* **20**: 119–129.

Balster, R. L., C. E. Johanson, R. T. Harris and C. R. Schuster. 1973. Phencyclidine self-administration in the rhesus monkey. *Pharmacol. Biochem. Behav.* **1**: 167–172.

Balster, R. L., C. R. Schuster and M. C. Wilson. 1971. The substitution of opiate analgesics in monkeys maintained on cocaine self-administration. Paper presented at the 33rd Ann. Meeting of the Committee on Problems of Drug Dependence, NAS-NRC.

Baxter, B. L., M. I. Gluckman, L. Stein and R. A. Scerni. 1974. Self-injection of apomorphine in the rat: positive reinforcement by a dopamine receptor stimulant. *Pharmacol. Biochem. Behav.* **2**: 387–391.

Blumberg, H., H. B. Dayton and P. S. Wolf. 1967. Analgesic and narcotic antagonist properties of noroxymorphone derivatives. *Toxicol. Appl. Pharmacol.* **10**: 406.

Burks, C. D. 1970. Schedule-induced polydipsia: are response-dependent schedules a limiting condition? *J. Exp. Anal. Behav.* **13**: 351–358.

Carlisle, H. J. 1971. Fixed-ratio polydipsia: Thermal effects of drinking, pausing, and responding. *J. Comp. Physiol. Psychol.* **75**: 10–22.

Crowder, W. F., S. G. Smith, W. M. Davis, J. T. Noel and W. R. Coussens. 1972. Effect of morphine dose size on the conditioned reinforcing potency of stimuli paired with morphine. *Psychol. Rec.* **22**: 441–448.

Davis, J. D. 1966. A method for chronic intravenous infusion in freely moving rats. *J. Exp. Anal. Behav.* **9**: 385–387.

Davis, J. D. and N. E. Miller. 1963. Fear and pain: Their effect on self-injection of amobarbital sodium by rats. *Science* **141**: 1286–1287.

Davis, J. D., G. C. Lulenski and N. E. Miller. 1968. Comparative studies of barbiturate self-administration. *Int. J. Addict.* **3**: 207–214.

Davis, W. M. and S. G. Smith. 1972. Alpha-methyltyrosine to prevent self-administration of morphine and amphetamine. *Curr. Ther. Res.* **14**: 114–121.

Davis, W. M. and S. G. Smith. 1974. Naloxone use to eliminate opiate-seeking behavior: Need for extinction of conditioned reinforcement. *Biol. Psychiat.* **9**: 181–189.

Davis, W. M. and S. G. Smith. 1975. Central cholinergic influence on self-administration of morphine and amphetamine. *Life Sci.* **16**: 237–246.

Deneau, G. A. and R. Inoki. 1967. Nicotine self-administration in monkeys. *Ann. N.Y. Acad. Sci.* **142**: 277–279.

Deneau, G., T. Yanagita and M. H. Seevers. 1969. Self-administration of psychoactive substances by the monkey. A measure of psychological dependence. *Psychopharmacologia* **16**: 30–48.

Dole, V. P. and M. E. Nyswander. 1968. Methadone maintenance and its implication for theories of narcotic addiction. *Res. Publ. Assoc. Res. Nerv. Ment. Dis.* **46**: 359–366.

Dougherty, J. and R. Pickens. 1973. Fixed-interval schedules of intravenous cocaine presentation in rats. *J. Exp. Anal. Behav.* **20**: 111–118.

Downs, D. A. and J. H. Woods. 1974. Codeine- and cocaine-reinforced responding in rhesus monkeys: effects of dose on response rates under a fixed-ratio schedule. *J. Pharmacol. Exp. Ther.* **191**: 179–188.

Downs, D. A. and J. H. Woods. 1975. Fixed-ratio escape and avoidance-escape from naloxone in morphine-dependent monkeys: effects of naloxone dose and morphine pretreatment. *J. Exp. Anal. Behav.* **23**: 415–427.

Eddy, N. B., H. Halback, H. Isbell and M. H. Seevers. 1965. Drug dependence: Its significance and characteristics. *Bull. WHO* **32**: 721–733.

Ellis, F. W. and J. R. Pick. 1970. Experimentally induced ethanol dependence in rhesus monkeys. *J. Pharmacol. Exp. Ther.* **175**: 88–93.

Everett, P. B. and R. A. King. 1970. Schedule-induced alcohol ingestion. *Psychon. Sci.* **18**: 278–279.

Falk, J. L. 1961. Production of polydipsia in normal rats by an intermittent food schedule. *Science* **133**: 195–196.

Falk, J. L., H. H. Samson and G. Winger. 1972. Behavioral maintenance of high concentrations of blood ethanol and physical dependence in the rat. *Science* **177**: 811–813.

Findley, J. D., W. W. Robinson and L. Peregrino. 1972. Addiction to secobarbital and chlordiazepoxide in the rhesus monkey by means of a self-infusion preference procedure. *Psychopharmacologia* **26**: 93–114.

Freed, E. X. 1974. Fluid selection by rats during schedule-induced polydipsia. *Quart. J. Alcohol Stud.* **35**: 1035–1043.

Freed, E. X., J. A. Carpenter and N. Hymowitz. 1970. Acquisition and extinction of schedule-induced consumption of alcohol and water. *Psychol. Rep.* **26**: 915–922.

Freedman, A. M. 1966. Drug addiction: An eclectic view. *J. Am. Med. Assoc.* **197**: 878–882.

Freund, G. 1969. Alcohol withdrawal syndrome in mice. *Arch. Neurol.* **21**: 315–320.

Gilbert, R. M. 1974. Schedule-induced ethanol polydipsia in rats with restricted fluid availability. *Psychopharmacologia* **38**: 151–157.

Goldberg, S. R. 1973. Comparable behavior maintained under fixed-ratio and second-order schedules of food presentation, cocaine injection or *d*-amphetamine injection in the squirrel monkey. *J. Pharmacol. Exp. Ther.* **186**: 18–30.

Goldberg, S. R. and C. R. Schuster. 1967. Conditioned suppression by a stimulus associated with nalorphine in morphine-dependent monkeys. *J. Exp. Anal. Behav.* **10**: 235–242.

Goldberg, S. R. and C. R. Schuster. 1970. Conditioned nalorphine-induced abstinence changes: Persistence in post morphine-dependent monkeys. *J. Exp. Anal. Behav.* **14**: 33–46.

Goldberg, S. R., F. Hoffmeister and U. U. Schlichting. 1972. Morphine antagonists: modification of behavioral effects of morphine dependence. *In* J. M. Singh, L. Miller, and H. Lal (eds.), *Drug Addiction:* I. *Experimental Pharmacology*. Futura Publishing Co., Mount Kisco, New York, pp. 31–48.

Goldberg, S. R., F. Hoffmeister, U. U. Schlichting and W. Wuttke. 1971a. Aversive properties of nalorphine and naloxone in morphine-dependent rhesus monkeys. *J. Pharmacol. Exp. Ther.* **179**: 268–276.

Goldberg, S. R., F. Hoffmeister, U. U. Schlichting and W. Wuttke. 1971b. A comparison of pentobarbital and cocaine self-administration in rhesus monkeys: Effects of dose and fixed-ratio parameter. *J. Pharmacol. Exp. Ther.* **179**: 277–283.

Goldberg, S. R., R. T. Kelleher and W. H. Morse. 1975. Second-order schedules of drug injection. *Fed. Proc.* **34**: 1171–1176.

Goldberg, S. R., J. H. Woods and C. R. Schuster. 1969. Morphine: Conditioned increases in self-administration in rhesus monkeys. *Science* **166**: 1306–1307.

Goldberg, S. R., J. H. Woods and C. R. Schuster. 1971c. Nalorphine-induced changes in morphine self-administration in rhesus monkeys. *J. Pharmacol. Exp. Ther.* **176**: 464–471.

Goldstein, D. B. and N. Pal. 1971. Alcohol dependence produced in mice by inhalation of ethanol: Grading the withdrawal reaction. *Science* **172**: 288–290.

Götestam, K. G. 1973. Intragastric self-administration of medazepam in rats. *Psychopharmacologia* **28**: 87–94.

Götestam, K. G. and B. E. Andersson. 1975. Self-administration of amphetamine analogues in rats. *Pharmacol. Biochem. Behav.* **3**: 229–233.

Hammond, A. L. 1971. Narcotic antagonists: New method to treat heroin addiction. *Science* **173**: 503–506.

Harris, R. T., J. L. Claghorn and J. C. Schoolar. 1968. Self administration of minor tranquilizers as a function of conditioning. *Psychopharmacologia* **13**: 81–88.

Harris, R. T., W. Waters and D. McLendon. 1974. Evaluation of reinforcing capability of delta-9-tetrahydrocannabinol in rhesus monkeys. *Psychopharmacologia* **37**: 23–29.

Heintzelman, M. E., J. Best and R. J. Senter. 1976. Polydipsia-induced alcohol dependency in rats: A reexamination. *Science* **191**: 482–483.

Hoffmeister, F. 1975. Negative reinforcing properties of some psychotropic drugs in drug-naive rhesus monkeys. *J. Pharmacol. Exp. Ther.* **192**: 468–477.

Hoffmeister, F. and S. R. Goldberg. 1973. A comparison of chlorpromazine, imipramine, morphine and *d*-amphetamine self-administration in cocaine-dependent rhesus monkeys. *J. Pharmacol. Exp. Ther.* **187**: 8–14.

Hoffmeister, F. and U. U. Schlichting. 1972. Reinforcing properties of some opiates and opioids in rhesus monkeys with histories of cocaine and codeine self-admininstration. *Psychopharmacologia* **23**: 55–74.

Hoffmeister, F. and W. Wuttke. 1973a. Negative reinforcing properties of morphine-antagonists in naive rhesus monkeys. *Psychopharmacologia* **33**: 247–258.

Hoffmeister, F. and W. Wuttke. 1973b. Self-administration of acetylsalicylic acid and combinations with codeine and caffeine in rhesus monkeys. *J. Pharmacol. Exp. Ther.* **186**: 266–275.

Hoffmeister, F. and W. Wuttke. 1975. Further studies on self-administration of antipyretic analgesics and combinations of antipyretic analgesics with codeine in rhesus monkeys. *J. Pharmacol. Exp. Ther.* **193**: 870–875.

Hoffmeister, F., S. R. Goldberg, U. U. Schlichting and W. Wuttke. 1970. Self-administration of *d*-amphetamine, morphine and chlorpromazine by cocaine "dependent" rhesus monkeys. *Naunyn-Schmiedebergs Arch. Pharmakol.* **266**: 359–360.

Holman, R. B. and R. D. Myers. 1968. Ethanol consumption under conditions of psychogenic polydipsia. *Physiol. Behav.* **3**: 369–371.

Hymowitz, N. 1971. Schedule-induced polydipsia and aggression in rats. *Psychon. Sci.* **23:** 226–228.

Iglauer, C. and J. H. Woods. 1974. Concurrent performances: Reinforcement by different doses of intravenous cocaine in rhesus monkeys. *J. Exp. Anal. Behav.* **22:** 179–196.

Irwin, S. and M. H. Seevers. 1952. Comparative study of regular and N-allylnormorphine-induced withdrawal in monkeys addicted to morphine, 6-methyldihydromorphine, Dromoran, methadone, and ketobemidone. *J. Pharmacol. Exp. Ther.* **106:** 397.

Jaffe, J. H. 1970. Narcotic analgesics. *In* L. Goodman and A. Gilman (eds.), *The Pharmacological Basis of Therapeutics*. Macmillan Co., New York, pp. 237–275.

Jasinski, D. R., W. R. Martin and C. A. Haertzen. 1967. The human pharmacology and abuse potential of N-allylnoroxymorphone (naloxone). *J. Pharmacol. Exp. Ther.* **157:** 420–426.

Johanson, C. E. and C. R. Schuster. 1975. A choice procedure for drug reinforcers: Cocaine and methylphenidate in the rhesus monkey. *J. Pharmacol. Exp. Ther.* **193:** 676–688.

Jones, B. E. and J. A. Prada. 1973. Relapse to morphine use in dog. *Psychopharmacologia* **30:** 1–12.

Kodluboy, D. W. and T. Thompson. 1971. Adjunctive self-administration of barbiturate solutions. *Proc. 79th Ann. Conv. APA*, pp. 749–750.

Kramer, J. C., V. S. Fischman and D. C. Littlefield. 1967. Amphetamine abuse. *J. Am. Med. Assoc.* **201:** 305–309.

Kumar, R. and I. P. Stolerman. 1972. Resumption of morphine self-administration by ex-addict rats: An attempt to modify tendencies to relapse. *J. Comp. Physiol. Psychol.* **78:** 457–465.

Lasagna, L. and H. K. Beecher. 1954. The analgesic effectiveness of nalorphine and nalorphine-morphine combinations in man. *J. Pharmacol. Exp. Ther.* **112:** 356–363.

Leander, J. D. and D. E. McMillan. 1973. Substantial oral morphine intake by the rat using schedule-induced polydipsia. *Fed. Proc.* **32:** 762.

Leander, J. D., D. E. McMillan and L. S. Harris. 1975. Schedule-induced oral narcotic self-administration: Acute and chronic effects. *J. Pharmacol. Exp. Ther.* **195:** 279–287.

Lester, D. 1961. Self-maintenance of intoxication in the rat. *Quart. J. Stud. Alcohol* **22:** 223–231.

Lester, D. 1966. Self-selection of alcohol by animals, human variation and the etiology of alcoholism. A critical review. *Quart. J. Stud. Alcohol* **27:** 395–438.

Lewis, M. J., D. L. Margules and O. B. Ward, Jr. 1975. Opioid-reinforced operant behavior: Selective suppression by alpha-methyl-para-tyrosine. *J. Comp. Physiol. Psychol.* **88:** 519–527.

Martin, W. R. 1967. Opioid antagonists. *Pharmacol. Rev.* **19:** 463–521.

Martin, W. R. and C. W. Gorodetzky. 1967. Cyclazocine an adjunct in the treatment of narcotic addiction. *Int. J. Addict.* **2:** 85–93.

Martin, W. R., C. W. Gorodetzky and T. K. McClane. 1966. An experimental study in the treatment of narcotic addicts with cyclazocine. *Clin. Pharmacol. Ther.* **7:** 455–465.

Martin, W. R., D. R. Jasinski and P. A. Mansky. 1973. Naltrexone, an antagonist for the treatment of heroin dependence. *Arch. Gen. Psychiat.* **28:** 784–791.

McMillan, D. E., J. D. Leander and F. W. Ellis. 1974a. Consumption of ethanol and water under schedule-induced polydipsia. *Pharmacologist* **16:** 637.

McMillan, D. E., J. D. Leander, T. W. Wilson, S. C. Wallace, T. Fix, S. Redding and R. T. Turk. 1976. Oral ingestion of narcotic analgesics by rats. *J. Pharmacol. Exp. Ther.* **196:** 269–279.

McMillan, D. E., F. B. Waddell and C. F. Cathcart. 1974b. Establishment of physical dependence in mice by oral ingestion of morphine. *J. Pharmacol. Exp. Ther.* **190:** 416–419.

Meisch, R. A. 1969. Self-administration of pentobarbital by means of schedule-induced polydipsia. *Psychon. Sci.* 16: 16–17.

Meisch, R. A. and P. Beardsley. 1975. Ethanol as a reinforcer for rats: Effects of concurrent access to water and alternate positions of water and ethanol. *Psychopharmacologia* 43: 19–23.

Meisch, R. A. and T. Thompson. 1971. Ethanol intake in the absence of concurrent food reinforcement. *Psychopharmacologia* 22: 72–79.

Meisch, R. A. and T. Thompson. 1972a. Ethanol intake during schedule-induced polydipsia. *Physiol. Behav.* 8: 471–475.

Meisch, R. A. and T. Thompson. 1972b. Ethanol reinforcement: Effects of concentration during food deprivation. *Finish Found. Alcohol Stud.* 20: 71–75.

Meisch, R. A. and T. Thompson. 1973. Ethanol as a reinforcer: Effects of fixed-ratio size and food deprivation. *Psychopharmacologia* 28: 171–183.

Meisch, R. A. and T. Thompson. 1974a. Ethanol intake as a function of concentration during food deprivation and satiation. *Pharmacol. Biochem. Behav.* 2: 589–596.

Meisch, R. A. and T. Thompson. 1974b. Rapid establishment of ethanol as a reinforcer for rats. *Psychopharmacologia* 37: 311–321.

Mello, N. K. 1973. A review of methods to induce alcohol addiction in animals. *Pharmacol. Biochem. Behav.* 1: 89–101.

Mello, N. K. and J. H. Mendelson. 1964. Operant performance by rats for alcohol reinforcement. A comparison of alcohol-preferring and nonpreferring animals. *Quart. J. Stud. Alcohol* 25: 226–234.

Mello, N. K. and J. H. Mendelson. 1971. Evaluation of a polydipsia technique to induce alcohol consumption in monkeys. *Physiol. Behav.* 7: 827–836.

Mendelson, J. H. and N. K. Mello. 1971. Effects of prolonged exposure to ethanol in infant monkeys. *Fed. Proc.* 30: 568.

Myers, R. D. and W. L. Veale. 1972. The determinants of alcohol preference in animals. *In* B. Kissin and H. Begleiter (eds.), *Biology of Alcoholism*, Vol. 2: *Physiology and Behavior.* Plenum Press, New York.

Nayak, P. K., A. L. Misra and S. J. Mulé. 1975. Physiological disposition and biotransformation of [^{3}H] cocaine in acute and chronically-treated rats. *Fed. Proc.* 34: 781.

Ogata, H., F. Ogata, J. H. Mendelson and N. K. Mello. 1972. A comparison of techniques to induce alcohol dependence and tolerance in the mouse. *J. Pharmacol. Exp. Ther.* 180: 216–230.

Pickens, R. 1968. Self-administration of stimulants by rats. *Int. J. Addict.* 3: 215–221.

Pickens, R. and W. C. Harris. 1968. Self-administration of *d*-amphetamine by rats. *Psychopharmacologia* 12: 158–163.

Pickens, R. and T. Thompson. 1967. Self-administration of amphetamine and cocaine by rats. Paper presented at the 29th Ann. Meeting of the Committee on Problems of Drug Dependence, NAS-NRC.

Pickens, R. and T. Thompson. 1968. Cocaine-reinforced behavior in rats: Effects of reinforcement magnitude and fixed-ratio size. *J. Pharmacol. Exp. Ther.* 161: 122–129.

Pickens, R. and T. Thompson. 1971. Characteristics of stimulant drug reinforcement. *In* T. Thompson and R. Pickens (eds.), *Stimulus Properties of Drugs.* Appleton-Century-Crofts, New York.

Pickens, R., R. A. Meisch and J. A. Dougherty, Jr. 1968. Chemical interactions in methamphetamine reinforcement. *Psychol. Rep.* 23: 1267–1270.

Pickens, R., R. A. Meisch and L. McGuire. 1967. Methamphetamine reinforcement in rats. *Psychon. Sci.* 8: 371–372.

Pieper, W. A., M. J. Skeen, H. M. McClure and P. G. Bourne. 1972. The chimpanzee as an animal model for investigating alcoholism. *Science* 176: 71–73.

Richter, C. P. and K. Campbell. 1940. Alcohol taste thresholds and concentrations of solution preferred by rats. *Science* 91: 507–508.

Risner, M. E. and K. A. Khavari. 1973. Morphine dependence in rats produced after five days of ingestion. *Psychopharmacologia* 28: 51–62.

Rosenblith, J. Z. 1970. Polydipsia induced in the rat by a second-order schedule. *J. Exp. Anal. Behav.* 14: 139–144.

Samson, H. H. and J. L. Falk. 1974a. Alteration of fluid preference in ethanol-dependent animals. *J. Pharmacol. Exp. Ther.* 190: 365–376.

Samson, H. H. and J. L. Falk. 1974b. Schedule-induced ethanol polydipsia: enhancement by saccharin. *Pharmacol. Biochem. Behav.* 2: 835–838.

Schlichting, U. U., S. R. Goldberg, W. Wuttke and F. Hoffmeister. 1971. *d*-Amphetamine self-administration by rhesus monkeys with different self-administration histories. Proc. Eur. Soc. for the Study of Drug Toxicity, 1970. *Excp. Med. Int. Cong. Ser.* 220: 62–69.

Schuster, C. R. 1970. Psychological approaches to opiate dependence and self-administration by laboratory animals. *Fed. Proc.* 29: 2–5.

Schuster, C. R. and R. L. Balster. 1973. Self-administration of agonists. *In* H. W. Kosterlitz, H. O. J. Collier and J. E. Villarreal (eds.), *Agonist and Antagonist Actions of Narcotic Analgesic Drugs.* University Park Press, Baltimore, pp. 243–254.

Schuster, C. R. and C. E. Johanson. 1974. The use of animal models for the study of drug abuse. *In* R. J. Gibbins, Y. Israel, H. Kalant, R. E. Popham, W. Schmidt and R. G. Smart (eds.), *Research Advances in Alcohol and Drug Problems.* Vol. 1. John Wiley & Sons, New York.

Schuster, C. R. and T. Thompson. 1969. Self administration of and behavioral dependence on drugs. *Ann. Rev. Pharm.* 9: 483–502.

Schuster, C. R. and J. E. Villarreal. 1968. The experimental analysis of opioid dependence. *In* D. Efron (ed.), *Psychopharmacology: A Review of Progress, 1968.* pp. 811–828. U.S. Government Printing Office, Washington, D.C.

Schuster, C. R. and J. H. Woods. 1968. The conditioned reinforcing effects of stimuli associated with morphine reinforcement. *Int. J. Addict.* 3: 223–230.

Segal, E. F. and W. M. Bandt. 1966. Influence of collateral water drinking on bar pressing under complex reinforcement contingencies. *Psychon. Sci.* 4: 377–378.

Segal, E. F. and S. M. Holloway. 1963. Timing behavior in rats with water drinking as a mediator. *Science* 140: 888–889.

Smith, S. G. and W. M. Davis. 1973. Haloperidol effects on morphine self-administration: Testing for pharmacological modification of the primary reinforcement mechanism. *Psychol. Rec.* 23: 215–221.

Stolerman, I. P., R. Kumar and H. Steinberg. 1971. Development of morphine dependence in rats: Lack of effect of previous ingestion of other drugs. *Psychopharmacologia* 20: 321–336.

Stretch, R., G. J. Gerber and S. M. Wood. 1971. Factors affecting behavior maintained by response-contingent intravenous infusions of amphetamine in squirrel monkeys. *Canad. J. Physiol. Pharmacol.* 49: 581–589.

Talley, W. H. and I. Rosenblum. 1972. Self-administration of dextropropoxyphene by rhesus monkeys to the point of toxicity. *Psychopharmacologia* 27: 179–182.

Thompson, T. 1968. Drugs as reinforcers: Experimental addiction. *Int. J. Addict.* 3: 199–206.

Thompson, T. and W. Ostlund, Jr. 1965. Susceptibility to readdiction as a function of the addiction and withdrawal environments. *J. Comp. Physiol. Psychol.* 60: 388–392.

Thompson, T. and R. Pickens. 1970. Stimulant self-administration by animals: Some comparisons with opiate self-administration. *Fed. Proc.* 29: 6–12.

Thompson, T. and C. R. Schuster. 1964. Morphine self-administration, food-reinforced, and avoidance behaviors in rhesus monkeys. *Psychopharmacologia* 5: 87–94.

Vitiello, M. V. and S. C. Woods. 1975. Caffeine: Preferential consumption by rats. *Pharmacol. Biochem. Behav.* 3: 147–149.

Wahlström, G. 1974. Withdrawal in the rat after long-term forced oral barbital administration. *Acta Pharmacol. Toxicol.* 35: 131–144.

Weeks, J. R. 1962. Experimental morphine addiction: Method for automatic intravenous injections in unrestrained rats. *Science* 138: 143–144.

Weeks, J. R. 1964. Experimental narcotic addiction. *Scientific American* 210: 46–52.

Weeks, J. R. and R. J. Collins. 1964. Factors affecting voluntary morphine intake in self-maintained addicted rats. *Psychopharmacologia* 6: 267–279.

Wikler, A. 1965. Conditioning factors in opiate addiction and relapse. *In* D. M. Wilner and G. G. Kassebaum (eds.), *Narcotics*. McGraw-Hill, New York.

Wikler, A. 1961. On the nature of addiction and habituation. *Brit. J. Addict.* 57: 73–79.

Wikler, A., W. R. Martin, F. T. Pescor and C. G. Eades. 1963. Factors regulating oral consumption of an opioid (etonitazene) by morphine-addicted rats. *Psychopharmacologia* 5: 55–76.

Wikler, A. and F. T. Pescor. 1967. Classical conditioning of a morphine abstinence phenomenon, reinforcement of opioid-drinking behavior and "relapse" in morphine-addicted rats. *Psychopharmacologia* 10: 255–284.

Wilson, M. C. and C. R. Schuster. 1972. The effects of chlorpromazine on psychomotor stimulant self-administration in the rhesus monkey. *Psychopharmacologia* 26: 115–126.

Wilson, M. C. and C. R. Schuster. 1973a. Cholinergic influence on intravenous cocaine self-administration by rhesus monkeys. *Pharmacol. Biochem. Behav.* 1: 643–649.

Wilson, M. C. and C. R. Schuster. 1973b. The effects of stimulants and depressants on cocaine self-administration behavior in the rhesus monkey. *Psychopharmacologia* 31: 291–304.

Wilson, M. C. and C. R. Schuster. 1974. Aminergic influences on intravenous cocaine self-administration by rhesus monkeys. *Pharmacol. Biochem. Behav.* 2: 563–571.

Wilson, M. C. and C. R. Schuster. 1975. Interactions between atropine, chlorpromazine and cocaine on food reinforced behavior. *Pharmacol. Biochem. Behav.* 3: 363–375.

Wilson, M. C., M. Hitomi and C. R. Schuster. 1969. Further studies of the self-administration of psychomotor stimulants in the rhesus monkey. Paper presented at the 31st Ann. Meeting of the Committee on Problems of Drug Dependence, NAS-NRC.

Wilson, M. C., M. Hitomi and C. R. Schuster. 1971. Psychomotor stimulant self administration as a function of dosage per injection in the rhesus monkey. *Psychopharmacologia* 22: 271–281.

Winger, G. D. and J. H. Woods. 1973. The reinforcing property of ethanol in the rhesus monkey: I. Initiation, maintenance and termination of intravenous ethanol-reinforced responding. *Ann. N.Y. Acad. Sci.* 215: 162–175.

Woods, J. H. and C. R. Schuster. 1968. Reinforcement properties of morphine, cocaine and SPA as a function of unit dose. *Int. J. Addict.* 3: 231–237.

Woods, J. H. and C. R. Schuster. 1970. Regulation of drug self-administration. *In* R. T. Harris, W. M. McIssac and C. R. Schuster (eds.), *Advances in Mental Science II: Drug Dependence*. University of Texas Press, Austin, pp. 158–169.

Woods, J. H. and R. E. Tessel. 1974. Fenfluramine: Amphetamine congener that fails to maintain drug-taking behavior in the rhesus monkey. *Science* 185: 1067–1069.

Woods, L. A. 1956. The pharmacology of nalorphine (N-allylnormorphine). *Pharmacol. Rev.* 8: 175–198.

Yanagita, T. and S. Takahashi. 1973. Dependence liability of several sedative-hypnotic agents evaluated in monkeys. *J. Pharmacol. Exp. Ther.* 185: 307–316.

Yanagita, T., K. Ando and S. Takahashi. 1970. A testing method for psychological dependence liability of drugs in monkeys. Paper presented at the 32nd Ann. Meeting of the Committee on Problems of Drug Dependence, NAS-NRC.

Yanagita, T., K. Ando, S. Takahashi and K. Ishida. 1969. Self-administration of barbiturates, alcohol (intragastrine) and CNS stimulants (intravenous) in monkeys. Paper presented at the 31st Ann. Meeting of the Committee on Problems of Drug Dependence, NAS-NRC.

Yanagita, T., G. A. Deneau and M. H. Seevers. 1965. Evaluation of pharmacological agents in the monkey by long-term intravenous self- or programmed-administration. *Excp. Med. Int. Cong. Ser.* 87: 453–457.

Yokel, R. A. and R. Pickens. 1971. Intravenous self-administration of dextro and levo isomers of amphetamine and methamphetamine by rats. *Pharmacologist* 13, Abstract.

Yokel, R. A. and R. Pickens. 1973. Self-administration of optical isomers of amphetamine and methylamphetamine by rats. *J. Pharmacol. Exp. Ther.* 187: 27–33.

Yokel, R. A. and R. Pickens. 1974. Drug level of *d*- and *l*-amphetamine during intravenous self-administration. *Psychopharmacologia* 34: 255–264.

Yokel, R. A. and R. A. Wise. 1975. Increased lever pressing for amphetamine after pimozide in rats: Implications for a dopamine theory of reward. *Science* 187: 547–549.

12
Drugs as Discriminative Stimuli

In Chapter 1 the term stimulus was defined as some aspect of the environment that can be related to a response. There are a variety of ways in which stimuli relate to behavior. These stimulus functions include (1) unconditioned stimuli which are capable of eliciting an unconditioned response, (2) conditioned stimuli which acquire the ability to elicit a conditioned response through the pairing of at least two stimuli presented in temporal contiguity, (3) reinforcing stimuli which increase the probability that the response they follow will recur and (4) discriminative stimuli which determine the availability of reinforcing stimuli.

While the stimuli which serve these functions are usually thought of as external stimuli, such as visual or auditory cues, drugs may also serve as stimuli in a variety of ways. The ability of drugs to act as both reinforcing stimuli and as unconditioned stimuli was reviewed in Chapter 11. Moreover, drugs have been shown to serve effectively as unconditioned stimuli in classical conditioning paradigms (Cameron and Appel, 1972; Pickens and Dougherty, 1971). In this chapter we will discuss the ability of drugs to function as discriminative stimuli.

A discriminative stimulus is said to set the occasion for the occurrence of a response. For example, if reinforcement follows a response only when a certain discriminative stimulus is present, responding usually occurs predominately in the presence of that stimulus. If this occurs, responding is said to be under *stimulus control* since the stimulus determines the probability of occurrence of the response. The stimulus can be any aspect of an organism's environment that controls its behavior. If drug administration is specifically associated with availability of reinforcement contingent upon some response, then the drug and any interoceptive cues associated with the administration of the drug become discriminative stimuli.

In general, two procedures have been used to examine the stimulus properties of drugs: (1) the *drug discrimination procedure* and (2) the *state-dependent learning procedure.* In the drug discrimination procedure, one response is followed by reinforcement in the presence of one stimulus (e.g., a dose of a drug) and another response is followed by reinforcement in the presence of another stimulus (e.g., a dose of another drug or of a vehicle control). In this case, the drug has a clear-cut discriminative function, setting the occasion for the response and reinforcement to follow. In the state-dependent learning procedure (which is also called a drug dissociation procedure), animals are trained to perform a task either after drug administration or under drug-free conditions. Performance of the task upon subsequent testing is said to depend on reinstating the same drug conditions or state that existed during training; hence the term *state-dependent*. For example, if training took place while the animals were drugged, optimum performance should occur only if the animals are also drugged during testing.

There is some question as to whether the function of a drug in the state-dependent learning paradigm is that of a discriminative stimulus. By definition, a discriminative stimulus is established by differentially reinforcing one response under one stimulus condition and another response under another stimulus condition. In the state-dependent learning procedure the subjects are given experience with only one stimulus (or drug) during training, and consequently do not have a history of being differentially reinforced in the presence or absence of the drug. While the function of a drug in the state-dependent learning paradigm may not represent clear-cut discriminative stimulus control by a drug, we will discuss this procedure along with some of the data generated by it since it plays an important role in the understanding of the stimulus function of drugs.

STATE-DEPENDENT LEARNING

The Procedure

In the state-dependent learning procedure, a response is first established under some specified condition. At a subsequent time, a test is given to determine if the response will recur. If the response was established while a subject was drugged, then recurrence of that response is expected to depend on reinstating the same drug conditions that were present during training. Similarly, if the response was established under conditions in which the animal did not receive a drug or received a vehicle control, performance of the response is expected to depend on reinstating the same non-drug conditions that were in effect during training. Performance decrements (i.e., failure to perform an established response) are presumed to be related to the degree of change in stimulus conditions between training and testing. This is essentially a go/no go task in which performance of the established response is a measure of retention, and nonperformance is a measure of lack of retention.

Since failure to perform a response can be due to a great many factors, it is important to demonstrate that performance decrements are the result of having trained an animal to make a response under conditions different from those in

TABLE 12-1. 2 × 2 Experimental design

		Testing	
		Drug	**Non-drug**
Training	Drug	D–D	D–ND
	Non-drug	ND–D	ND–ND

effect during testing and not simply the result of factors such as motor disability. A 2 × 2 factorial design is usually employed (Miller, 1957) to provide this control. Two groups of subjects are used. One group is *trained* under drug (D) conditions, and the other group is trained without a drug [i.e., non-drug (ND) conditions]. These two groups are further divided into two more groups; each of these groups is *tested* either under drug (D) or non-drug (ND) conditions. Therefore, four groups are used: one group trained and tested in the drug state (D-D); another group trained and tested in the non-drug state (ND-ND); another group trained in the drug state but tested in the non-drug state (D-ND); and finally a group trained under non-drug conditions but tested under drug conditions (ND-D). Table 12-1 identifies these four groups.

The use of four groups enables experimenters to differentiate effects attributable to changes in the stimulus conditions between training and testing from effects attributable to factors which may influence the animal's ability to perform the response (e.g., motor disability). If, for example, performance during testing in the ND-D group is poor compared to performance during testing in the ND-ND group, it is possible that the poor performance is due to the fact that the ND-D group was tested under stimulus conditions (where the stimulus is the drug) different from those in effect during training. If the change in drug conditions accounts for poor performance, then one should also see poor performance upon testing in the D-ND group, since the drug condition during testing of this group is also different from that in effect during training. On the other hand, it is possible that the drug directly affects performance of the task. This effect should appear when the performance of the D-D and ND-D groups is compared. Therefore, by using these four groups, the effect of a change in drug conditions between training and testing can be separated from other drug effects. However, even with this design, a mixture of effects can lead to difficulties of interpretation, and several additional control experiments may be required to demonstrate the effect conclusively. Overton (1974) has discussed the limitation of these designs and proposed some alternative strategies.

The Data

The first study of state-dependent learning was done by Girden and Culler in 1937. Girden and Culler were originally interested in investigating the question of whether conditioning was possible when the conditioned response was not actually performed by the subject. Early investigators (Harlow and Stagner, 1933) failed to condition a response in a curarized dog or cat, but later Light and Gantt (1936) succeeded. Although Girden and Culler initiated their work in order to investigate this question, they also discovered that animals conditioned under curare only maintained the response under curare, whereas animals conditioned in the absence of curare only maintained the response in the absence of curare.

The following preparation was used: Animals were curarized and presented with a shock applied to their hind paw which produced a leg flexion response (unconditioned response). The response was then conditioned to occur to a bell which preceded the shock (see Chapter 1 for an explanation of classical conditioning procedures). Since the semitendinosus muscle responds when shock is applied to the hind paw, this muscle was dissected out from nearby muscles and tissue. The muscle was also temporarily ligated, i.e., the blood supply to the semitendinosus muscle was blocked. Therefore, an iv infusion of curare did not reach the semitendinosus muscle in sufficient quantities to produce paralysis. The nerve was left intact. Girden and Culler showed that the conditioned response to a bell paired with shock could be established in curarized animals. When the curare wore off, however, the conditioned response did not occur. The unconditioned response to the shock was still present, indicating that failure to respond was not due to paralysis. Upon recurarization, the conditioned response reappeared. Girden and Culler (1937) showed that the converse was also true. A conditioned response established under non-drug conditions vanished under curare but reappeared after recovery from the drug.

Although subsequent researchers have modified the procedure used by Girden and Culler, a number of studies have been done along these lines. Those of Overton (1964) are perhaps best known. Overton trained rats to escape from shock in a t-maze using a spatial discrimination. On each trial a rat was dropped into the start box of a t-maze in which the grid floor was electrified. The rat was then allowed to run freely in the maze until it reached the correct goal box (i.e., where no shock was present). On training trials only one goal box was accessible. Two groups of rats were used. Group I received 25 mg/kg of pentobarbital and was trained to go to the left goal box; Group II received saline and was trained to go to the right goal box. After ten such training trials, both groups were tested. Only one test trial was given each day. Each rat was tested under both drug and non-drug conditions, which alternated each day. The rats in Group I (trained under pentobarbital to turn left) turned left when tested under pentobarbital, but responded randomly when tested with saline. Similarly, the rats in Group II (trained under saline to go right), turned right under saline conditions, but turned randomly under pentobarbital.

Other drugs have been reported to produce similar effects. State-dependent learning has been demonstrated with ethanol (Grossman and Miller, 1961;

Holloway, 1972; Crow, 1966; Deutsch and Roll, 1973; Richardson, 1972), amobarbital (Miller, 1964), chlorpromazinc (Otis, 1964; Lal, 1969), scopolamine (Carlton and Vogel, 1965), chlordiazepoxide (Sachs *et al.*, 1966; Goldberg *et al.*, 1973; Iwahara and Matsushita, 1971), meprobamate (Barnhart and Abbot, 1967), pentobarbital (Holmgren, 1964; Mayse and DeVietti, 1971; Chute and Wright, 1973), atropine (Paskal, 1962), morphine and amphetamine (Belleville, 1964; Lal, 1969; Roffman and Lal, 1972; Carey, 1973), as well as Δ^9-THC, Δ^8-THC (Henriksson and Järbe, 1971; Goldberg *et al.*, 1973) and mescaline (Siegel and Jarvik, 1971).

In summary these studies have shown that a behavior learned while an organism is drugged sometimes fails to appear under non-drug conditions, yet will reliably reappear when the animal is given drug again. This fact may play an important part in the understanding of human drug consumption. Alcohol is one drug whose stimulus properties are widely known. Though the literature is small, the general conclusion is that moderate doses of alcohol produce a partial dissociation of some types of learning such as discriminated avoidance, visceral learning tasks and verbal learning tasks (Bustamante *et al.*, 1968; Diethelm and Barr, 1962; Goodwin *et al.*, 1969; Storm and Caird, 1967; Weingartner and Faillace, 1971; Goodwin, 1974). These studies have shown that the performance of either a sober or an intoxicated subject on a variety of tasks was best when the drug condition during testing was the same as that in effect during training. The task was performed less well when the drug condition was different in training from that in testing. Overton (1972) has reviewed some of this work and discusses its implications for the treatment of alcoholism. Similar findings have been reported for marijuana (Rickles *et al.*, 1973).

The stimulus properties of drugs may also have special implications in clinical settings. For example, many forms of therapy take place while patients are drugged. Whether these behaviors will transfer to new situations and to non-drug conditions is an important consideration.

Finally, this work also suggests some considerations for experimental design. Many experiments are designed in such a way that the animals are trained in non-drug conditions and tested in drug conditions. Any behavioral changes seen during testing are often attributed to direct effects of the drug. Impaired performance, however, may be due to the change in stimulus conditions between training and testing.

DRUG DISCRIMINATION

The Procedure

While the state-dependent learning paradigm generated interesting data about the stimulus properties of drugs, the drug discrimination procedure is more commonly used today to examine these properties. In a drug discrimination study, animals are trained to respond differentially under different drug conditions. For example, one response is reinforced in the presence of one drug condition; another response is reinforced in the presence of a different drug condition. Performance is then tested in each drug condition, and the animal's response choice is measured. The advantage of the discrimination procedure over the go/no go task used in the state-dependent learning procedure is that drug-induced performance deficits do not bias any one response over another response since each response is topographically similar (i.e., a right vs. a left turn rather than turning or failing to turn). Moreover, the same four conditions are used in the drug discrimination procedure as in the state-dependent learning procedure, the difference being that in the drug discrimination procedure, each animal is tested in each of the four conditions. First of all, an animal is trained in *both* the drug and non-drug conditions; however, the response trained in each condition is different. Second, an animal is tested in both drug and non-drug conditions. A variety of responses and a variety of drug comparisons (drug vs. saline, one drug vs. another drug, one dose of a drug vs. a different dose of the same drug) have been examined with this procedure.

The Data

Probably the earliest work in this area is that of Culler and associates. Culler *et al.* (1939) demonstrated that differential responding could be obtained under curare and non-drug conditions. They first conditioned right leg flexion of one dog to the sound of a bell paired with the occurrence of shock. The animal was then curarized. Under curare, the unconditioned response occurred when shock was applied to the paw, but the conditioned response to the bell was not present. While still under curare the left leg of the same dog was then conditioned to the bell, just as the right leg had been. Upon recovery from curare, conditioning was tested. The conditioned response in the right leg, which was established when the dog was *not* curarized, could be elicited with the bell. The unconditioned response in the left leg appeared when shock was applied to the paw, but the conditioned response was not present. When the animal was curarized again, reversal occurred, i.e., the right-leg conditioned response was not present while the left-leg conditioned response occurred.

It has also been shown that rats can be trained to respond differentially in a t-maze on the basis of a drug stimulus. Overton (1964) trained rats to escape shock by running to one side of a t-maze when given pentobarbital and to the opposite side when given saline. Each rat was given a daily 10-trial training session. All trials during a daily training session took place under one drug condition (either pentobarbital or saline). Drug conditions alternated on successive days. The side of the maze selected by the rat on the first trial of each training session was used as a measure of the amount of discriminative control exerted by pentobarbital.   In a later study (1966) Overton showed that a variety of drugs (ethanol, ethyl carbamate, phenobarbital, chlordiazepoxide, meprobamate, atropine and scopolamine) could be discriminated from saline with this procedure.

Similar findings have been shown with other procedures. Kubena and Barry (1969a,b) used two different procedures to demonstrate that animals could discriminate between the presence and absence of various drugs. One of the procedures is similar to an approach/avoidance task. Rats were trained to press a lever. Lever pressing was followed by either food or shock, depending on whether the animal received drug or saline. For example, in one group of animals responding was followed by food in the presence of a drug and by shock in the presence of saline. Following training with this procedure, the rats in this group generally responded on the lever (i.e., approached it) on days on which they received a drug, and withheld responding (i.e., avoided the lever) on days on which they received saline.

Kubena and Barry (1969a,b) also utilized a two-lever choice procedure. Two levers were present in the box and lever pressing was followed by food on only one of the two levers. Whether the rats received drug or saline determined which lever produced food. For example, right-lever responses were followed with food on a VI 1-min schedule only when the animal had received a certain dose of a specific drug. Left-lever responses were followed by food when the animal received saline. The first 5 min of each session without food presentation provided a test of the rat's choice between the two levers. Kubena and Barry showed that rats could discriminate between 1200 mg/kg of alcohol and saline and between 10 mg/kg of atropine sulfate and saline with both procedures. Further work by Barry and Kubena (1972) has shown that rats can also discriminate between 4.0 mg/kg of tetrahydrocannabinol and saline in the approach/avoidance procedure.

Procedures similar to Overton's t-maze and Kubena and Barry's choice procedure are now routinely used to examine drug discriminations. The t-maze procedure is sometimes modified so that responding is maintained by food presentation rather than escape from shock. Various schedules are used to maintain responding in the two-lever choice procedure. All procedures, however, are similar in that a drug cue determines which of two responses produces reinforcement. They are also similar in that test periods take place in the absence of reinforcement so that drug discriminative control can be assessed independently of the effects of reinforcement. In t-maze experiments the animal's choice is measured on the first trial of a test session, before reinforcement occurs. In the choice procedure, testing takes place in extinction. Some investigators run the first minutes of each training session in extinction and use only the data from this period as a measure of drug discriminability. Others intersperse brief extinction sessions between two training sessions and remove the animal from the experiment after the brief extinction session.

A number of drugs have been examined with these procedures and have been shown to serve as effective discriminative stimuli in the control of differential responding. Table 12-2 presents some of these drugs and lists the doses examined and discrimination procedures employed. Sometimes the range of doses examined is very broad. For example, Overton (1966) used a dose of 150 mg/kg of atropine as a discriminative stimulus in the control of t-maze responding, while others (Kubena and Barry, 1969a,b; Harris and Balster, 1971) have used much lower doses with procedures involving lever pressing. While most of the work with drug discrimination has involved discriminations between some drug and saline, a few attempts have been made to establish discriminations between two different drugs and between different doses of one drug. Tables 12-3 and 12-4 present some of these comparisons. Moreover, Overton (1967) has shown

TABLE 12-2. Studies demonstrating discriminative control between drug and non-drug conditions[1]

Drug and dose	Task	Reference
Alcohol		
2400 mg/kg	t-maze	Overton (1966)
1200 mg/kg	approach-avoidance (lever press)	Kubena and Barry (1969a, b)
1200 mg/kg	2-lever choice	Kubena and Barry (1969a, b)
1200 mg/kg	multiple schedule	Harris and Balster (1971)
Amphetamine		
4.0 mg/kg d-.	3-compartment escape	Schecter and Rosecrans (1973)
0.8 mg/kg d-	2-lever choice	Jones et al. (1974)
0.8 mg/kg l-	2-lever choice	Jones et al. (1974)
1.0 mg/kg d-	2-lever choice	Kuhn et al. (1974)
1.0 mg/kg dl-	multiple schedule	Harris and Balster (1968, 1970, 1971)
0.3 and 2.5 mg/kg dl-	2-lever choice	Waters et al. (1972)
0.8 mg/kg d-	2-lever choice	Huang and Ho (1974)
Atropine sulfate		
150 mg/kg	t-maze	Overton (1966)
10 mg/kg	approach-avoidance (lever press)	Kubena and Barry (1969a, b)
10 mg/kg	2-lever choice	Kubena and Barry (1969a, b)
10 mg/kg	multiple schedule	Harris and Balster (1971)
Chlordiazepoxide		
30 mg/kg	t-maze	Overton (1966)
15 mg/kg	conditional discrimination	Brown et al. (1968)
25 mg/kg	multiple schedule	Harris and Balster (1971)
Diazepam		
8.0 mg/kg	t-maze	Johansson and Järbe (1975)

Drug and dose	Task	Reference
Lysergic acid diethylamide		
0.048 mg/kg	t-maze	Schecter and Rosecrans (1972a)
0.120 mg/kg	2-lever choice	Hirschhorn and Winter (1971)
0.04–0.08 mg/kg	2-lever choice	Cameron and Appel (1973)
0.01–0.08 mg/kg	2-lever choice	Greenberg et al. (1975a)
0.072 mg/kg	2-lever choice	Hirschhorn and Rosecrans (1974a)
Marijuana extract		
10 mg/kg	2-lever choice	Bueno and Carlini (1972)
Meprobamate		
200 mg/kg	t-maze	Overton (1966)
Mescaline		
9.9 mg/kg	2-lever choice	Hirschhorn and Winter (1971)
10 mg/kg	S^D-S^Δ discrimination	Winter (1973)
Morphine		
4.5, 9, 18 and 36 mg/kg	t-maze	Hill et al. (1971)
20 mg/kg	3-compartment escape	Rosecrans et al. (1973)
10 mg/kg	2-lever choice	Hirschhorn and Rosecrans (1974a, b)
Nicotine		
0.4 mg/kg	t-maze	Schecter and Rosecrans (1971, 1972b, c)
0.2 mg/kg	lever choice	Morrison and Stephenson (1969)
Pentazocine		
10 mg/kg	2-lever choice	Kuhn et al. (1976)
Pentobarbital		
10–25 mg/kg	t-maze	Overton (1964, 1966)
20 mg/kg	t-maze	Hill et al. (1971)
20 mg/kg*	conditional discrimination	Bliss et al. (1971)
15 mg/kg	3-compartment escape	Rosecrans et al. (1973)
7.0 mg/kg	S^D-S^Δ discrimination	Winter (1974b)
Phenobarbital		
60–80 mg/kg	t-maze	Overton (1966)
Psilocybin		
0.4 mg/kg	multiple schedule	Harris and Balster (1971)
Scopolamine		
300 mg/kg	t-maze	Overton (1966)
Tetrahydrocannabinol (Δ^9)		
4.0 mg/kg	approach-avoidance (lever press)	Kubena and Barry (1972)
5.0 and 10 mg/kg	t-maze	Henriksson and Järbe (1972)
3.0 or 4.0 mg/kg*	2-lever choice	Ferraro et al. (1974)
4.0 mg/kg	2-lever choice	Hirschhorn and Rosecrans (1974b)
1.0 mg/kg	2-lever choice	Greenberg et al. (1975b)

*Rhesus monkeys.
[1] All studies done in rats, except where indicated with an asterisk

TABLE 12-3. Studies examining discriminative control between two drugs

Drugs and doses	Discriminative control found	Reference
9.9 mg/kg mescaline vs. 0.03 mg/kg LSD	No	Hirschhorn and Winter (1971)
8.0 mg/kg mescaline vs. 0.08 mg/kg LSD	Yes, but poor control	Cameron and Appel (1973)
0.8 mg/kg psilocybin vs. 0.08 mg/kg LSD	Yes, but poor control	Cameron and Appel (1973)
1.0 mg/kg d-amphetamine vs. 0.08 mg/kg LSD	Yes	Cameron and Appel (1973)
1.0 mg/kg Δ^9-THC vs. 1.0 mg/kg psilocybin	Yes	Greenberg et al. (1975b)
20 mg/kg pentobarbital vs. 70 mg/kg phenobarbital	No	Overton (1966)
5.0 mg/kg chlorpromazine vs. 20 mg/kg pentobarbital	Yes	Overton (1966)
10 mg/kg pentobarbital vs. 150 mg/kg atropine	Yes	Overton (1966)
60 mg/kg phenobarbital vs. 300 mg/kg scopolamine	Yes	Overton (1966)
150 mg/kg atropine vs. 300 mg/kg scopolamine	No	Overton (1966)

that rats can be trained to respond differentially to three different drug states. Overton demonstrated differential responding to 150 mg/kg atropine, 40 mg/kg phenobarbital and saline with a three-alley maze.

Attempts have also been made to quantify the ability of a drug to serve as a discriminative stimulus (called drug discriminability). One way to measure drug

TABLE 12-4. **Studies demonstrating discriminative control between two doses of the same drug**

Drug and doses	Reference
10 mg/kg vs. 20 mg/kg pentobarbital	Overton (1968b)
2.0 mg/kg vs. 10 mg/kg pentobarbital	Trost and Ferraro (1974)
0.3 mg/kg vs. 2.5 mg/kg *dl*-amphetamine	Waters *et al.* (1972)

discriminability is to examine the speed of acquisition of a drug discrimination. Another way to measure drug discriminability is to determine the minimum dose of a drug that an animal can learn to discriminate from saline. This measure is often presented as the ED_{50} or the dose of a drug which produces drug-appropriate responding 50% of the time. When any of these or other measures of drug

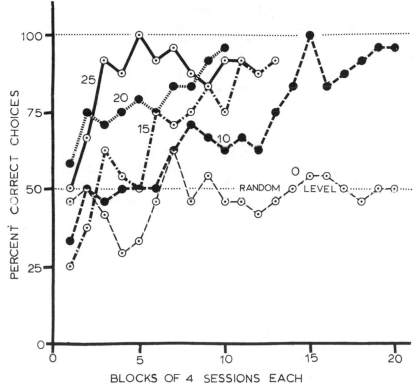

Fig. 12-1. Acquisition of a pentobarbital-saline discrimination. Percent correct responses as a function of the number of training sessions. Each curve represents a different training dose of pentobarbital. (From Overton, 1964.)

discriminability are used, it must be emphasized that the degree of discriminability exerted by any stimulus depends on the intensity of that stimulus and the particular task used to measure discriminability. Drugs may have different effective intensities, depending on the dose of the drug examined. For example, Overton (1964) has shown that the speed with which a pentobarbital-saline discrimination is acquired depends on the dose of pentobarbital examined (see Fig. 12-1). Drugs also have different onsets and durations of action that may affect the drugs' effective intensity at any one time. Therefore, when comparisons are made between drugs, a broad range of doses with appropriate pretreatment times must be examined.

DRUG GENERALIZATION STUDIES

One of the characteristics of behavior which has been brought under stimulus control is that it may also occur in the presence of other similar stimuli. This phenomenon is termed stimulus generalization (or transfer). Generalization usually occurs to stimuli which are similar to the stimuli used to establish the discrimination (i.e., the training stimuli). (See Chapter 10, p. 341 for a discussion of generalization procedures.) One way to examine generalization is with the following procedure: First, a discrimination is established between two stimuli (e.g., a drug and saline). Then stimuli other than those used during discrimination training (test stimuli) are presented. These test stimuli may be different doses of the training drug, or they may be different drugs. Responding is observed in the presence of the test stimuli. Testing is usually carried out under extinction so that drug cues are not confounded with reinforcement cues. The function that relates the animal's response characteristics to different values of the test stimuli is termed a generalization gradient. For example, following training on a 1.0 mg/kg amphetamine-saline discrimination, an animal, when tested in extinction, will respond on the amphetamine lever a high percentage of the time following amphetamine (1.0 mg/kg) administration and on the saline lever a high percentage of the time following saline administration. In a generalization test, lower or higher doses of amphetamine are administered to the animal, and the percentage of responding on the amphetamine lever is observed. One might expect to see a gradient of responding on the amphetamine lever, with a high percentage of responding on the amphetamine lever following doses close to the training dose and with progressively less responding on that lever as the dose of amphetamine is reduced or increased. Similarly, generalization testing is used to examine the discriminable properties of other drugs. For example, animals trained on an amphetamine-saline discrimination might be tested with another drug such as methylphenidate. Responding on the amphetamine lever a high percentage of the time would suggest a similarity between amphetamine and methylphenidate.

Comparisons Between Different Doses
and Administration Times of the Same Drug

Overton (1966) examined the relationship between the dose of a drug and the rat's ability to discriminate between drug and non-drug conditions with a generalization procedure. Rats were trained to respond differentially in a t-maze on the basis of a 10 mg/kg dose of pentobarbital or saline. Then they were tested at various doses of pentobarbital (2.5–15 mg/kg). The percentage of responding on the pentobarbital side of the t-maze decreased as the dose of pentobarbital decreased (see Fig. 12-2). At a dose of pentobarbital higher than the 10 mg/kg training dose, the percentage of responding on the pentobarbital side of the t-maze did not decrease: indeed, it was higher than following the training dose. There have been other reports that test doses higher than the training dose produce percentages of responding greater than at the training dose. This has been demonstrated for THC (Barry and Kubena, 1972) and mescaline (Hirschhorn and Winter, 1971).

Kuhn *et al.* (1974) examined generalization to various doses of *d*-amphetamine with a two-lever choice procedure. Rats were trained to press a right or left lever, depending on whether they had received 1.0 mg/kg of *d*-amphetamine or saline. Testing took place with lower and higher doses of *d*-amphetamine. It was found that the number of responses on the drug lever decreased as the dose of *d*-am-

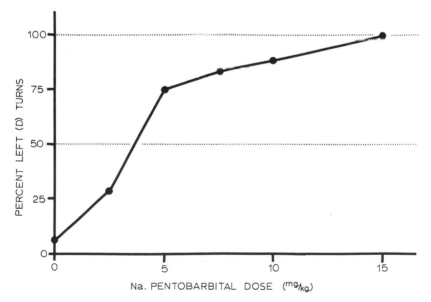

Fig. 12-2. Percent of total responding on the pentobarbital side of the t-maze as a function of dose. (From Overton, 1966.)

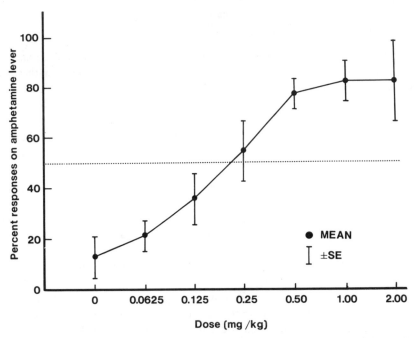

Fig. 12-3. Percent responding on the *d*-amphetamine lever as a function of dose. Each novel dose was given twice to all rats in a random order, and all injections were given 30-min before the session. Each point represents the average of 12 scores. (From Kuhn *et al.*, 1974.)

phetamine decreased (see Fig. 12-3). Responding on the drug lever did not fall off at a dose of amphetamine higher than the training dose. In this respect, generalization gradients produced by drug stimuli may differ from generalization gradients produced by exteroceptive stimuli such as lights and tones that generally peak at or near the training stimulus and fall off rapidly in either direction. Since only one dose higher than the training dose is usually examined, however, it is difficult to draw general conclusions about the shape of this part of the generalization gradient. Table 12-5 presents the results of various studies in which rats were initially trained to make a discrimination between a drug and some vehicle and then were tested for generalization to various other doses of the training drug.

While the data obtained by varying dose of a training drug have been shown to produce consistent generalization gradients, it is important to recall that the degree to which any stimulus exerts control over responding is dependent upon training conditions. For example, Waters *et al.* (1972) showed that the dose of a drug used during training is an important determinant of the generalization gradient. They trained two groups of rats on a two-lever discrimination task.

TABLE 12-5.   Studies examining generalization to different doses of a drug

| Training drug | Generalization | | References |
	Yes	No	
1200 mg/kg alcohol	600 mg/kg	300 mg/kg	Kubena and Barry (1969a)
			Barry and Kubena (1972)
1.0 mg/kg d-amphetamine	0.25–2.0 mg/kg	0–0.125 mg/kg	Kuhn et al. (1974)
0.8 mg/kg l-amphetamine	2.4 mg/kg		Jones et al. (1974)
1.0 mg/kg dl-amphetamine	0.3–0.7 mg/kg		Harris and Balster (1971)
0.8 mg/kg d-amphetamine	1.6–2.4 mg/kg	0.2–0.4 mg/kg	Huang and Ho (1974)
10 mg/kg atropine sulfate	2.5–5.0 mg/kg		Kubena and Barry (1969a)
			Barry and Kubena (1972)
4.0 mg/kg chlor-promazine	5.0, 6.0 mg/kg	2.0 mg/kg	Stewart (1962)
0.25 μM/kg LSD (0.12 mg/kg)	0.03–0.25 μM/kg	0.01–0.02 μM/kg	Hirschhorn and Winter (1971)
0.08 mg/kg LSD	0.02–0.06 mg/kg	0.01 mg/kg	Greenberg et al. (1975a)
0.01 mg/kg LSD	0.0025–0.6 mg/kg		Greenberg et al. (1975a)
0.08 mg/kg LSD	0.04 mg/kg	0.02 mg/kg	Cameron and Appel (1973)
40 μM/kg mescaline (9.9 mg/kg)	40–80 μM/kg	5.0, 10, 20 μM/kg	Hirschhorn and Winter (1971)
10 mg/kg mescaline	6.0 mg/kg	0–3.0 mg/kg	Winter (1973)
0.2 mg/kg nicotine	0.10–0.15 mg/kg	0.05 mg/kg	Morrison and Stephenson (1969)
0.4 mg/kg nicotine	0.18–0.26 mg/kg	0.04–0.07 mg/kg	Schecter and Rosecrans (1971)
10.0 mg/kg pentazocine	6.0–12 mg/kg	2.0–4.0 mg/kg	Kuhn et al. (1976)
10 mg/kg pentobarbital	5.0–15 mg/kg	2.5 mg/kg	Overton (1966)
4.0 mg/kg THC	2.0 and 16 mg/kg	0.25–1.0 mg/kg	Kubena and Barry (1972)
			Barry and Kubena (1972)

One group was trained to discriminate between saline and 2.5 mg/kg of dl-amphetamine. Another group was trained to discriminate between 2.5 and 0.3 mg/kg of dl-amphetamine. Generalization testing was then carried out with the two training doses and intermediate doses of dl-amphetamine. The group trained to discriminate between 2.5 and 0.3 mg/kg of dl-amphetamine responded to amphetamine doses of 1.0 mg/kg or greater as if these doses were the same as 2.5 mg/kg of dl-amphetamine. Rats trained to discriminate between saline and

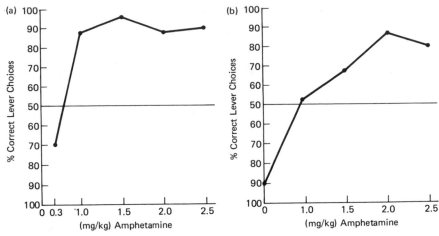

Fig. 12-4. Percent of correct lever choices as a function of five doses of *dl*-amphetamine. (a) Animals were trained to discriminate between 2.5 and 0.3 mg/kg *dl*-amphetamine prior to the generalization test. (b) Animals were trained to discriminated between saline and 2.5 mg/kg *dl*-amphetamine prior to the generalization test. (From Waters *et al.*, 1972.)

2.5 mg/kg of *dl*-amphetamine responded randomly at the 1.0 mg/kg dose (see Fig. 12-4a, b).

Greenberg *et al.* (1975a) report a similar finding with LSD. They trained rats to discriminate LSD (80 μg/kg) from saline in a two-lever choice task. A dose-response curve was obtained for LSD following training. Doses of LSD from 20–60 μg/kg produced 65% or more responding on the LSD lever. LSD at a dose of 10 μg/kg produced responding on the saline lever. Training was then carried out between 10 μg/kg of LSD and saline. Following training, the same dose of LSD (10 μg/kg) produced a high percentage of responding on the LSD lever (Fig. 12-5).

Attempts have also been made to examine the onset and duration of action of drugs as stimuli. Schecter and Rosecrans (1971) tested the discriminative control of a single dose of nicotine (0.4 mg/kg) given at varying times prior to test sessions with animals trained to discriminate nicotine (given just before the session) from saline. At 5, 10 and 20 minutes postinjection, over 85% of the subjects made drug choices. From 30 minutes through 50 minutes, the animals' drug choices were random. Kuhn *et al.* (1974) made a similar investigation of the duration of the stimulus properties of *d*-amphetamine by varying the interval between drug injection and testing. They found that the stimulus effects of *d*-amphetamine dissipated between 60 and 90 minutes postinjection (see Fig. 12-6).

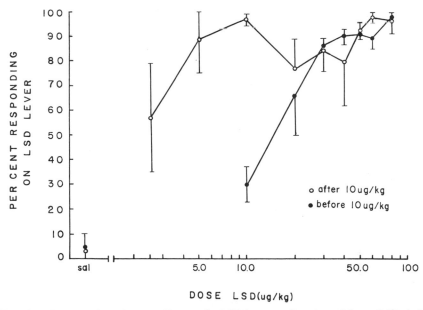

Fig. 12-5. Percent of total responding on the LSD lever as a function of dose. Solid circles represent lever choice after rats had been trained to discriminate between 80 µg/kg of LSD and saline. Open circles represent lever choice after rats had been trained to discriminate between 10 µg/kg of LSD and saline. Vertical lines represent ±SD. All injections were administered ip 30-min before testing. Each data point represents the average of six animals. (From Greenberg *et al.*, 1975a.)

Comparisons Between Different Drugs

Generalization gradients have also been obtained by training rats to make a drug-saline discrimination and then testing for generalization with other drugs (of the same or different pharmacological classes), and observing the percentage of responding appropriate to the training drug. Overton (1966) examined five drugs that have similar pharmacological properties for generalization among them. Animals were trained to run to one goal box when drugged either with pento-barbital, phenobarbital, ethyl alcohol, ethyl carbamate or meprobamate and to the opposite goal box when given saline. In order to examine the similarity of these drugs, generalization tests were given, i.e., animals trained with one of the five drugs were given one of the other four drugs on the test day and their choice of goal box was observed. Almost all the animals ran to the drug side of the maze when test drugs were given, suggesting that the drugs had similar stimulus properties.

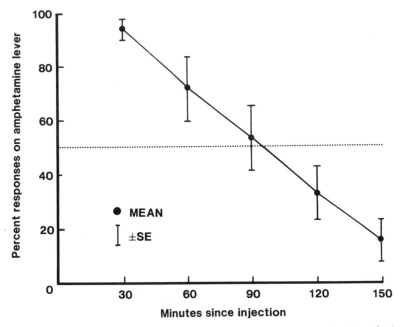

Fig. 12-6. Percent of total responding on the *d*-amphetamine lever as a function of minutes since injection. Rats were returned to home cages after injections for the allotted time before testing was carried out. All rats were tested twice at each time delay. Each point represents the average of 12 scores. (From Kuhn *et al.*, 1974.)

Similarly, Kubena and Barry (1969a) trained animals to make either an alcohol-saline or an atropine sulfate–saline discrimination and then tested for generalization to various other drugs. It was shown that pentobarbital and chlordiazepoxide produced the alcohol response in the groups trained to discriminate alcohol and saline. Chlorpromazine and amphetamine produced saline responses. Figure 12-7 shows the percentage of alcohol responses in tests following several doses of alcohol, pentobarbital and chlordiazepoxide. Similarly, Figure 12-8 shows the percentage of atropine responses in rats following several doses of atropine and scopolamine for the atropine-saline group.

In general, generalization has been shown to occur between drugs with similar pharmacological actions if equally effective doses are compared (Barry, 1974). Table 12-6 presents the results of generalization studies in which comparisons were made between different drugs. In general, doses of test drugs that produced over 50% responding appropriate to the training drug, were considered to produce generalization. It should be noted that these conclusions are often based on only one test dose. Failure to demonstrate generalization between drugs in the absense of dose-response curves cannot be considered evidence that

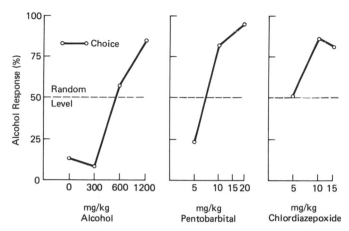

Fig. 12-7. Percent of total responding on the alcohol lever as a function of the dose of alcohol, pentobarbital or chlordiazepoxide. (From Kubena and Barry, 1969a.)

the stimulus properties of the training drug and the test drug would be discriminable if different doses were examined. Moreover, each study used different training procedures and different doses of the training drug. In addition, the times between drug administration and training or test sessions were usually held constant, whereas each drug (and each dose of a drug) may produce varying onsets and durations of action.

For example, Schecter and Rosecrans (1972a) report that animals trained to respond differentially in the presence of 0.048 mg/kg of LSD and saline respond

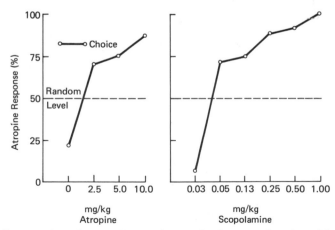

Fig. 12-8. Percent of total responding on the atropine lever as a function of dose of atropine or scopolamine. (From Kubena and Barry, 1969a.)

TABLE 12-6.   Studies examining generalization across drugs

Training drug	Generalization		References
	Yes	No	
Alcohol, 1200 mg/kg	pentobarbital, 10–20 mg/kg chlordiazepoxide, 10–15 mg/kg chloral hydrate, 90–120 mg/kg	pentobarbital, 5.0 mg/kg chlordiazepoxide, 5.0 mg/kg chlorpromazine, 2.0 mg/kg d-amphetamine, 1.0 mg/kg atropine, 10 mg/kg	Kubena and Barry (1969a) Barry and Kubena (1972)
d-Amphetamine, 4.0 mg/kg	l-amphetamine, 4.0–8.0 mg/kg	nicotine, 0.4 mg/kg mescaline, 7.4–29.7 mg/kg fenfluramine, 4.0–8.0 mg/kg lysergic acid diethylamide, 0.048 mg/kg	Schecter and Rosecrans (1973)
d-Amphetamine, 1.0 mg/kg	methamphetamine, 1.0 mg/kg	lysergic acid diethylamide, 0.04–0.08 mg/kg psilocybin, 0.5–1.0 mg/kg tetrahydrocannabinol, 0.5–1.0 mg/kg mescaline, 5.0–10 mg/kg caffeine, 6.0–20 mg/kg	Kuhn et al. (1974)

d-Amphetamine, 0.8 mg/kg	methylphenidate, 2.5 mg/kg; cocaine, 7.5 mg/kg; methamphetamine, 0.8–1.6 mg/kg; l-amphetamine, 0.8–1.6 mg/kg	methylphenidate, 0.5–1.0 mg/kg; mescaline, 12.5–25 mg/kg; tyramine, 1.0–4.0 mg/kg	Huang and Ho (1974)
d-Amphetamine, 0.8 mg/kg	l-amphetamine, 1.6–2.4 mg/kg	l-amphetamine, 0.4–0.8 mg/kg; para-hydroxyamphetamine, 1.01 mg/kg	Jones et al. (1974)
l-Amphetamine, 0.8 mg/kg	d-amphetamine, 0.8 mg/kg; methylphenidate, 3.5 mg/kg	para-hydroxyamphetamine, 1.01 and 2.02 mg/kg	Jones et al. (1974)
dl-Amphetamine, 1.0 mg/kg	d-amphetamine, 1.5 mg/kg	chlorpromazine, 2.0 mg/kg; atropine, 9.0 mg/kg; lysergic acid diethylamide, 0.04 mg/kg; psilocybin, 0.2 mg/kg; phenobarbital, 4.0 mg/kg	Harris and Balster (1970)
Atropine sulfate, 10 mg/kg	scopolamine, 0.06–1.0 mg/kg	scopolamine, 0.03 mg/kg; atropine methyl bromide, 5.0 mg/kg	Kubena and Barry (1969a)
Atropine sulfate, 150 mg/kg	homatropine, 100–150 mg/kg; cyclopentolate, 150 mg/kg; scopolamine,	homatropine methyl bromide, 50 mg/kg; atropine methylnitrate, 65 mg/kg	Overton (1966)

TABLE 12-6 (Continued)

Training drug	Generalization		References
	Yes	No	
	75–300 mg/kg	pentobarbital, 5.0–20 mg/kg erythroidine, 20 mg/kg	Stewart (1962)
Chlorpromazine, 4.0 mg/kg	acepromazine, 2.0–8.0 mg/kg perphenazine, 2.0–6.0 mg/kg prothipendyl, 12 mg/kg	imipramine, 10–30 mg/kg prochlorperazine, 1.0–6.0 mg/kg prothipendyl, 4.0–8.0 mg/kg	
Imipramine, 20 mg/kg		chlorpromazine, 3.0–7.0 mg/kg acepromazine, 8.0 mg/kg	Stewart (1962)
Lysergic acid diethylamide, 0.1 μM/kg	mescaline, 60–120 μM/kg psilocybin, 3.0–9.0 μM/kg	d-amphetamine, 14.8–29.6 μM/kg	Schecter and Rosecrans (1972a)
Lysergic acid diethylamide, 0.072 mg/kg	mescaline, 8.0 mg/kg THC, 2.5–10 mg/kg	morphine, 5.0–20 mg/kg mescaline, 4.0–6.0 mg/kg d-amphetamine, 1.0 mg/kg chlorpromazine, 0.5 mg/kg	Hirschhorn and Rosecrans (1974a)
Lysergic acid diethylamide, 0.08 mg/kg	l-LSD, 0.25 mg/kg	l-LSD, 0.08 mg/kg	Cameron and Appel (1973)

Training drug	Test drugs	Reference
Mescaline, 10 mg/kg	PCPA, 50–100 mg/kg	Winter (1973, 1974a)
2,3,4-trimethoxy-phenethylamine, 6 and 10 mg/kg	psilocybin, 0.4–0.8 mg/kg	
	scopolamine, 4.0 mg/kg	
Morphine, 10 mg/kg	3,4-dimethoxy-phenylethylamine, 1.0–60 mg/kg	Hirschhorn and Rosencrans (1974a)
Nicotine, 0.2 mg/kg	lysergic acid diethylamide, 0.07–0.60 μM/kg	Morrison and Stephenson (1969)
	d-amphetamine, 0.4 mg/kg	
	apomorphine, 0.06 or 0.025 mg/kg	
	norepinephrine, 0.025 or 0.05 mg/kg	
	pentobarbital, 2.0 mg/kg	
	physostigmine, 0.05 or 0.1 mg/kg	
	chlordiazepoxide, 20.0 mg/kg	
	caffeine, 20.0 mg/kg	
	gallamine, 10.0 mg/kg	
Nicotine, 0.4 mg/kg	nicotine isomethonium, 0.4 mg/kg	Schecter and Rosecrans (1972b)
	lobeline, 0.4–10 mg/kg	
	d-amphetamine, 2.0–4.0 mg/kg	

TABLE 12-6 (Continued)

Training drug	Generalization		References
	Yes	No	
Pentazocine, 10 mg/kg	morphine, 5.0–7.5 mg/kg	arecoline, 0.25–2.0 mg/kg; morphine, 0.75, 1.5, 3.0 mg/kg; naloxone, 0.4 mg/kg	Kuhn et al. (1976)
Pentobarbital, 20 mg/kg	phenobarbital, 80 mg/kg; alcohol, 2400 mg/kg; ethyl carbamate, 750 mg/kg; meprobamate, 200 mg/kg; amobarbital, 30 mg/kg; secobarbital, 15–20 mg/kg; barbital, 150 mg/kg; chloral hydrate, 150–200 mg/kg; ether, (subanaesthetic doses); paraldehyde, (300–400 mg/kg	d-amphetamine, 2.5–10 mg/kg; bemegride sulfate, 1.0–7.5 mg/kg; gallamine, 2.5–7.5 mg/kg; lysergic acid diethylamide, 0.2 mg/kg; physostigmine, 1.0 mg/kg; erythroidine, 20.0 mg/kg	Overton (1966)

Tetrahydrocannabinol
(Δ^9-THC),
4.0 mg/kg

chloralose,
30 mg/kg
Δ^3-THC,
4.0 mg/kg

alcohol,
500–1000 mg/kg
pentobarbital,
10 mg/kg
chlordiazepoxide,
15 mg/kg
chlorpromazine,
2.0–4.0 mg/kg
morphine,
4.0–8.0 mg/kg
atropine,
5.0–10 mg/kg
cocaine,
10–20 mg/kg
scopolamine,
0.25 mg/kg
lysergic acid diethylamide,
0.1–0.2 mg/kg
cannabinol,
10 mg/kg
mescaline,
15–30 mg/kg

Kubena and Barry (1972);
Barry and Kubena (1972)

on the LSD lever following administration of mescaline and psilocybin. On the other hand, Cameron and Appel (1973) do not report generalization to psilocybin in animals trained to discriminate 0.08 mg/kg LSD from saline. It should be noted however, that these two studies differ in many ways. First, different doses of LSD (0.048 vs. 0.08 mg/kg) were used in training. Second, different doses of psilocybin were used in generalization testing. Schecter and Rosecrans examined psilocybin in a dose range from 0.85 to 2.65 mg/kg while Cameron and Appel examined a lower range (0.4–0.8 mg/kg). Third, the training procedures were different. Schecter and Rosecrans used a t-maze procedure in which correct responses provided access to sweetened milk and incorrect responses were followed by shock. Cameron and Appel employed a two-lever choice procedure maintained by a DRL 20-sec schedule of water presentation.

Aside from the various procedural variations from experiment to experiment which make comparisons between drugs difficult, there are other problems with using generalizaion procedures to investigate the similarity or dissimilarity of two drug stimuli. One of these problems is what Overton (1974) calls "transfer test overinclusiveness." In the generalization test (or transfer test), the animal is essentially required to compare a test drug with two training conditions and then indicate which of the training conditions is most similar to the test drug. Note that the animal is forced to make some response, even if the test drug differs significantly from both training conditions. The animal has no way to indicate that the test drug is not similar to either of the training conditions. For example, Schecter and Rosecrans (1973) showed that animals trained to make a 4.0 mg/kg amphetamine-saline discrimination responded on the saline side of a compartment when tested in a generalization study with 0.4 mg/kg nicotine, 7.4–29.7 mg/kg mescaline or 0.05 mg/kg LSD. All these drugs have, however, been shown to be discriminable from saline in other tests. This illustrates the need for further comparisons to determine if two drugs that show generalization are in fact nondiscriminable. Overton (1974) presents a thorough discussion of these problems.

MECHANISMS OF DRUG STIMULUS CONTROL

While numerous theoretical explanations have been advanced to account for drug stimulus control (see Overton, 1968a; Brown et al., 1968; Bliss, 1974; Wright, 1974, for a discussion of these), the ability of certain drugs to serve as discriminative stimuli is usually explained on the basis of drug-induced interoceptive cues. Drug cues appear to operate in a fashion analogous to other physical stimuli. The formal rules that describe the characteristics of discriminative control by drugs and by exteroceptive stimuli are similar. For example, we have seen that generalization takes place with the same drug when it is administered at various dose levels and also with drugs of similar pharmacological action. Discrimination between dissimilar drugs has also been shown. Moreover, it has been shown that drug stimuli are just as effective in controlling behavior as shock stimuli or as visual stimuli (Overton, 1964). Harris and Balster (1971) have also shown that drugs are just as effective as external stimuli in controlling schedules of reinforcement.

It has also been suggested that drug discriminations are probably *not* the result of drug induced alterations in the perception of environmental stimuli. Overton (1966) has investigated this position and eliminated the possibility that at least the basis of a pentobarbital-saline discrimination is the alteration of footshock or a change in visual perception. Overton obtained differential responding based on the presence or absence of pentobarbital (15 mg/kg) in a t-maze. Choice in the t-maze was maintained even when animals were blinded or when large variations in shock intensity were used.

Examination of the mechanisms underlying drug cues has received considerable experimental attention. Drug cues have been challenged by a variety of pharmacological and biochemical manipulations, thus enabling the investigation of CNS mechanisms and/or sites of action responsible for the cue.

Central vs. Peripheral Drug Cues

Recent evidence indicates that a drug has to act centrally to be discriminable. For example, rats trained to discriminate either *d*- or *l*-amphetamine from saline respond on the saline-related lever when tested with hydroxyamphetamine, a drug that is devoid of central activity but mimics the peripheral effects of amphetamine (Jones *et al.*, 1974). Moreover, it has been shown (Overton, 1966; Kubena and Barry, 1969a) that when rats that have been trained on an atropine sulfate–saline discrimination are tested with peripherally acting cholinergic blockers such as atropine methyl bromide and atropine methyl nitrate, they respond on the saline side of the t-maze. These drugs do not pass the blood-brain barrier in appreciable quantities, and thus produce peripheral but no central anticholinergic effects, indicating that the stimulus properties of atropine are central rather than peripheral.

Similar effects have been shown with nicotine (Schecter and Rosecrans, 1972b). Schecter and Rosecrans trained rats to make a saline-nicotine discrimination. When the animals were given nicotine isomethonium iodide-hydroiodide—a quaternary salt of nicotine which does not penetrate the blood-brain barrier at low doses—it was found that this drug did not produce a nicotine response. Moreover, the stimulus control exerted by nicotine can be antagonized only by nicotinic blocking agents with central nervous system activity. Peripherally active nicotinic blocking agents fail to have the same effect. Morrison and Stephenson (1969) trained rats to make a saline-nicotine discrimination. Nicotine in combination with the centrally active blocker mecamylamine produced saline choices (i.e., effective antagonism), whereas the peripherally active blocker chlorisondamine when combined with nicotine still resulted in nicotine choices. These results have been confirmed by Schecter and Rosecrans (1971) in a t-maze choice procedure with mecamylamine and another peripherally active nicotinic blocking agent, hexamethonium.

While curare, a peripheral neuromuscular blocker, has been shown to produce discriminative control (Girden and Culler, 1937; Culler et al., 1939), it should be pointed out that the curare used in these experiments was in a crude form. In this form, curare also has CNS effects. Purified d-tubocurarine, which has little, if any, CNS effect, has not been shown to produce differential responding (Solomon and Turner, 1962). Gallamine, another peripheral neuromuscular blocking agent which lacks CNS effects but produces marked muscle flaccidity has also been shown to be ineffective as a discriminative stimulus (Overton, 1966).

Taken together, these results suggest that centrally active drugs are more effective as drug stimuli than compounds which are only active peripherally. On the other hand, it should be noted that some drugs with CNS activity have not been shown to be effective discriminative stimuli. Most attempts to obtain discriminative control with chlorpromazine and with imipramine have failed (Overton, 1966; Harris and Balster, 1971); however, Stewart (1962) did report some discriminative control with these drugs, but only after very extensive training procedures.

Pharmacological and Biochemical Mechanisms

Drug stimuli have also been used as a means for studying mechanisms of drug action. Two general strategies are used in this investigation. One strategy is to obtain discriminative control by some drug and then attempt to obliterate the discrimination with an antagonist drug. For example, it has been shown that naloxone can antagonize discriminative control by morphine (Rosecrans et al., 1973; Hirschhorn and Rosecrans, 1974a; Kuhn et al., 1976) and by pentazocine (Kuhn et al., 1976). Table 12-7 presents the effect of naloxone on a morphine-saline discrimination.

Schecter and Rosecrans (1971) examined the effect of various cholinergic blockers on the discriminative properties of nicotine. In their studies, they first obtained discriminative control in a t-maze with 0.4 mg/kg of nicotine vs. saline. They then performed the following manipulations: (1) pretreatment with atropine (0.1 mg/kg), which blocks muscarinic-cholinergic neurons (see Chapter 3); and (2) pretreatment with one of two nicotinic blockers, either mecamylamine (0.5 mg/kg), which produces CNS blockade, or hexamethonium (0.75 mg/kg), which is predominately a peripheral blocker. They found that atropine could not block the nicotine-saline discrimination. Mecamylamine, a CNS

TABLE 12-7.   Effects of naloxone on a discrimination between 20 mg/kg morphine and saline

Drug	(n)	No. of trials	% Responses into morphine compartment
Morphine and saline	12	12	75.0
Morphine and naloxone (0.2 mg/kg)	12	12	58.3
Morphine and naloxone (0.4 mg/kg)	12	12	25.0[1]
Morphine and naloxone (0.8 mg/kg)	12	12	25.0[1]

[1]Probability of difference from morphine score being due to chance: $P < 0.05$, χ^2-test.
From Rosecrans *et al.* (1973).

nicotinic blocker, could block the nicotine-saline discrimination, but hexamethonium, a peripheral nicotinic blocker, could not.

Another strategy for examining drug stimuli is to modify the biochemical systems presumed to mediate certain drug effects. If, for example, nicotine produces some of its behavioral effects by altering brain concentrations of either the catecholamines or serotonin, then a depletion of these biogenic amines should influence the ability of nicotine to serve as a discriminative stimulus. Schecter and Rosecrans (1972c) examined the biochemical systems which might be responsible for nicotine's stimulus properties. They first obtained discriminative control in a t-maze with 0.4 mg/kg of nicotine vs. saline. They then performed the following biochemical manipulations: (1) pretreatment with parachlorophenylalanine (PCPA, 350 mg/kg), a tryptophan hydroxylase inhibitor (see p. 91); and (2) pretreatment with alpha-methylparatyrosine methylester (AMPT-methylester, 90 or 135 mg/kg), a tyrosine hydroxylase inhibitor (see p. 77). Parachlorophenylalanine has been shown to reduce brain serotonin content by about 85% at 72 hours after drug administration and alpha-methylparatyrosine has been shown to reduce brain norepinephrine content by about 50% (Rosecrans *et al.*, 1973). Inhibition of serotonin synthesis by PCPA had no effect on the ability of nicotine to act as a discriminative stimulus. On the other hand, the AMPT—methylester significantly decreased nicotine-appropriate responding, while having no effect on saline responses (see Fig. 12-9). These results suggest that the nicotine stimulus is dependent upon normal levels of norepinephrine and/or dopamine in the brain.

Preliminary investigations have also been made of the biochemical system underlying the discriminative properties of amphetamine (Kuhn *et al.*, 1974; Roffman and Lal, 1972; Schecter and Rosecrans, 1973; Schecter and Cook, 1975),

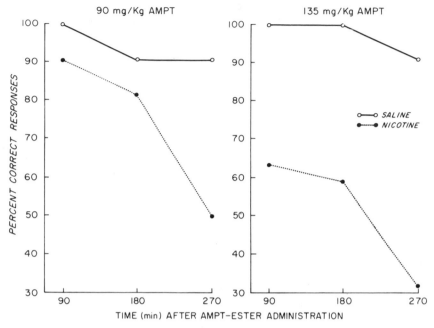

Fig. 12-9. Percent of total correct responses in a saline-nicotine discrimination following pretreatment with 90 or 135 mg/kg alpha-methylparatyrosine methyl ester as a function of time after administration of the AMPT-methylester. Each point represents 12 trials, with each of six rats receiving both saline and nicotine twice at each dose, and at each time after AMPT-methylester. (From Schecter and Rosecrans, 1972c.)

morphine (Rosecrans *et al.*, 1973; Hirschhorn and Rosecrans, 1974a), LSD (Hirschhorn and Rosecrans, 1974a; Cameron and Appel, 1973) and mescaline (Browne and Ho, 1975).

Tolerance

When drugs are administered chronically, tolerance is often observed. That is, there is a progressive diminution of the magnitude of the drug effect. Drug discrimination may provide a way to examine development of tolerance to drug effects. Bueno and Carlini (1972) trained rats to climb a rope and then injected them daily with a marijuana extract (10 mg/kg). Initially, performance was impaired by marijuana's effect on rope climbing, but tolerance developed to this disruption. They were then trained to press either one of two bars in a Skinner box, depending on whether they were given 10 mg/kg of marijuana extract or saline. After 30 injections the discrimination was established, indicating that marijuana could still serve as a discriminative stimulus long after a series of daily injections had produced tolerance in another behavioral situation (i.e., rope climbing).

Hirschhorn and Rosecrans (1974b) made a similar investigation of tolerance with morphine and Δ^9-THC. First, they established a two lever discrimination between 10 mg/kg of morphine and between 4.0 mg/kg of Δ^9-THC and saline. Then training was continued with daily injections of both drugs. In spite of repeated daily injections of morphine, up to 16 times the training dose, and Δ^9-THC to 8 times the training dose, discriminated responding was still observed, suggesting that tolerance does not develop to the stimulus effects of Δ^9-THC or morphine.

Since much of the work discussed thus far has questioned the possibility that drug discriminations are based on peripheral cues, this work indicates that marijuana, Δ^9-THC and morphine are probably still active in the central nervous system even after tolerance has been shown to a specific behavioral measure.

SUMMARY

Data have been examined which show that animals can be trained to respond differentially in the presence or absence of various drug conditions, suggesting that drugs can act as discriminative stimuli. A variety of drugs have been shown to obtain discriminative control. Generalization between similar drugs and between different doses of a drug has been shown, as well as discrimination between pharmacologically dissimilar drugs. Some mechanisms of drug stimulus control were discussed, and it was shown that drugs acting in the central nervous system are more effective discriminative stimuli than peripherally acting drugs.

REFERENCES

Barnhart, S. S. and D. W. Abbott. 1967.   Dissociation of learning and meprobamate. *Psychol. Rep.* **20:** 520–522.

Barry, H., III. 1974. Classification of drugs according to their discriminable effects in rats. *Fed. Proc.* **33:** 1814–1824.

Barry, H., III, and R. K. Kubena. 1972. Discriminative stimulus characteristics of alcohol, marijuana and atropine. *In* J. M. Singh, L. Miller and H. Lal (eds.), *Drug Addiction: Experimental Pharmacology.* Futura Publishing Co., Inc., Mt. Kisco, New York.

Belleville, R. E. 1964. Control of behavior by drug-produced internal stimuli. *Psychopharmacologia* **5:** 95–105.

Bliss, D. K. 1974. Theoretical explanations of drug-dissociated behaviors. *Fed. Proc.* **33:** 1787–1796.

Bliss, D. K., M. Sledjeski and A. L. Leiman. 1971. State-dependent choice behavior in the rhesus monkey. *Neuropsychologia* **9:** 51–59.

Brown, A., R. S. Feldman and J. W. Moore. 1968. Conditional discrimination learning based upon chlordiazepoxide: Dissociation or cue? *J. Comp. Physiol. Psychol.* **66:** 211–215.

Browne, R. G. and B. T. Ho. 1975. Role of serotonin in the discriminative stimulus properties of mescaline. *Pharmacol. Biochem. Behav.* **3:** 429–435.

Bueno, O. F. and E. A. Carlini. 1972. Dissociation of learning in marijuana tolerant rats. *Psychopharmacologia* 25: 49–56.

Bustamante, J. A., A. Rossello, A. Jordan, E. Pradera and A. Insua. 1968. Learning and drugs. *Physiol. Behav.* 3: 553–555.

Cameron, O. G. and J. B. Appel. 1972. Conditioned suppression of bar-pressing behavior by stimuli associated with drugs. *J. Exp. Anal. Behav.* 17: 127–137.

Cameron, O. G. and J. B. Appel. 1973. A behavioral and pharmacological analysis of some discriminable properties of *d*-LSD in rats. *Psychopharmacologia* 33: 117–134.

Carey, R. J. 1973. Disruption of timing behavior following amphetamine withdrawal. *Physiol. Psychol.* 1: 9–12.

Carlton, P. L. and J. R. Vogel. 1965. Studies of the amnesic properties of scopolamine. *Psychon. Sci.* 3: 261–262.

Chute, D. L. and D. C. Wright. 1973. Retrograde state dependent learning. *Science* 180: 878–880.

Crow, L. T. 1966. Effects of alcohol on conditioned avoidance responding. *Physiol. Behav.* 1: 89–91.

Culler, E., J. D. Coakley, P. S. Shurrager and H. W. Ades. 1939. Differential effects of curare upon higher and lower levels of the central nervous system. *Am. J. Psychol.* 52: 266–273.

Deutsch, J. A. and S. K. Roll. 1973. Alcohol and asymmetrical state-dependency: A possible explanation. *Behav. Biol.* 8: 273–278.

Diethelm, O. and R. M. Barr. 1962. Psychotherapeutic interviews and alcohol intoxication. *Quart. J. Stud. Alcohol* 23: 243–251.

Ferraro, D. P., J. P. Gluck and C. W. Morrow. 1974. Temporally-related stimulus properties of Δ^9-tetrahydrocannabinol in monkeys. *Psychopharmacologia* 35: 305–316.

Girden, E. and E. Culler. 1937. Conditioned responses in curarized striate muscle in dogs. *J. Comp. Psychol.* 23: 261–274.

Goldberg, M. E., M. A. Hefner, R. C. Robichaud and B. Dubinsky. 1973. Effects of Δ^9-tetrahydrocannabinol (THC) and chlordiazepoxide (CDP) on state-dependent learning: Evidence for asymmetrical dissociation. *Psychopharmacologia* 30: 173–184.

Goodwin, D. W. 1974. Alcoholic blackout and state-dependent learning. *Fed. Proc.* 33: 1833–1835.

Goodwin, D. W., B. Powell, D. Bremer, H. Hoine and J. Stern. 1969. Alcohol and recall: State-dependent effects in man. *Science* 163: 1358–1360.

Greenberg, I., D. M. Kuhn and J. B. Appel. 1975a. Behaviorally induced sensitivity to the discriminable properties of LSD. *Psychopharmacologia* 43: 229–232.

Greenberg, I., D. Kuhn and J. B. Appel. 1975b. Comparison of the discriminative stimulus properties of Δ^9-THC and psilocybin in rats. *Pharmacol. Biochem. Behav.* 3: 931–934.

Grossman, S. P. and N. E. Miller. 1961. Control for stimulus-change in the evaluation of alcohol and chlorpromazine as fear-reducing drugs. *Psychopharmacologia* 2: 342–351.

Harlow, H. F. and R. Stagner. 1933. Effect of complete striate muscle paralysis upon the learning process. *J. Exp. Psychol.* 16: 283–294.

Harris, R. T. and R. L. Balster. 1968. Discriminative control by *dl*-amphetamine and saline of lever choice and response patterning. *Psychon. Sci.* 10: 105–106.

Harris, R. T. and R. L. Balster. 1970. An analysis of psychological dependence. *In* R. T. Harris, W. M. McIsaac and C. R. Schuster, Jr. (eds.), *Advances in Mental Science II: Drug Dependence.* University of Texas Press, Austin, Texas, pp. 214–226.

Harris, R. T. and R. L. Balster. 1971. An analysis of the function of drugs in the stimulus control of operant behavior. *In* T. Thompson and R. Pickens (eds.), *Stimulus Properties of Drugs.* Appleton-Century-Crofts, New York, pp. 111–132.

Henriksson, B. G. and T. Järbe. 1971. The effects of two tetrahydrocannabinols, (Δ^9-THC and Δ^8-THC) on conditioned avoidance learning in rats and its transfer to normal state conditions. *Psychopharmacologia* 22: 23–30.

Henriksson, B. G. and T. Järbe. 1972. Δ^9-tetrahydrocannabinol used as discriminative stimulus for rats in position learning in a T-shaped water maze. *Psychon. Sci.* 27: 25–26.

Hill, H. E., B. E. Jones and E. C. Bell. 1971. State dependent control of discrimination by morphine and pentobarbital. *Psychopharmacologia* 22: 305–313.

Hirschhorn, I. D. and J. A. Rosecrans. 1974a. A comparison of the stimulus effects of morphine and lysergic acid diethylamide (LSD). *Pharmacol. Biochem. Behav.* 2: 361–366.

Hirschhorn, I. D. and J. A. Rosecrans. 1974b. Morphine and Δ^9-tet.a. drocannabinol: Tolerance to the stimulus effects. *Psychopharmacologia* 36: 243–253.

Hirschhorn, I. D. and J. C. Winter. 1971. Mescaline and lysergic acid diethylamide (LSD) as discriminative stimuli. *Psychopharmacologia* 22: 64–71.

Holloway, F. A. 1972. State-dependent effects of ethanol on active and passive avidance learning. *Psychopharmacologia* 25: 238–261.

Holmgren, B. 1964. Conditioned avoidance reflex under pentobarbital. *Bol. Inst. Estud. Med. Biol.* 22: 21–38.

Huang, J. and B. T. Ho. 1974. Discriminative stimulus properties of d-amphetamine and related compounds in rats. *Pharmacol. Biochem. Behav.* 2: 669–673.

Iwahara, S. and K. Matsushita. 1971. Effects of drug-state changes upon black-white discrimination learning in rats. *Psychopharmacologia* 19: 347–358.

Johansson, J. O. and T. U. C. Järbe. 1975. Diazepam as a discriminative cue: its antagonism by bemegride. *Eur. J. Pharmacol.* 30: 372–375.

Jones, C. N., H. F. Hill and R. T. Harris. 1974. Discriminative response control by d-amphetamine and related compounds in the rat. *Psychopharmacologia* 36: 347–356.

Kubena, R. K. and H. Barry, III. 1969a. Generalization by rats of alcohol and atropine stimulus characteristics to other drugs. *Psychopharmacologia* 15: 196–206.

Kubena, R. K. and H. Barry, III. 1969b. Two procedures for training differential responses in alcohol and nondrug conditions. *J. Pharm. Sci.* 58: 99–101.

Kubena, R. K. and H. Barry, Ill. 1972. Stimulus characteristics of marijuana components. *Nature* 235: 397–398.

Kuhn, D. M., J. B. Appel and I. Greenberg. 1974. An analysis of some discriminative properties of d-amphetamine. *Psychopharmacologia* 39: 57–66.

Kuhn, D. M., l. Greenberg and J. B. Appel. 1976. Stimulus properties of the narcotic antagonist pentazocine: Similarity to morphine and antagonism by naloxone. *J. Pharmacol. Exp. Ther.* 196: 121–127.

Lal, H. 1969. Control of learned conditioned-avoidance responses (CAR) by amphetamine and chlorpromazine. *Psychopharmacologia* 14: 33–37.

Light, J. S. and W. H. Gantt. 1936. Essential part of reflex arc for establishment of conditioned reflex. Formation of conditioned reflex after exclusion of motor peripheral end. *J. Comp. Psychol.* 21: 19–36.

Mayse, J. F. and T. L. DeVietti. 1971. A comparison of state dependent learning induced by electroconvulsive shock and pentobarbital. *Physiol. Behav.* 7: 717–721.

Miller, N. E. 1957. Objective techniques for studying motivational effects of drugs on animals. *In* S. Garattini and V. Ghetti (eds.), *Psychotropic Drugs.* Elsevier, Amsterdam, pp. 83–103.

Miller, N. E. 1964. The analysis of motivational effects illustrated by experiments on amylobarbitone sodium. *In* H. Steinberg, A. V. S. DeReuck and J. Knight (eds.), *Animal Behavior and Drug Action.* Little, Brown and Co., Boston, pp. 1–18.

Morrison, C. F. and J. A. Stephenson. 1969. Nicotine injections as the conditioned stimulus in discrimination learning. *Psychopharmacologia* **15**: 351–360.

Otis, L. S. 1964. Dissociation and recovery of a response learned under the influence of chlorpromazine or saline. *Science* **143**: 1347–1348.

Overton, D. A. 1964. State-dependent or "dissociated" learning produced with pentobarbital. *J. Comp. Physiol. Psychol.* **57**: 3–12.

Overton, D. A. 1966. State-dependent learning produced by depressant and atropine-like drugs. *Psychopharmacologia* **10**: 6–31.

Overton, D. A. 1967. Differential responding in a three choice maze controlled by three drug states. *Psychopharmacologia* **11**: 376–378.

Overton, D. A. 1968a. Dissociated learning in drug states (state dependent learning). *In* D. H. Efron (ed.), *Psychopharmacology: A Review of Progress 1957–1967.* U.S. Government Printing Office, Washington, D.C.

Overton, D. A. 1968b. Visual cues and shock sensitivity in the control of T-maze choice by drug conditions. *J. Comp. Physiol. Psychol.* **66**: 216–219.

Overton, D. A. 1972. State dependent learning produced by alcohol and its relevance to alcoholism. *In* B. Kissen and H. Begleiter (eds.), *The Biology of Alcoholism, Physiology and Behavior.* Plenum Press. New York, pp. 193–217.

Overton, D. A. 1974. Experimental methods for the study of state dependent learning. *Fed. Proc.* **33**: 1800–1813.

Paskal, V. 1962. Dissociative effects of atropine on a simple learned task in the rat. *Undergraduate Research Reports in Psychology.* McGill University, Toronto, pp. 37–43.

Pickens, R. and J. A. Dougherty. 1971. Conditioning of the activity effects of drugs. *In* T. Thompson and R. Pickens (eds.), *Stimulus Properties of Drugs.* Appleton-Century-Crofts, New York, pp. 39–50.

Richardson, E. J. 1972. Alcohol state-dependent learning: acquisition of a spatial discrimination in the goldfish (*Carassuis auratus*). *Psychol. Rec.* **22**: 545–553.

Rickles, W. H., Jr., M. J. Cohen, C. A. Whitaker and K. E. McIntyre. 1973. Marijuana-induced state-dependent verbal learning. *Psychopharmacologia* **30**: 349–354.

Roffman, M. and H. Lal. 1972. Role of brain amines in learning associated with "amphetamine-state." *Psychopharmacologia* **25**: 195–204.

Rosecrans, J. A., M. H. Goodloe, Jr., G. J. Bennett and I. D. Hirschhorn. 1973. Morphine as a discriminative cue: Effects of amine depletors and naloxone. *Eur. J. Pharmacol.* **21**: 252–256.

Sachs, E., M. Weingarten and N. W. Klein, Jr. 1966. Effects of chlordiazepoxide learning and its transfer to the normal state and other drug conditions. *Psychopharmacologia* **9**: 17–30.

Schechter, M. D. and J. A. Rosecrans. 1971. C.N.S. effect of nicotine as the discriminative stimulus for the rat in a T-maze. *Life Sci.* **10**: 821–832.

Schechter, M. D. and J. A. Rosecrans. 1972a. Lysergic acid diethylamide (LSD) as a discriminative cue: Drugs with similar stimulus properties. *Psychopharmacologia* **26**: 313–316.

Schechter, M. D. and J. A. Rosecrans. 1972b. Nicotine as a discriminative cue in rats: inability of related drugs to produce a nicotine-like cueing effect. *Psychopharmacologia* **27**: 379–387.

Schechter, M. D. and J. A. Rosecrans. 1972c. Nicotine as a discriminative stimulus in rats depleted of norepinephrine or 5-hydroxytryptamine. *Psychopharmacologia* **24**: 417–429.

Schechter, M. D. and J. A. Rosecrans. 1973. *d*-Amphetamine as a discriminative cue: Drugs with similar stimulus properties. *Eur. J. Pharmacol.* **21**: 212–216.

Schechter, M. D. and P. G. Cook. 1975. Dopaminergic mediation of the interoceptive cue produced by *d*-amphetamine in rats. *Psychopharmacologia* **42**: 185–193.

Siegel, R. K. and M. E. Jarvik. 1971. Evidence for state-dependent learning with mescaline in a passive avoidance task. *Psychon. Sci.* **26**: 260–261.

Solomon, R. L. and L. H. Turner. 1962. Discriminative classical conditioning in dogs paralyzed by curare can later control discriminative avoidance responses in the normal state. *Psychol. Rev.* **69**: 202–219.

Stewart, J. 1962. Differential responses based on the physiological consequences of pharmacological agents. *Psychopharmacologia* **3**: 132–138.

Storm, T. and W. K. Caird. 1967. The effects of alcohol on serial verbal learning in chronic alcoholics. *Psychon. Sci.* **9**: 43–44.

Trost, J. G. and D. P. Ferraro. 1974. Discrimination and generalization of drug stimuli in monkeys. *In* J. M. Singh and H. Lal (eds.), *Drug Addiction,* Vol. 3. Symposia Specialists, Miami, Florida.

Waters, W. H., D. W. Richards, III and R. T. Harris. 1972. Discriminative control and generalization of the stimulus properties of *d,l*-amphetamine in the rat. *In* J. M. Singh, L. Miller and H. Lal (eds.), *Drug Addiction: Experimental Pharmacology.* Futura Publishing Co., Mt. Kisco, New York.

Weingartner, H. and L. A. Faillace. 1971. Alcohol state-dependent learning in man. *J. Nerv. Ment. Dis.* **153**: 395–406.

Winter, J. C. 1974a. The effects of 3,4-dimethoxyphenylethylamine in rats trained with mescaline as a discriminative stimulus. *J. Pharmacol. Exp. Ther.* **189**: 741–747.

Winter, J. C. 1974b. Hallucinogens as discriminative stimuli. *Fed. Proc.* **33**: 1825–1832.

Winter, J. C. 1973. A comparison of the stimulus properties of mescaline and 2,3,4-trimethoxyphenylethylamine. *J. Pharmacol. Exp. Ther.* **185**: 101–107.

Wright, D. C. 1974. Differentiating stimulus and storage hypotheses of state-dependent learning. *Fed. Proc.* **33**: 1797–1799.

Index

seizure susceptibility, 110
self-stimulation, 184
sleep, 105–106
stereotyped behavior, 178–179
history and general effects of, 57–59, 86,
135, 197–198
interaction of, with other drugs, 174–175,
177–179, 205
neurochemical effects of, 78, 92–93, 125
Reserve pool, 74, 131–132. *See also* Granules; Storage
Respondent conditioning. *See* classical
conditioning
Response dependent shock. *See* Shock
maintained responding
Response-shock interval, 21
Reticular activating system (RAS), 104
Retrieval, 245
Retrograde amnesia. *See* Amnesia,
retrograde
Reuptake
drugs which block, 77, 92, 123–124, 174,
190–191, 194
occurrence of, 72, 74, 77, 88, 215
Ribonucleic acid (RNA), 34–35, 40 (Table
2-3), 247, 256–267, 272–274
Ribosomes, 257
RNA. *See* Ribonucleic acid
Ro 4-4602
behavioral effects of, 129, 146–151
neurochemical effects of, 77, 92, 123
Rotorod, 4. *See also* Locomotor activity
Route of administration. *See* administration route
Running wheel, 4. *See also* Locomotor
activity

S-100, 263–265
Salicylates. *See* Acetylsalicylic acid
Schedule-controlled behavior
definition of, 13–23
drug effects upon, Chapter 9
role of acetylcholine in, 224–231
role of catecholamines in, 143–157, 161–164
role of serotonin in, 99–103
See also Conditioned suppression; Negative reinforcement; Positive reinforcement; Punished responding
Schedule-induced polydipsia, 22–23, 361–363

Schizophrenia. *See* Psychosis
Scintillation counting. *See* Liquid scintillation counting
Scopolamine
behavioral effects of, on
conditioned suppression, 314 (Table
9-4)
discrimination, 354
drug discrimination, 401, 405–406, 417,
419, 421
food and water intake, 224
learning, 232–234, 236–237, 254 (Table
8-2)
locomotor behavior, 220
negative reinforcement, 307 (Table 9-3)
positive reinforcement, 230, 288 (Table
9-1), 297–299
punished responding, 314 (Table 9-4)
neurochemical effects of, 83, 218, 219
Scotophobin, 273–274
Secobarbital, 303, 354, 367 (Table 11-1),
420. *See also* Barbiturates
Second order schedule, 18, 374
Seizure susceptibility, 110
Self-administration of drugs. *See* Chapter 11
Self-stimulation, 184–186, 230–231
Sensory function, 5–6, 282. *See also* Analgesia; Discrimination
Septal area, 93, 97, 108, 118, 214
Septum. *See* Septal area
Serotonergic, 37. *See also* Serotonin
Serotonin
distribution and metabolism of, 40 (Table
2-3), 86–89 (Figs. 4-1; 4-2)
drugs affecting
amphetamine, 187–191
aromatic-L-amino acid decarboxylase inhibitor (Ro 4-4602), 92
benzodiazepines, 195, 197
chloroamphetamine, para, 92
chlorophenylalanine, para, 91–92, 97,
100–103, 105–110
chlorpromazine, 92
cycloheximide, 98
5,6-dihydroxytryptamine, 93–94, 102,
109
6-hydroxydopamine, 125
5-hydroxytryptophan, 95–96, 99–101,
102, 104–106, 109–110
lysergic acid diethylamide, 92
methysergide, 92